HEALTH CARE IN TRANSITION

MOBILE HEALTH

ADVANCES IN RESEARCH AND APPLICATIONS

HEALTH CARE IN TRANSITION

Additional books and e-books in this series can be found on Nova's website under the Series tab.

HEALTH CARE IN TRANSITION

MOBILE HEALTH

ADVANCES IN RESEARCH AND APPLICATIONS

GAURAV GUPTA
NAGESH KUMAR
YASHWANT SINGH
AND
VARUN JAISWAL
EDITORS

nova
Medicine & Health
New York

Additional color graphics may be available in the e-book version of this book.

Library of Congress Cataloging-in-Publication Data

ISBN: 978-1-53619-420-3

Published by Nova Science Publishers, Inc. † New York

CONTENTS

Preface		**vii**
Chapter 1	Role of IoT in Healthcare: An Overview *Sachin Kashyap, Brij Bhushan Sharma, Nagesh Kumar, Pankaj Vaidya and Gaurav Gupta*	**1**
Chapter 2	Wearable Devices: Pros and Cons *Pankaj Vaidya and Brij Bhushan Sharma*	**17**
Chapter 3	Decision Support Algorithms for Data Analysis *Ajay Sharma, Sameer, Tarun Pal and Varun Jaiswal*	**31**
Chapter 4	Innovation Insight for Healthcare Provider Digital Twins: A Review *Chitresh Sharma and Gaurav Gupta*	**97**
Chapter 5	LASIK Innovation Technology for Disease Identification During Lactation *G. S. Pradeep Ghantasala and Anuradha Reddy*	**129**
Chapter 6	A Prospective and Comparative Study of Machine and Deep Learning Techniques for Smart Healthcare Applications *Ahmad Waleed Salehi, Gaurav Gupta and Sonia*	**163**

Chapter 7 Context-Aware Mobile Healthcare for Smart Health Services in Nursing Homes **191**
Kalpana Verma

Chapter 8 Machine Learning Techniques to Fight against Pandemic: A Review **217**
Bharti Thakur and Nagesh Kumar

Chapter 9 Computational Approaches for Malaria Diagnosis Using Machine Learning: A Review **231**
Vandana, Kapil Sethi and Ankit Gupta

Chapter 10 Can Mobile Health Technology Improve Health Related Quality of Life of Chronic Disease Patients in Emerging Economies?: "Happy Heart" A Randomized Controlled Trial in India **257**
Yojna Sah Jain, Vaishali M. Patil, Praful Jain and Omar Nada

About the Editors **317**

Index **321**

PREFACE

Smart health technologies continue to gain research interest across the globe in this digital era. Researchers are focusing on advancements in healthcare systems to make human life better. Also, such advancements help in early disease diagnosis and prevention of the worst diseases. Designing smart healthcare systems is possible only because of recent developments in artificial intelligence, machine learning and IoT technologies. Though mHealth refers to all mobile devices which can communicate data, mobile phones are presently the most popular platform for mHealth delivery. Ninety-four percent of the world population owns/uses a mobile phone, making mobile phones an optimal delivery platform for mHealth interventions. mHealth may catalyse the healthcare delivery model from a historical/episodic model into a tangible/patient-centric model. mHealth is being viewed progressively by many as an essential technology metaphor to achieve rich, vigorous patient engagement, ultimately achieving a patient-centric paradigm change.

This book will discuss diverse topics to explain the rapidly emerging and evolving mobile health and artificial perspective, the emergence of integrated platforms and hosted third-party tools, and the development of decentralized applications for various research domains. It presents various applications that are helpful for research scholars and scientists who are working toward identifying and pinpointing the potential of as well as the hindrances to mHealth. The wide variety in topics it presents offers readers multiple perspectives on a variety of disciplines.

The aim of this edited book is to publish the latest research advancements in the convergence of automation technology, artificial intelligence, biomedical engineering and health informatics. This will help readers to grasp the extensive point of view and the essence of recent advances in this field. This book solicits contributions which include theory, case studies and computing paradigms pertaining to healthcare applications. The prospective audience would be researchers, professionals, practitioners, and students from academia and industry who work in this field. We hope the chapters presented will inspire future research from both theoretical and practical viewpoints to spur further advances in the field. A brief introduction about each chapter follows.

Chapter 1 focuses on the role of Internet of Things (IoT) technologies in healthcare which provides an overview of the various types of IoT devices and data generating equipment for medical information.

In Chapter 2, the objective is to provide a brief discussion about the advantages and disadvantages of using IoT based technologies in healthcare such as wearable devices.

Chapter 3 deals with important aspects of data science for healthcare systems, which includes various algorithms for decision support system algorithms.

Chapter 4 discusses various innovative technologies like digital twins for healthcare and medical diagnosis.

Chapter 5 discusses research investigating the long-term effects of pregnancy and lactation on the female body.

Chapter 6 summarizes recent advances in machine and deep learning techniques for smart healthcare applications.

Chapter 7 presents a review on context-aware mobile healthcare for smart health services in nursing homes.

Chapter 8 focuses on certain machine learning methods that can help in early prediction of pandemics.

Chapter 9 explores techniques and methods based on machine learning for malaria diagnosis.

Chapter 10 is a complete discussion about mobile health technology to improve health-related quality of life of chronic disease patients in emerging economies.

We are grateful to the authors and reviewers for their excellent contributions for making this book possible.

In: Mobile Health
Editors: G. Gupta, N. Kumar et al.
ISBN: 978-1-53619-420-3

Chapter 1

ROLE OF IOT IN HEALTHCARE: AN OVERVIEW

Sachin Kashyap, Brij Bhushan Sharma*, Nagesh Kumar, Pankaj Vaidya and Gaurav Gupta
Yogananda School of A. I., Computers and Data Sciences,
Shoolini University of Biotechnology and Management Sciences,
Solan, Himachal Pradesh, India

ABSTRACT

As IoT's role in providing solutions to many fields is increasing day by day. Sensors are playing a significant role in medical and medicine field. The remote monitoring of the patients is possible with the use of IoT enabled devices. Interactions of the patients and doctor are easier. IoT can play a vital role in patients, Physicians, hospitals, and healthcare insurance companies. IoT devices include Sensor, Actuators, Detectors, Monitors and Cameras etc. These devices are used for the data collections. IoT is one of the most trending fields in research nowadays, and it is attracting researcher due to its extensive coverage in almost every field from healthcare to defence and from industries to agriculture.

* Corresponding Author's Email: brijbhushan@shooliniuniversity.com.

In this paper, we have studied the role and importance of IoT in healthcare. Various IoT applications have been discussed with the procedures, pros and cons of the particular application. This chapter will contribute to the literature for the new researchers.

Keywords: Internet of Thing, sensors, fog computing, medical, medicine, smart healthcare

1. Introduction

The human population is growing at a rapid pace. Even primary healthcare will become out of reach to most people in our nearby time. Healthcare is one of the main priorities of human. However, population growth, population ageing, unbalanced food resource utilization (Sharma & Kumar, 2020) that will lead to the malnutrition among many peoples, increase in the pollution level of our surroundings, i.e., a severe threat to our health are some significant problems that have become apparent in our healthcare field (Nagesh Kumar & Sharma, 2020). To combat these problems, we will have to upgrade our healthcare system using a technological method such as "Internet of Things" (Rani, Kumar, & Bhushan, 2019).

1.1. What Is the Internet of Things (IoT)?

The Internet of things commonly known as IoT is a technological method of interconnecting the physical devices over a network (Rasooli, Bhushan, & Kumar, 2020). They all can share the analyzed-collected data, without requiring human to human or human to computer interaction. "Internet" in IoT refers to the worldwide network of interconnected computer networks, while "things" refers to a physical device with an I. P. address assigned and can transfer data over a network. An IoT device could be as simple as a health-tracking wearable or as complex as a network of the sensors deployed in the city to check the pollution level. While IoT cannot prevent humans from catching diseases or ageing, it can redefine the healthcare system by making it more comfortable in terms of accessibility.

1.2. Aim of IoT in Healthcare

Firstly, to make healthcare accessible to all the people from all over the places. Secondly, to improve the treatments' quality and efficiency and to deduct the time and cost of transportation and hospital stays for the patients.

2. LITERATURE SURVEY

Table 1. Literature survey

Sr. No.	Year	Authors	Title	Key Findings
1.	2017	S. Anand and S. K. Routray	Issues and Challenges in Healthcare Narrowband IoT (Anand & Routray, 2017)	Authors have provided a detailed study in this article, and they have provided information regarding the issues and challenges available in current IoT devices operating in the healthcare industry. Some of the essential points they have pointed regarding the issues and challenges are: Hospital Security Client satisfaction Cost Regulatory standards Moreover, if an IoT needs to be implemented in hospitals, hospitals must upgrade the services according to the IoT devices' standards, which is impossible for hospitals, especially in rural areas.
2.	2017	Aysha K. Alharam, and Wael El-madany	The complexity of Cyber Security Architecture for IoT Healthcare Industry: A Comparative Study (Alharam & El-Madany, 2017)	In this paper, authors have discussed the thorny cybersecurity architecture available for the IoT based healthcare systems. They have compared various resources of various architectures.

Table 1. (Continued)

Sr. No.	Year	Authors	Title	Key Findings
3.	2016	Jinyoung an & Wan-Young Chung	A Novel Indoor Healthcare with Time Hopping-based Visible Light Communication (An & Chung, 2017)	In this paper, authors have developed and implemented a VLC visible light communication system for E. M. wave indoor healthcare. They have conducted an experiment in which they have transmitted multiple medical data in real-time.
4.	2017	Sudhir K. Routray & Sharath Anand	Narrowband IoT for Healthcare (Routray & Anand, 2017)	It can offer cost-effective services necessary for both provincial and metropolitan zones. Medical care is a crucial help area; furthermore, it needs keen advances for better administrations. Authors have shown the main application of Narrowband IoT.
5.	2017	Parag Chatterjee, Leandro J. Cymberknop, Ricardo L. Armentano	IoT-based Decision Support System for Intelligent Healthcare – Applied to Cardiovascular Diseases (Chatterjee, Cymberknop, & Armentano, 2018)	Authors have provided suggestions that IoT can be a vital asset in smart healthcare systems. One of the most crucial goals of such technology devices is to empower the clinicians by providing them with better data to understand the particular disease at a certain level. Reports generated by such machinery can easily be analyzed. The paper majorly highlighting the following points in IoT Healthcare: Decision based system, predictive analytics
6.	2017	Niharika Kumar	IoT Architecture and System Design for Healthcare Systems (Niharika Kumar, 2018)	It a survey paper and in this author have provided a comprehensive survey of architecture and system design regarding the IoT in the healthcare system. Various hardware related to the same technology has been discussed.
7.	2019	Feisal Hadi Masmali & Shah Jahan Miah	Adoption of IoT based innovations for healthcare service delivery in Saudi Arabia (Miah, 2019)	In this paper, authors have discussed and stated that nowadays, only a few technologies like android have the upper hand in IoT as they are the standalone application providers in the sector. Bus once the IoT platform is introduced to it. It will revolutionize a particular sector. It will integrate all the platforms to one. IoT can be beneficial in monitoring applications.

Sr. No.	Year	Authors	Title	Key Findings
8.	2018	Priyanka Jangra & Monish Gupta	A Design of Real-Time Multilayered Smart Healthcare Monitoring Framework using IoT (Jangra & Gupta, 2018)	Authors have implemented and simulated a smart healthcare monitoring framework using the Internet of things; they have provided enough material in this paper to be a beneficial asset in the healthcare industry to handle appropriately. They have proposed a framework in this paper that can handle and utilize the bio-sensor-based data.
9.	2018	Dr. Malti Bansal & Bani Gandhi	IoT Based Development Boards for Smart Healthcare Applications (Bansal & Gandhi, 2018)	Various boards have been discussed in this paper and authors have provided good literature, in this paper regarding these boards and discussed the role of IoT with its importance to the healthcare system in day to day life.
11.	2015	Nuria Pazos et. al.	connection – Automatic Integration of IoT Devices (Pazos, Muller, Aeberli, & Ouerhani, 2015)	This paper provided a complete, IoT based platform. This paper contributed in two ways: it addressed the issues and challenges of IoT fragmentation regarding the communication protocols and data formats. It will be contributing to data parsing, protocol interpretation etc. they have developed an Eclipse plug-in which can generate the OSGi Bundles implementing the three modules of communication agents.
12.	2019	Inderpreet Singh & Deepak Kumar	Improving IoT Based Architecture of Healthcare System (Singh & Kumar, 2019)	In this paper, the authors added literature and suggested a comprehensive overview of IoT device manufacturing and Framework development for clinical services. Role of various sensors has also been discussed how they are creating IoT devices useful in healthcare.
13.	2014	Felipe Fernandez & George C. Pallis	Opportunities and challenges of the Internet of Things for healthcare Systems engineering perspective (Fernandez & Pallis, 2014)	Various opportunities and challenges regarding IoT in healthcare sectors have been discussed in this paper by the authors. Moreover, it suggested that a structured based engineering methodology for the manufacturing of useful IoT has been required.

Table 1. (Continued)

Sr. No.	Year	Authors	Title	Key Findings
14.	2015	Yvette E. Gelogo et. al.	Internet of things (IoT) Driven U-healthcare System Architecture (Gelogo, Oh, Park, & Kim, 2015)	In this paper, authors have discussed The IoT, and it can be utilized in clinical consideration where hospitalized patients whose physiological status requires close consideration can be continually observed utilizing IoT - driven, noninvasive checking This expects sensors to gather extensive physiological data and utilizations entryways and the cloud to dissect and store the data and afterwards send the investigated information remotely to guardians for additional examination and audit. This paper considers the u-medical service framework as for the Internet of Things (IoT) point of view.
15.	2017	S. LAVANYA et. al.	Remote Prescription and IN-HOME healthcare based on IoT (Lavanya, Lavanya, & Divyabharathi, 2017)	An IoT-based wise home-driven medical services stage (iHome medical care framework), which consistently associates intelligent sensors, joined the human body for physiological checking for the day by day medicine the executives. It additionally offers various occasions to adjust a wide assortment of e-health applications with least changes, and it improves client effectiveness.
16.	2017	Adarsh Kumar et. al.	A Novel Smart Healthcare Design, Simulation, and Implementation using Healthcare 4.0 Processes (A. Kumar et al., 2020)	In this paper, The benefits of coordinating blockchain innovation and Industry 4.0 patterns are progressively investigated these days. Most of the keen medical care frameworks either focus on information security issues or huge information the board without understanding the ground truth to make it achievable for end-clients. The combination of blockchain innovation, Industry 4.0 and medical care framework (named Healthcare 4.0) gives different capacities including robotization, permanence, straightforwardness, security, information alter insurance, dispersed and very much oversaw approach, adaptation to non-critical failure, nature of-administration, information excess, and so forth to applications like medical care. The proposed approach exploits Healthcare 4.0 in insurance from the disappointment of

				focal specialists and applies a decentralized methodology, framework and information security, execution improvement, simple information support and so on and proposes savvy medical care functionalities in detail. A reproduction streamlining approach is proposed to improve the general framework and sub-frameworks presentation. The proposed approach is tried, checked and approved through reenactment and execution. Various boundaries are taken in recreation and execution to assess the framework's presence and its reliant and free factors. Execution and reenactment results show a mistake variety of - 0.55 (least) to 4.24 (most significant) because of an adjustment in climate and test system limitations. This close examination approves the proposed approach. In future ways examination, it very well may be inferred that countless mediums to huge organizations in medical services areas are advancing toward Healthcare 4.0 patterns based methodology and it is before long reflected to be the progressive methodology by supplanting the present conventional or computerized medical services frameworks
17.	2018	Anali Yeole & D. R. Kalbande	Change Management Approach for Integrating IoT Technology in Healthcare System (Yeole & Kalbande, 2018)	This paper provided various techniques for embracing new advancements to improve medical care administrations. After diverse various executives' speculations, we proposed a change the board model for Integrating IoT Technology in Healthcare (CMM-IoT). Our proposed model spotlights on sway examination before instilling innovation in the work process. The second significant point discussed was preparing workers to utilise innovation better at all levels. Another significant point discussed is that nimble strategy should be utilized while instilling IoT in the medical services area. While planning IoT, the most important truth was that we should centre concerning the security and protection of all the framework investors.

Table 1. (Continued)

Sr. No.	Year	Authors	Title	Key Findings
18.	2020	Vidya Priya Darcini. S, et. al.	A Comprehensive Review on the Emerging IoTCloud based Technologies for Smart Healthcare (Vidya Priya Darcini, Isravel, & Silas, 2020)	The medical services area receives numerous advantages acquired from the Internet of Things (IoT). Specialists over the world have investigated numerous advances for improving the improvements in IoT based medical services hardware. The headways in wearable innovation give the consideration suppliers with a cost-sparing treatment technique, continually observing and practical help to both ordinary and impaired individuals. Since IoT can change the economy and society universally, making medical services areas more also associated, arranged in will help E-wellbeing applications. This paper presents a nitty-gritty study of the current IoT based medical services observing frameworks with various IoT structures and the advantages and difficulties of IoT and cloud frameworks. This examination showed the advantages of utilizing IoT in-home and emergency clinic conditions. Likewise, the paper talks about the A. I. calculations that can be utilized with the IoT framework. These frameworks are discovered to be easy to use and savvy. The framework utilizes numerous sensors to observe the individual's well-being boundaries and Think to speak IoT stages to gather and envision the information. To perform information investigation, A. I. calculations are utilized. The finding from the information investigation will play out the characterization furthermore, forecast of information for distinguishing the potential illnesses.

3. Applications of IoT in Healthcare Field

Table 2. Applications of IoT in the healthcare field

Sr. No.	Applications	Procedure	Pros	Cons
1	Remote Patient Monitoring: It is an IoT based technological method used to monitor patients outside the conventional clinical settings, such as in-home or in remote areas.	Like the smart band, health trackers will collect the patient's data at home and send it to the doctor over a connected network.	(i) Helps move the regular routines of medical checkups from hospitals to the patient home. (ii)Reduces travel and hospitalization costs. (iii)Helps to make the healthcare easier in terms of accessibility, by breaking the geographic barriers for peoples living in remote areas.	(i). It requires a good network connection. (ii) Accuracy of the data collected is doubtful. (iii) Security and privacy of the sensitive data, as remote patient monitoring works over digital networks prone to many attacks.
2	Medical waste management: It is the procedure of disposing of the waste properly to ensure the safety of the general population. (Smart dustbins with embedded sensors.)	Sensors will be embedded inside the hospital's dustbins, and their location will be traced. If the amount of waste is beyond the threshold inside the dustbin, then cleaning staff will be notified immediately.	(i) Reduces the risk factor of mass infection inside the hospital. (ii) Provides a healthy working environment. (iii) Extra work of hospital decreases.	(i) Sensor nodes used in the dustbins have limited memory size. (ii) Wireless technologies used in a system such as Zigbee and WIFI have a shorter range and lower data speed. RFID based systems are affected by surrounding metal objects.
3	Patient monitoring at the hospital:	Health status of patients like B. P. etc., and another status like glucose inside the bottle, oxygen in-cylinder etc., are going to finish, will be sent to doctor and caretaking staff.	(i). Health monitoring of patients admitted to hospitals will be easy for doctors. (ii) No need for caretakers to be around patients by all time.	It requires a steady and fast network connection.

Table 2. (Continued)

Sr. No.	Applications	Procedure	Pros	Cons
4	Patient location monitoring:	Location status of patients inside an asylum will be sent to the staff.	(i)Location of patients will be traced easily. (ii)No need for staff to be around patients all the time.	Accuracy of data is the problem.
5	Record keeping of patients:	All patients' data is digitally sent to the doctors and will be stored in a computer or cloud.	(i)Quick and easy access. (ii) Reduces paper records filing costs. (iii) Makes it possible to easily backup documents in case of disaster.	Security threat of stealing and manipulating of sensitive data.
6	Inventory of medicines and equipment:	RFID tags will be installed to the equipment types for noting their check-in and out time from inventory. The same method will be applied to keep	Helps in maintaining the record of pieces of equipment and medicine consumption in a hospital. Helps to decrease the extra work of staff.	RFID based systems are affected by surrounding metal objects. Security threat of manipulation of the data.
7	Efficient drug management: It is a procedure following from production to the usage of drug by the patient without being misused.	Checking and reporting appropriate parameters like temperature for drug production. The usage of smart tags in drug utilization monitoring by smart devices.	(i) Improves the quality of drugs produced. (ii)Immediate reporting to the regulatory body if anywhere is wrong distribution.	The security risk is high as the devices are connected over a network; therefore, the information can be manipulated.
8	Robotic surgery:	For more precise surgeries, IoT enabled robotic devices should be used, and the doctor's commands should operate them.	(i). It enables doctors to operate with more control and precision. (ii) It can save many lives as it makes it possible to operate from a distant place, in an emergency like in warzone.	(i)Security risk is high as the devices are connected over a network. Therefore the commands can be manipulated. (ii)It requires a steady and fast network connection.

4. Security Concerns

All the devices are connected over the networks for communication purposes; therefore, IoT healthcare could become a target for hackers. Security concerns for IoT-based healthcare are similar to standard communication protocols.

- *Confidentiality* – To ensure the inaccessibility of medical data for unauthorized users.
- *Authentication* – to ensure that the person is verified with which the patient is communicating.
- *The authorization ensures* that only authorized nodes are accessible for network services or resources.
- *Privacy* is a mandatory issue because sensitive data is exchanged across the network. It can be achieved by the end to end encryption of the data.

4.1. Challenges

IoT also have some growing challenges with the advancement in technologies.

- *Processing Limitations* – The processors embedded in IoT health devices are not very powerful in speed. Moreover, these devices are not designed to perform computations, i.e., they simply act as a sensor or actuator.
- *Memory Limitations* – IoT healthcare devices collect either small or massive amount of data, and most have low memory. So based on the amount of data, storage has to be allocated.
- *Energy Limitations* - IoT healthcare network includes the devices having limited battery power, e.g., smart bands. Such devices energy has to be conserved by switching on the power- saving

mode when no sensor reading needs to be reported. They operate at a low CPU speed if there is nothing essential to be processed.

- *Security Scalability* - Spontaneous growth of IoT devices connected to local and global networks has led to the security breach as Low scale security methods are not sufficient to secure each device. Therefore, designing a highly scalable security method is a challenge to obtain the security requirements for the devices.
- *Communication* - IoT health devices are connected through a wide range of wireless network links like BLE (Bluetooth Low Energy), WIFI, Zigbee and 3G/4G. Therefore, obtaining a secure communication protocol for the wireless channel is challenging.
- *Devices Multiplicity* - There is diversity in the IoT healthcare devices, ranging from fully computational devices to simple RFID tags. Each device varies in term of their capabilities like memory, processing, software and power. Therefore, designing a security method protocol that can accommodate even simple devices is challenging.
- *A Multi-Protocol Network* - IoT healthcare devices rather than only communicating with the external network devices may also communicate with the devices inside the local network. Therefore, designing of a multi-protocol network system is a challenge.
- *Data confidentiality* - Medical data is sensitive information. So in order, to protect the data from the unauthorized persons, we need to build the information and identity management system.
- *Availability* - of all IoT healthcare services (either local or global/cloud services) to authorized parties when needed even under denial-of-service attacks.
- *Ubiquitous data exchange through wireless technologies* – Maintaining the data's integrity during the transmission process between devices is a challenge. Because each IoT healthcare network provides some time-varying measurements, there is a need to ensure that each message is fresh.

Conclusion

In this chapter, we have studied various papers that can have covered literature regarding the role of the Internet of Things in healthcare. After completing the literature on smart healthcare technologies, we found that IoT can be useful, and it can play a vital role, especially in those conditions where monitoring of a particular patient is complicated. This paper provides a critical point regarding the work of various authors and this paper can be contributed as the literature in the field of healthcare and can help author who is implementing the IoT in the field of smart healthcare devices.

References

Alharam, A. K., & El-Madany, W. (2017). The complexit cybersecurity architecture for IoT healthcare industry: A comparative study. *Proceedings - 2017 5th International Conference on Future Internet of Things and Cloud Workshops*, W-Fi Cloud 2017, 2017-Janua, 246–250. https://doi.org/10.1109/FiCloudW.2017.100.

An, J., & Chung, W. Y. (2017). ANovelindoor healthcare with time hopping-based visible light communication. *2016 IEEE 3rd World Forum on Internet of Things, WF-IoT* 2016, 19–23. https://doi.org/10.1109/WF-IoT.2016.7845438.

Anand, S., & Routray, S. K. (2017). Issues and challenges in healthcare narrowband IoT. *Proceedings of the International Conference on Inventive Communication and Computational Technologies, ICICCT 2017,* (Icicct), 486–489. https://doi.org/10.1109/ICICCT.2017.7975247.

Bansal, M., & Gandhi, B. (2018). IoT based development boards for smart healthcare applications. 2018 4th International Conference on Computing Communication and Automation, *ICCCA* 2018, 1–7. https://doi.org/10.1109/CCAA.2018.8777572.

Chatterjee, P., Cymberknop, L. J., & Armentano, R. L. (2018). IoT-based decision support system for intelligent healthcare - Applied to cardiovascular diseases. *Proceedings - 7th International Conference on Communication Systems and Network Technologies*, *CSNT* 2017, 362–366. https://doi.org/10.1109/CSNT.2017.8418567.

Fernandez, F., & Pallis, G. (2014). *Opportunities and challenges of the Internet of Things for healthcare.* 263–266. https://doi.org/10.4108/icst.mobihealth.2014.257276.

Gelogo, Y. E., Oh, J. W., Park, J. W., & Kim, H. K. (2015). Internet of Things (IoT) Driven U-Healthcare System Architecture. *Proceedings - 8th International Conference on Bio-Science and Bio-Technology, BSBT* 2015, 24–26. https://doi.org/10.1109/BSBT.2015.17.

Jangra, P., & Gupta, M. (2018). A Design of Real-Time Multilayered Smart Healthcare Monitoring Framework Using IoT. International Conference on Intelligent and Advanced System, *ICIAS* 2018, 1–5. https://doi.org/10.1109/ICIAS.2018.8540606.

Kumar, A., Krishnamurthi, R., Nayyar, A., Sharma, K., Grover, V., & Hossain, E. (2020). A Novel Smart Healthcare Design, Simulation, and Implementation Using Healthcare 4.0 Processes. *IEEE* Access, 8, 118433–118471. https://doi.org/10.1109/ACCESS.2020.3004790.

Kumar, Nagesh, & Sharma, B. (2020). Opportunities and Challenges with WSN's in Smart Technologies: A Smart Agriculture Perspective. *Advances in Intelligent Systems and Computing*, 1132, 441–463. https://doi.org/10.1007/978-3-030-40305-8_22.

Kumar, Niharika. (2018). IoT architecture and system design for healthcare systems. Proceedings of the 2017 International Conference on Smart Technology for Smart Nation, *SmartTechCon* 2017, 1118–1123. https://doi.org/10.1109/SmartTechCon.2017.8358543.

Lavanya, S., Lavanya, G., & Divyabharathi, J. (2017). Remote prescription and I-Home healthcare based on IoT. *IEEE International Conference on Innovations in Green Energy and Healthcare Technologies* - 2017, IGEHT 2017, 1–3. https://doi.org/10.1109/IGEHT.2017.8094069.

Miah, F. H. M. & S. J. (2019). Adoption of IoT based innovations for healthcare service delivery in Saudi Arabia. *IEEE CSDE Conf,* 1–2. https://doi.org/10.1109/CSDE48274.2019.9162390.

Pazos, N., Muller, M., Aeberli, M., & Ouerhani, N. (2015). ConnectOpen - Automatic integration of IoT devices. *IEEE World Forum on Internet of Things, WF-IoT 2015 - Proceedings,* 640–644. https://doi.org/10.1109/WF-IoT.2015.7389129.

Rani, D., Kumar, N., & Bhushan, B. (2019). Implementation of an Automated Irrigation System for Agriculture Monitoring using IoT Communication. *5th IEEE International Conference on Signal Processing, Computing and Control* (ISPCC 2k19), 138–143.

Rasooli, M. W., Bhushan, B., & Kumar, N. (2020). Applicability of wireless sensor networks & IoT in saffron & wheat crops: A smart agriculture perspective. *International Journal of Scientific and Technology Research,* 9(2), 2456–2461.

Routray, S. K., & Anand, S. (2017). Narrowband IoT for Healthcare. International Conference on Information, Communication & Embedded Systems. *IEEE,* (Icices), 0–3.

Sharma, B. B., & Kumar, N. (2020). Internet of things-based hardware and software for smart agriculture: A review. *Lecture Notes in Electrical Engineering*, 597, 151–157. https://doi.org/10.1007/978-3-030-29407-6_13.

Singh, I., & Kumar, D. (2019). Improving IOT Based Architecture of Healthcare System. 2019 4th International Conference on Information Systems and Computer Networks, *ISCON* 2019, 113–117. https://doi.org/10.1109/ISCON47742.2019.9036287.

Vidya Priya Darcini, S., Isravel, D. P., & Silas, S. (2020). A Comprehensive Review on the Emerging IoT-Cloud based Technologies for Smart Healthcare. *2020 6th International Conference on Advanced Computing and Communication Systems*, *ICACCS* 2020, 606–611. https://doi.org/10.1109/ICACCS48705.2020.9074457.

Yeole, A., & Kalbande, D. R. (2018). Change Management Approach for Integrating IoT Technology in Healthcare System. 2018 International

Conference on Smart City and Emerging Technology, *ICSCET* 2018, 1–4. https://doi.org/10.1109/ICSCET.2018.8537335.

In: Mobile Health
Editors: G. Gupta, N. Kumar et al.
ISBN: 978-1-53619-420-3

Chapter 2

WEARABLE DEVICES: PROS AND CONS

Pankaj Vaidya* and Brij Bhushan Sharma
Yogananda School of AI, Computer and Data Sciences,
Shoolini University of Biotechnology and Management Sciences,
Solan, Himachal Pradesh, India

ABSTRACT

In today's busy schedule everyone is moving towards technology, where the role of internet-connected devices has increased at sudden and with huge impact. Technology is taking care of almost everything in day-to-day life, from smart homes to smart industries and intelligent hospitals to intelligent healthcare. Wearable devices play a vital role in keeping track of one's fitness. These devices are internet-connected provides you with the data regarding your health parameters without disturbing you from doing your daily jobs. This chapter has discussed the pros and cons of wearable devices in detail. Moreover, we have compared various devices and their functions and features so that everyone can easily understand the importance of these such devices.

Keywords: IoT devices, wearable devices, Internet of Thing, Smart Technologies

---

* Corresponding Author's Email: pankaj.vaidya@shooliniuniversity.com.

INTRODUCTION

This chapter discusses the role of wearable devices in healthcare. Wearable devices are in trend from the past few years. In 2014, wearable devices usage was only 9%, and within four years, it rises from 9% to 33%. These devices are powered by various modern technologies like machine learning, big data, AI & Cloud Computing, etc. These devices' essential features are tracking, remote monitoring of the patient, gathering data, and providing new patterns to enhance the health and lifestyle etc. As modern technology is involved with these devices, the accuracy is quite lovely and offers a straightforward user interface.

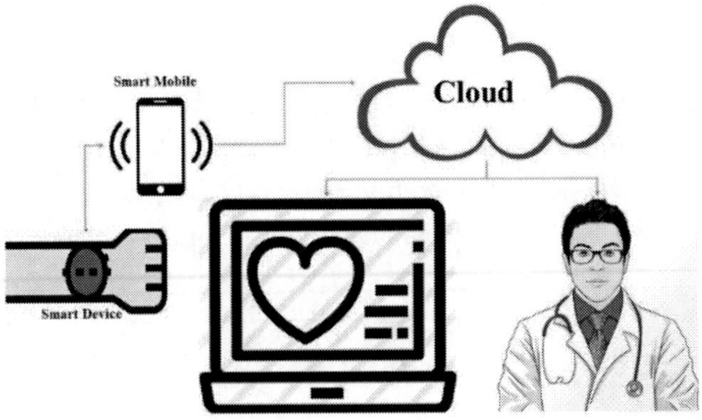

Figure 1. Process of remote monitoring.

The internet of things is a recent technology used to collect data using sensors and then transfer it. This allows every device to communicate (Sharma & Kumar, 2020). IoT provides opportunities for electronic devices to share the gathered data using the internet (Kumar & Sharma, 2020). benefits offered by these smart wearable devices are:

- Reduces medical errors and cost
- Users are better aware of his/her health status
- Users can maintain their health to the best of their ability
- These devices can help in responding to the life-threatening conditions like cardiac diseases or some other medical emergency.

LITERATURE SURVEY

Table 1. Literature survey

Sr. No.	Title	Authors	Year	Findings
1	Apps and wearables for monitoring physical activity and sedentary behaviour: A qualitative systematic review protocol on barriers and facilitators (Wilde, Ward, Sewell, Müller, & Wark, 2018)	Laura J Wilde et al. (Wilde et al., 2018)	2018	The methods provided in the article will help in guiding the researcher how to plan and design better research which aims towards the activity and behaviour of the wearable devices and mobile phone applications.
2	Enabling Technologies for the Internet of Health Things (Rodrigues et al., 2018)	Joel j. p. c. Rodrigues et al. (Rodrigues et al., 2018)	2018	Authors stated that IoT is the most emerging technology, and the internet of things is providing innovations to the industries. One of the biggest industries which are taking full benefits of the internet of things is the healthcare industry. Authors have identified few healthcare-related devices which include wearable devices. A proper detailed analysis was performed in the available devices with accurate description. This paper contributes an excellent knowledge to the students/ research to embrace society with new modern technology.
3	A Web-Based System for Home Monitoring of Patients With Parkinson's Disease Using Wearable Sensors (Bor-Rong Chen, Shyamal Patel, Thomas Buckley, Ramona Rednic, Douglas J. McClure, Ludy Shih & Matt Welsh, 2016)	Bor-Rong Chen (Bor-Rong Chen, Shyamal Patel, Thomas Buckley, Ramona Rednic, Douglas J. McClure, Ludy Shih & Matt Welsh, 2016)	2016	Authors have introduced device mercury live, which monitors the patients' status suffering from the disease known as Parkinson at their homes. They placed sensors on the patient's body and provided him/her with the laptop to interact with the clinician. The mercury life is an integrated platform which includes a wearable sensor which is going to placed on the patient body, and then it captures accelerometer data. The other part of the system is the web-based application which allows the user full-duplex communication with the clinician. With the proposed method, the clinician can access all the stored data.

Table 1. (Continued)

Sr. No.	Title	Authors	Year	Findings
4	Improving the efficiency and reliability of wearable based mobile eHealth applications (Garcia-perez, Diaz-zayas, Rios, & Merino, 2017)	Cesar Garcia-Perez et al. (Garcia-perez et al., 2017)	2017	In this paper, the authors improved mobile health applications using the software-defined network and NVF, including real-time monitoring and traffic polarization to meet emergency and security services' reliability. An approach is presented to a wearable application in case of emergency services. An API is also introduced to increase health application improvement and acceleration.
5	A demand for wearable devices in health care(K. Vijayalakshmi 1 *, S. Uma 1, R. Bhuvanya 1, 2018)	A. Suresh et al. (K. Vijayalakshmi 1 *, S. Uma 1, R. Bhuvanya 1, 2018)	2018	In the most recent couple of years, wearable gadgets are generally famous in everyday life. Authors provided a survey in this paper; they studied concerning different wearable items and its health advantages. Additionally, they looked at potential security issues in these sorts of wearable gadgets. Finally, they summed up the exploration advancement in the commercial centre and future difficulties on the wearable device in the clinical field.
6	Body sensor networks, wearables, and the Internet of Things. (Benny P. L. Lo, Henry Ip, 2016)	Benny P. L. et al. (Benny P. L. Lo, Henry Ip, 2016)	2016	In this paper, the authors stated that we are already using so many advanced technological devices, including IoT wearable devices. People nowadays rely on these new technologies. These gadgets influence people to like initially, people used to share their exercise images, but now they share the information of exercises utilizing the wrist bands. Alarm clocks have been replaced with the same wristbands. So the authors suggested that these such technologies can be used to enhance the clinical activities. They provide long and continuous measurement of the action, physiological, and behavioural information. As these gadgets come at a reasonable price, they can revolutionize clinical activities.

Sr. No.	Title	Authors	Year	Findings
7	Wearable, interconnected devices promise more efficient and comprehensive health care. (Metcalf, Milliard, Gomez, & Schwartz, 2016)	D. Metcalf et al. (Metcalf et al., 2016)	2016	The IoT is a potential rising arrangement that comprises of interconnected gadgets. These organized gadgets offer better, quicker, and less expensive client-driven advancements in wellbeing are utilization just as account Arranged wearable gadgets and applications assume a fundamental job, filling in as establishing the ever-developing act of the IoT in medical services. There might be a significant expansion in things like embeddable little, and effectively controlled CPU embeds that can be put anyplace inside an individual's body. Regarding the medical care area, they might have the option to gauge fundamental signs without intrusive medical procedure. Embeddable, for example, electronic tattoos, for instance, might be furnished with sensors that can send through remote innovation. Additionally, three-dimensional printed clinical gadgets are exceptionally encouraging increments to the IoT, in that, each article embedded in the human body might be searchable or then again identifiable through organizations.
8	The literature on Wearable Technology for Connected Health: Scoping Review of Research Trends, Advances, and Barriers (Loncar-turukalo, Zdravevski, & Chouvarda, 2019)	T. Loncar-turukalo et al. (Loncar-turukalo et al., 2019)	2019	In this literature, survey authors have provided scientific literature on wearable technology in health care they have covered articles from January 2010 to February 2019. They covered enabling technologies and trends and addressed both at user end and technological end. This literature's primary critical findings are Applications of all wearable devices in the health domains are growing mature day by day; however, more R&D is required to increase the accuracy, reliability, dependability, and comfortability.

Table 1. (Continued)

Sr. No.	Title	Authors	Year	Findings
	Wearable Health Technology and Electronic Health Record Integration: Scoping Review and Future Directions (Dinh-Le, Chuang, Chokshi, & Mann, 2019)	C. Dinh-Le et al. (Dinh-Le et al., 2019)	2019	Authors have presented vital challenges and emerging technologies solutions to the rapidly growing field. They developed a process to search and document the current state of the wearable device's technological advancements in the field of health care.
9	Designing, Implementing, and Evaluating Mobile Health Technologies for Managing Chronic Conditions in Older Adults: A Scoping Review (Matthew-Maich et al., 2016)	Nancy Matthew-Maich et al. (Matthew-Maich et al., 2016)	2016	This paper presents a few shared characteristics over these extraordinary settings utilizing topical develops to illuminate interconnected cycles of the plan, usage, and assessment when creating mHealth arrangements most appropriate to the necessities of more seasoned grown-ups living at home. During a brief mechanical advancement period, rules for innovative work in mHealth should be versatile to persistent change as new instruments become accessible, even as the medical care conveyance framework itself encounters advance toward network care. With the improvement of compelling and productive proof-based advancements, mHealth arrangements offer the extraordinary potential for streamlining a maturing populace's wellbeing.
10	Ambient Assisted Living Healthcare Frameworks, Platforms, Standards, and Quality Attributes (Memon, Wagner, Pedersen, Aysha Beevi, & Hansen, 2014)	M. Memon et al. (Memon et al., 2014)	2014	The user has done the wealthy review and provided many industries and research organizations currently working in field ambient assisted living. They covered almost 12 projects in this review, and these projects are only those beyond the pilot phase and had deployed the projects and the solutions they provided into the real world.

Sr. No.	Title	Authors	Year	Findings
11	Active and Assisted Living Ecosystem for the Elderly(Marcelino et al., 2018)	I. Marcelino et al. (Marcelino et al., 2018)	2018	The author has performed experiments using the prototype they developed; additionally, they have added three complementary services: medical category, leisure category, and call centre category. Total of 23 interviews was conducted, including 19 senior and four young adults to validate the prototype. Majorly two aspects were appreciated by the seniors that are 1. The free video phone calls and the second one is that they felt that they are reliving days from their past.
12	wearable technology for biomechanics: e-textile or micromechanical sensors? (Veltink & De Rossi, 2010)	P. H. Veltink (Veltink & De Rossi, 2010)	2010	Authors have stressed to the conclusions that fully wearable, user-friendly and accurate systems are not available to be that as it may, they are presently predictable in an imminent future. On the textile side, an ongoing field of examination, significantly more work should be performed, either at the degree of innovation improvement or the level of calculation improvement for reverse kinematics. The best possible designation of material sensors exhibits is additionally and the issue to be additionally tended to for additional exact and computationally effective reproduction of appendages positions when it is to be acted progressively. Incorporating micromechanical with e-material sensors have never endeavoured to date; this synergistic methodology must be researched, and proper tangible combination techniques and calculations need to be executed.

WEARABLE DEVICES WITH THEIR PROS AND CONS

AVA Bracelet

Specially designed for the women provides better insights to the user about their health. The device is night-only wearable. Helpful for the pregnant women, key parameters to keep an eye on are Skin Temperature, pulse rate (resting), breathing rate. Heart rate, sleep quality, movement, heat loss, hydration and sweating etc. The device offers a perfect accuracy percentile about around 89% ("AVA Bracelet," n.d.).

Table 2. AVA bracelet

Sr. No.	Pro's	Con's
1.	User Interface	Cost is high
2.	Database details up to five nights can be stored	Connectivity issues
3.	Accuracy 89%	It sometimes not shows the correct results

AliveCor

It is a portable device that can easily be carried in pockets. The device takes medical-grade EKG recordings. It measures normal heart rhythm within just 30 seconds. The devices connect with smartphone and deliver all data to it. Easy to use the device. Users are only required to put their fingers on the device's sensor unit, and that is it information will be processed within 30 seconds, and you can check it on your smartphone and share it with medical professional ("alive or," n.d.).

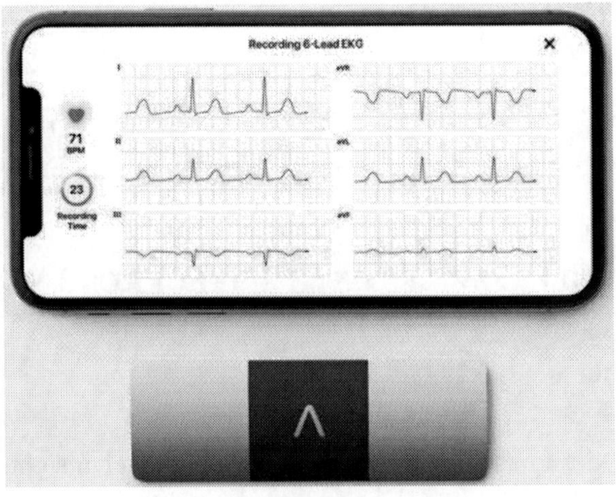

Figure 2. Alivecor device ("Alivecor," n.d.).

Table 3. AlivCor

Sr. No.	Pro's	Con's
1	Easy to use	Limited Connectivity mostly compatible with iPhone or Samsung galaxy
2	Affordable (19.19$)	
3	Portable	
4	Reliable	

TEMPTRAQ

A new device that is a Monitoring Sensor for Babies and Children. Easy to use no difficulties offered by the device in terms of usage as everyone faces traditional thermometers. The TEMPRAQ is available with a soft patch including Bluetooth sensor. It can easily be placed under the child's arm. The device is highly accurate. Moreover, parents can keep an eye on the temperature for 24 hours ("Temptraq," n.d.).

Table 4. TEMPTRAQ

Sr. No.	Pro's	Con's
1	Only available smart device	Single time use only Connectivity range 40 feet
2	Highly accurate	
3	Water-resistant	
4	Reliable	

Smart Sleep Wearable

This device is introduced by a well-renowned company, Philips, a soft headband with sensors inbuilt. It identifies individuals sleep needs and accordingly provides a medically approved solution. It also produces audio tones which provide strength to your sleep. Similar to any other smart device, it also comes with app connectivity. Where you can check the log of sleep metrics, also this app offers you tips and guidance for better sleep ("Philips," n.d.).

Bio Patch MC100

It is the latest wearable non-invasive device. It helps medical professionals to monitor their patients. It provides data regarding heart rate, variability in heart rate, ECG, respiration rate etc. introduced by SEER. Usage is also straightforward. The user only must connect this device to the left side of the chest. Multi-algorithm criteria are followed to calculate the vital signs. After that, all the gathered data is sent to the cloud platform. Doctors or medical professionals can analyze the parameters ("Bio Patch MC100," n.d.)

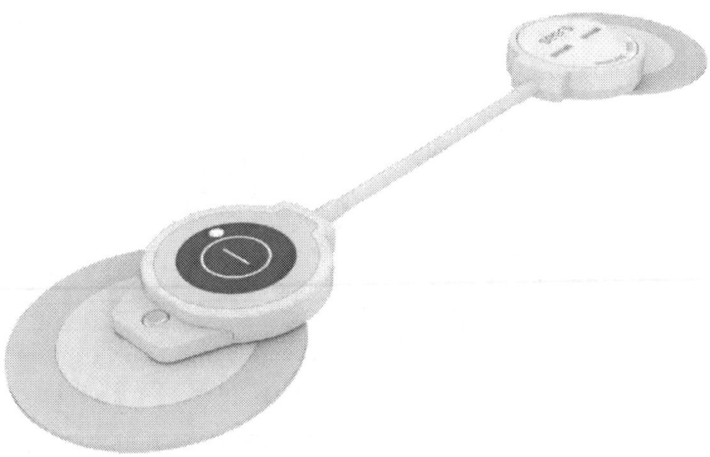

Figure 3. Bio Patch MC100 ("Bio Patch MC100," n.d.).

CONCLUSION

In this paper, we have studied the role of wearable devices in healthcare. We covered five world-class wearable devices in this chapter with their pro's and cons. with the use of new advanced technologies like IoT, Machine Learning, and AI, these devices impact the healthcare industries. An easy, fast and reliable method for the clinicians to keep an eye on their patient's health remotely. Although we also found that there are some modifications still required in such kind of devices. This chapter will provide literature to the researcher who is willing or working in the field of healthcare.

REFERENCES

Alivecor. (n.d.). Retrieved from https://store.alivecor.in/cart.

Alivecor. (n.d.). Retrieved from https://store.alivecor.in/products/kardiamobile-6l?variant=33258427285592.

AVA Bracelet. (n.d.). Retrieved from https://www.avawomen.com/how-ava-works/.

Benny P. L. Lo, Henry Ip, and G.-Z. Y. (2016). Body sensor networks, wearables, and the Internet of Things. *Transforming Health Care Ieee Pulse*, (February 2016), 4–8. https://doi.org/10.1109/MPUL.2015.2498474.

Bio Patch MC100. (n.d.). Retrieved from https://seerstech.com/wearable-bio-patch/.

Bor-Rong Chen, Shyamal Patel, Thomas Buckley, Ramona Rednic, Douglas J. McClure, Ludy Shih, D. T., & Matt Welsh, and P. B. (2016). *A Web-Based System for Home Monitoring of Patients with Parkinson's Disease Using Wearable Sensors*. 58(3), 831–836.

Dinh-Le, C., Chuang, R., Chokshi, S., & Mann, D. (2019). Wearable health technology and electronic health record integration: Scoping review and future directions. *Journal of Medical Internet Research,* 21(9), 1–13. https://doi.org/10.2196/12861.

Garcia-perez, C., Diaz-zayas, A., Rios, A., & Merino, P. (2017). Improving the efficiency and reliability of wearable based mobile eHealth applications. *Pervasive and Mobile Computing*. https://doi.org/10.1016/j.pmcj.2017.06.021.

Kumar, N., & Sharma, B. (2020). Opportunities and Challenges with WSN's in Smart Technologies: A Smart Agriculture Perspective. *Advances in Intelligent Systems and Computing*, 1132, 441–463. https://doi.org/10.1007/978-3-030-40305-8_22.

Loncar-turukalo, T., Zdravevski, E., & Chouvarda, I. (2019). The literature on Wearable Technology for Connected Health : Scoping Review of Research Trends, Advances, and Barriers Corresponding Author : *Journal of Medical Internet Research*, 21, 1–23. https://doi.org/10.2196/14017.

Marcelino, I., Laza, R., Domingues, P., Gómez-Meire, S., Fdez-Riverola, F., & Pereira, A. (2018). Active and assisted living ecosystem for the elderly. *Sensors* (Switzerland), 18(4), 1–18. https://doi.org/10.3390/s18041246.

Matthew-Maich, N., Harris, L., Ploeg, J., Markle-Reid, M., Valaitis, R., Ibrahim, S., … Isaacs, S. (2016). Designing, implementing, and evaluating mobile health technologies for managing chronic conditions in older adults: A scoping review. *JMIR MHealth and UHealth*, 4(2), 1–18. https://doi.org/10.2196/mhealth.5127.

Memon, M., Wagner, S. R., Pedersen, C. F., Aysha Beevi, F. H., & Hansen, F. O. (2014). Ambient Assisted Living healthcare frameworks, platforms, standards, and quality attributes. *Sensors* (Switzerland), 14(3), 4312–4341. https://doi.org/10.3390/s140304312.

Metcalf, D., Milliard, S. T. J., Gomez, M., & Schwartz, and M. (2016). Wearable, interconnected devices promise more efficient and comprehensive health care. *Wearables and the Internet of Things for Health Ieee Pulse* 35, 35, 1–5. https://doi.org/10.1109/MPUL.2016.2592260.

Philips. (n.d.). Retrieved from https://www.usa.philips.com/c-e/smartsleep.html.

Rodrigues, J. J. P. C., De Rezende Segundo, D. B., Junqueira, H. A., Sabino, M. H., Prince, R. M. I., Al-Muhtadi, J., & De Albuquerque, V. H. C. (2018). Enabling Technologies for the Internet of Health Things. *IEEE Access*, 6, 13129–13141. https://doi.org/10.1109/ACCESS.2017.2789329.

Sharma, B. B., & Kumar, N. (2020). Internet of things-based hardware and software for smart agriculture: A review. *Lecture Notes in Electrical Engineering*, 597, 151–157. https://doi.org/10.1007/978-3-030-29407-6_13.

Temptraq. (n.d.). Retrieved from https://www.temptraq.com/FAQs.

Veltink, P. H., & De Rossi, D. (2010). Conversations in BME. *IEEE Engineering in Medicine and Biology Magazine*, (June), 37–43.

Vijayalakshmi, K., S. Uma, R. Bhuvanya, A. S. (2018). A demand for wearable devices in health care. *International Journal of Engineering & Technology*, (January), 1–4. https://doi.org/10.14419/ijet.v7i1.7.9377.

Wilde, L. J., Ward, G., Sewell, L., Müller, A. M., & Wark, P. A. (2018). Apps and wearables for monitoring physical activity and sedentary behaviour: A qualitative systematic review protocol on barriers and facilitators. *Digital Health*, 4, 205520761877645. https://doi.org/10.1177/2055207618776454.

In: Mobile Health
Editors: G. Gupta, N. Kumar et al.
ISBN: 978-1-53619-420-3

Chapter 3

DECISION SUPPORT ALGORITHMS FOR DATA ANALYSIS

Ajay Sharma[1,*], Sameer[2], Tarun Pal[3] and Varun Jaiswal[4]
[1]Dept of Biotechnology and Bioinformatics,
Jaypee University of Information Technology JUIT
[2]Dept of Mathematics Jaypee University of Information Technology
JUIT Sloan, H. P
[3]Department of Biotechnology (Bioinformatics)
Vignan's Foundation for Science, Technology and Research
(Deemed to be University, NAAC- A), Vadlamudi, Guntur,
Andhra Pradesh
[4]Centre for Disease Control (NCDC) New Delhi India
Gachon University, Bokjeong-dong, Sujeong- gu,
Seongnam-si, Gyeonggi-do, South Korea

ABSTRACT

A decision support systems (DSS) are computer-based application that collects and puts together, and examine the business information to

* Corresponding Author Email: ajaysharmadharmani@gmail.com.

encourage and facilitate the quality of business. A very much planned DSS helps leaders in aggregating and grouping of data in various sources. Raw data, information and records from the employees, the board and heads plan the DSS business model. DSS network and analysis framework help the administration, organizations to recognize, solve problems, and make a decision. It is a framework that permits a human-machine interface, whereas the administrators have control all through the decisions process. Decision-making data straightforwardly related to the managers, yet besides goes above and beyond common administration systems by allowing decision-makers to interact with the computer. The capacity of a person to retail command over the decision-making process isn't simply enough to tackle very much organized structured problems yet besides helps in taking care of semi-organized and unstructured issues. This book chapter is focused on the different aspects of a decision support system ranging from the introductory part of the DSS network followed by the development and deployment of a support system. The article covers diverse topics related to support systems including web-based systems, user interfaces, software engineering approaches, etc. The last section of this article covers the machine learning-based case studies which could help in gaining visibility that how the machine learning is incorporated in the decision-making process.

Keywords: machine learning, decision support system, deep learning, algorithm, data analysis, data mining

1. INTRODUCTION

A decision support system (DSS) network is that framework that helps the administration in captivating the business choices and to take decisions. It is a framework that permits a human-machine interface where the leaders have control all through the dynamic process of decision-making. It has one essential target objective that is to give the managerial/administrative staff with fundamental data for setting up intelligent choices directly to the stakeholders, executives for making better decisions (Eom, Lee, et al. 1998). DSS not only helps in bringing dynamic decision-making information straightforwardly to the heads, additionally it goes above and beyond common place traditional administration data framework, by permitting the chief managers to connect with the computers. Hence, the computer used in DSS is just a device, which helps in the assessment, execution, and evaluation of other options so that they may get an authoritative choice (Hoogenboom, Jones et al. 2004). The capacity of a person to retail command over the decision-making process the decision cycle isn't simply valuable to tackle all-around organized well-structured issues yet additionally helps in taking care of semi-organized and unstructured issues. In this way, the Decision-Support System (DSS) is a particular information management system intended to help the managers abilities in all phases of decision making, *for example,* problem identification, choosing significant information, relevant data, picking the way to deal with be utilized in dynamic and assessing the elective course of action(Eom, Lee et al. 1998). A decision support system network must create data in such a structure that chief executives may comprehend and when such data is required, they place this data under the immediate control of the heads. Accordingly, the DSS empowers the business heads to take productive, efficient, economic, and financial decisions when required (Eom and Kim 2006). With regards to good decision making, depending too intensely on programmed decision making coming from recognition or relying a lot upon feeding of data in the system from every side can be hazardous. In some cases, you neglect one or the other notification, search out vital data that uphold and support the decision making. This might be a result of our biasness, absence, lack of time, and various other resources (Alavi and Henderson 1981). Notwithstanding, with regards to hierarchical decision making, maybe you wouldn't have any desire to face any challenge. The reasons are self-evident. One wrong decision could make various things go awry, including company product image, product development phase lifecycle, permanent monetary, and company brand. By and large, you can't master the essentials of financial aspects, measurements, and task exploration to settle on clear decisions (Wikström, Edenius et al. 2011). Apart from these, you need some information-based frameworks that help business and strengthens the decision-making in an organization. This is the place where a choice based DSS network comes into the picture. It is a computer-based electronic framework that causes you to make arranging, assembling, activities, operations, and the executive's management decision choices, in light of data accessible, available in the system (Wikström, Edenius et al. 2011). However, you should recall that these frameworks are not the decision-makers. They simply help in decision making, by offering experiences that you might be missing and giving accurate computations. A definitive leader is just you, a Decision support system(DSS) networks have picked up colossal prevalence in different spaces, including: military operations, security, medication, assembling, manufacturing, designing, engineering, and business (Turban, Sharda et al. 2010). These can uphold and support the process of decision making in circumstances where precision is significant. Moreover, they give admittance to applicable information by incorporating different structured forms and sources of information, supporting human intellectual insufficiencies (Galimore 2011). While DSS utilizes AI to address issues, you shouldn't overestimate its significance importance. It's a method to get relative figures to premise a few or Say, for example, you need to devise a store supply chain network development system. For implementing this, the DSS examines a load of stock and production development. Premise the information accessible, it looks at the results of various decisions, encouraging you to sort out what may work best at present. It encourages you to set up a flexibility of supply chain development that ultimately works very well (Turban, Sharda et al. 2010).

Let's take *another example*: Assume you need to upgrade and optimize your sales. For this purpose, you'll make a few suspicions, assumptions, gather information about statistical facts, data points, generate reports, inspect design patterns, and lastly make a decision. At the point when you do it physically, no one can tell what errors you're submitting (Turban, Sharda et al. 2010). A DSS, in such a circumstance, can accumulate and break down information and make predictions by checking an existing example. Its momentum up the entire cycle, giving you bits of knowledge into how you can advance and enhance your business sales processes.

Since we understand what a DSS supportive network does, how about we comprehend what precisely it is, and how it functions. A decision support system is:

- Computer-based application or program that assembles, compiles, joins, and investigate the raw data information, records, basics of sociology, applied science, arithmetic and managerial science, and individual information of decision-makers to recognize issues and decide their answers which leads to facilitate the prime decision making (Bonczek, Holsapple et al. 2014).
- A DSS network is an intelligent computer application that has total access to data about your organization's structure. It offers comparative figures between one period and the accompanying. Its activity income figures are subject to speculations related to things with item deals, product sales. A DSS is sufficiently smart enough to assist you with understanding the expenses and results from coming consequences because of various decisions and other choices (Bonczek, Holsapple et al. 2014).

A decision support system network provides the barriers to good decision making, including:

- Lack of experience/expertise
- Biasness in the system
- Shortage of time, delay
- Wrong calculations/system computations

1.1. Brief History of Decision Support System

The excursion expedition of the DSS to establish the network started in late 1960s with model-driven DSS. The 1970's saw hypothesis advancement around there and it was in the mid-1980s when the usage of accounting-based spreadsheets DSS, monetary financial planning arranging, and group DSS occurred (Neustadt 2011). The late 1980s and mid-1990s saw the development of business intelligence, Data warehouses, ODSS (Organization Decision Support System), and EIS (Executive Information System). The mid-1990s signified the beginning of data-based and online web-based decision support system networks. The support systems can be isolated into accompanying different arrangements and classifications as follows:

- *Model-driven DSS:* M-DSS depends upon basic quantitative models. It utilized restricted information and stressed control financial models. A model-driven DSS was utilized underway arranging, production planning, scheduling, and board management. It gives the most rudimentary usefulness to assembling and the manufacturing areas (Boza, Alemany et al. 2014).
- *Data-driven DSS:* Information based DSS underscored the entrance and control of information customized to explicit undertakings utilizing general instruments, tools. While it likewise gives rudimentary functionality and usefulness to the business organizations, it depends vigorously on time-series information. It had the option to help via making a dynamic decision in a scope of different circumstances (Zada, Guirguis et al. 2012).
- *Communication-driven DSS (C-DSS):* As the name proposes, communication driven DSS utilizes correspondence communication and organization-based network technologies advance to encourage decision making. The significant difference between this and the past classes of DSS was that it upheld and supports cooperation, collaboration, and correspondence communication. It utilized and used a variety of tools incorporating a Computer-based release datasheets record, sound, and video for the analysis (Stanek, Drosio et al. 2014).
- *Document-driven DSS:* A document-driven DSS uses enormous document database information that stores documents, pictures, sounds, recordings, and hypertext docs. It has an essential web-based search engine instrument related to looking through the information when required. The data put away can be raw facts and figures, historical data information, minutes of the meeting,

catalogs, trade correspondences, product requirements (Chen and Dong 2010; Abdullah, Kabir et al. 2015).

- *Knowledge-driven DSS:* Information based DSS are human-computer system frameworks that accompany critical thinking skill. These systems combine artificial intelligence with human psychological limits and can propose activities to clients. The notable point is that these frameworks have the ability in a specific space, domain (Baumeister and Striffler 2015).
- *Web-based DSS:* Web-based DSS is observed as the most modern refined decision-based network that expands its capacities by utilizing world wide web and internet (Gudigantala, Song et al. 2011). The improvement continues with advancement, evolution in web innovation. As it should be obvious, already the attention was on accelerating the decision making. However, by way of the idea developed, it moved and shifted to building an intuitive computer-based system that network that could use the information and offer experiences insights to handle badly organized issues. The definition, plan, design, knowledge, intelligence, and extent of DSS keep on advancing with time. The current DSS is equipped and prepared to help settle on additional intricate complex decision choices (Gudigantala, Song et al. 2011; Zhang, Chen et al. 2015).

1.2. Characteristics of Decision Support System Network (DSS) (Campion Jr, Waitman et al. 2010; Tripathi 2011)

- It is an approach to consolidate information from data proposed to be used in decision making. A decision support system does not automate or robotize modification accomplished on data nor fundamentally gives the output as a report, rather it supports a decision-maker to solve critical thinking approach.

- A DSS authorized the leader to associate in a characteristic neutral way because of the careful design plan of user interface.
- Decision support systems networks are anticipated to assist in decision choices that are planned as semi-organized, complex problems. These issues remain impenetrable to complete computerization.
- A DSS might be developed to help one-time decisions, those are rare, infrequent; regardless, the sort of issue or opportunity best tended to through usage of a DSS in anyone that involves human-based judgment.
- An organizational network is conventionally expected to perform, as desired for either a particular decision-maker or a group of decision-makers. This permits the system architect to design, modify the important system features and highlights different kinds of representations in the form of results generated through the software.
- Rather than building a particular DSS from scratch, a DSS system developer can utilize, look into a bundle of interconnected equipment, hardware, and programming software's need to develop a DSS.
- A decision support system is a network that is best conceptualized as a cycle process rather than a product.
- It is an approach to arrange data planned for use in dynamic decision making. Its envelopes the utilization of an information-based database for a particular decision-making process.
- A DSS network doesn't mechanize or automate change, transformations performed on information, nor just give yield as a report, rather than it supports the leaders' critical thinking and problem-solving approach.
- A DSS permits the leader to communicate and interact in a characteristic neutral way since a careful design plan of the UI is developed.

- Decision support system networks are intended, designed to help and support decisions that are defined as semi-organized, complex issues. These issues stay impervious to finish computerization.
- A DSS might be built to help and support one-time decision, those are inconsistent; notwithstanding, the sort of issue or opportunity best addressed through usage of a DSS is one that necessitates human judgment.
- A decision support system network is normally intended, designed for either a specific decision-maker or a group of managers. This permits the system software designer to design and customize significant system framework that highlight to adjust the sort of representations.
- Slightly than building a specific DSS with no pre-preparation, a system analyst can utilize a bundle of interrelated hardware equipment and programming software called DSS developer.

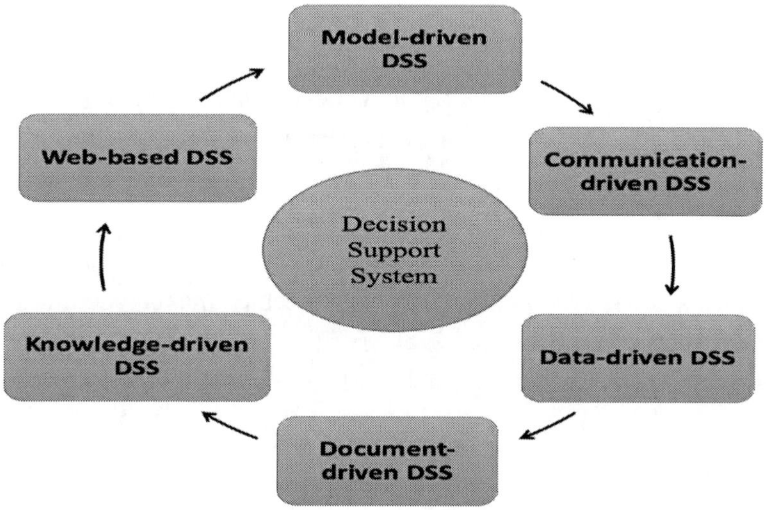

Figure 1. Different categories of available decision support system to facilitate the decision-maker.

1.3. Elements of Decision Support System

Decision support system networks are first planned as data-based information organization structures that are joined together with mathematical, numerical modelling systems framework to give the amazing, versatile, adaptable instruments for quantitative investigation of the heads administration-based choices decisions. Decision support systems were at first planned as an information base administration system joined with numerical based mathematical modelling to give incredible, adaptable apparatuses for quantitative examination of organization based decisions choices (Asemi, Safari et al. 2011).

All the supplementary as the DSS idea has been stretched out by joining thoughts, ideas from a master expert system and psychological brain science, which manages how individuals take the decision and decide to solve the problem. Information is essential for settling on administrative managerial choices however information data alone isn't adequate to settle on to make the decision. Different components are to be considered over while building administrative managerial decisions (Galimore 2011).

Even starting late, the DSS thought has been connected by joining considerations from world-class intelligent systems and intellectual brain science, which oversees how people tackle issues and decide. Data, information is basic for making administrative decisions. Sometimes in most of the cases, only data isn't satisfactory to make the decision. Various components are to be contemplated over while making administrative regulatory decisions (Juan, Gao et al. 2010).

Total factors that are responsible as an element of a support system:

1. Data
2. Decision-based rules
3. Human-based judgment
4. Managerial knowledge
5. Mathematical models for making the rules

Decisions are based on the arrangement of choice rules by an information-based framework. Since the rules rely upon data in an information database: net benefits, in any case, that it depends upon the executive to choose which rule should be applied. A conservative information database base doesn't realize whether a net benefit is normal, better than average, or below normal. Determination of the suitable decision guideline depends upon the manager's judgment on if a year-ago net benefit was typical normal. Exact DSS principle rules could be set up for deciding this also. The arrangement of decision rules, guidelines is impressively different because it requires historical and current data for the next year (Accorsi, Manzini et al. 2014). The sorts of information-based networks contain record and current information, not estimates. Estimates are frequently founded on numerical, mathematical, and statistical simulations that need authentic historical data. In this manner, an information-based database can provide the relevant data on which such prediction takes place. The modelling segment of the DSS gives the anticipating model. Mathematical based numerical forecast is not without errors, notwithstanding and they may not consider every significant factor. Consequently, a human judgment must be utilized to decipher, adjust, and change the estimated forecast. Administrative managerial decisions depend upon information on the association and its current environment. This information is excluded from the databases management system is only here and there found in and manipulate the data by any means (Seidling, Phansalkar et al. 2011).

Expert systems attempt to catch master information on the problematic domain, particular problem area and utilize that information to make the decision. Information is put away as a different element called an information base, which is comparable to the database in an information-based database system. In an information-based framework, the information-based database management system (DBMS) is software that controls data in the form of tables within a database (Beheshti 2010; Asemi, Safari et al. 2011).

In an expert system, the interference engine is an intricate program that controls the information base which is once in a while called an information base database in the expert system literature. Data in the database will in general, numeric, with some character information. Data in information bases are more subjective or literary, and interference engines may utilize subjective qualitative thinking as opposed to quantitative models to make a decision. There is now an unmistakably perceptible pattern toward the advancement of DSS networks that coordinates the information bases, mathematical models, and main DSS framework deduction incorporated into frameworks for the executives to make a decision. The expected effect of these decision-support systems networks is enormous (Beheshti 2010).

2. User Involved in Developing a Decision Support System

The definitive client of a decision support system network are the managers, executives, or decision-makers; be that as it may or may not run the system. Founded on his examination on Decision Support Systems, Alter recognized after four unmistakable utilization designs (Power 2007; Костин 2020).

1. Terminal mode
2. Clerk mode
3. Subscription mode
4. Intermediary mode

- *Terminal mode:* The leader, decision-maker is an immediate client of the system framework through which user accesses the root-based mode of the system.
- *Clerk mode:* The decision control creator utilizes the system framework straightforwardly however offline/disconnected, planning contribution on programming based DSS software. The essential contrast differentiation between this approach and the

terminal mode is in the innovation utilized batch versus on the web online.

- *Subscription mode:* The decision-maker got the reports which were created naturally and checked consistently. This is the regular method of use for the management reporting systems. Though some information, data analysis systems, or accounting models might be utilized along these report lines. It isn't ordinary for choice-based decision support systems (DSS) networks to use reports.
- *Intermediary mode:* The executives utilize the system framework through many mediators, who play out and perform the analysis, decipher, and report the results of the outcome. The executive leader doesn't realize the intermediary utilization of the framework to show up at the mentioned requested information.

The part of an intermediary is regular in the utilization of DSS networks and merits separate consideration. It has regularly been contended that decision support system networks will be opposed because administrators will refuse to utilize the terminals. The job role of executive, manager or CEO is exceptionally divided with regular interferences. Such an example of action is a significant requirement on the utilization of a framework requiring fixation throughout some sort of time. The utilization of intermediary users permits the supervisor, executive to get the profit from the support system network without really executing it.

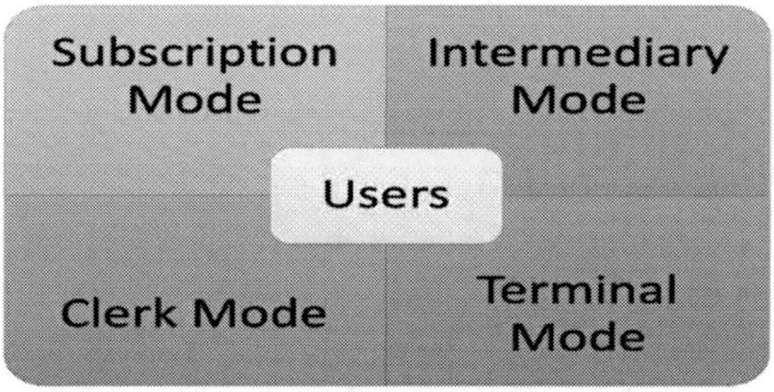

Figure 2. Type of users involved in the DSS.

3. Components Involved in the Developpent of a Decision Support System

Like some other programming frameworks, DSS likewise has also components and periods of advancement in development. Regardless of what sort of decision support network you re considering to create, you should design about these four segments and took these into the consideration (Turban, Sharda et al. 2010; Bonczek, Holsapple et al. 2014):

- *Input:* What sort type of input does it need for the complete analysis. As it is already mentioned that, it may be very well devised rules, problem, spreadsheets, pages/text, or information-based database arrangements.
- *User Knowledge/Expertise:* Regardless of whether sources of input will necessitate the manual examination by the end-user client or not.
- *Output:* What type of output will be displayed and the output should be comparatively correct or original for making the decision.
- *Decisions:* Regardless of whether it should be a suggestion support system network then again you simply need it to examine, analyze the information and result of various activities. There are two sorts of intermediates that reflect various kinds of help for the administrator, executives.
  - *Expert tool user:* This individual has skills in the presentation of at least one or more types to handle the specialized problem-solving available software. The expert tools user, clients perform the task that the professionals can't do without having the right skills or training to perform, analyze the problem.
  - *Staff analyst/Staff assistant:* This individual has specified understanding about issues and some involvement in the DSS network technology. The staff collaborator extends the

managerial capabilities by taking over a large number of the problem-solving approaches such as, setting up the issue in the problem, acquiring information, and building the underlying model. The staffing assistance performs the work and the supervisor might fix it if time will remain accessible.

Some additional middle people are the staff collaborators. There is additionally a continuous requirement for the expert tools used to handle the DSS. The utilization of go-betweens grants the DSS system to be more modern, sophisticated, amazing, and powerful. On line, intuitive system frameworks are as yet attractive with mediators since they permit them to work more quickly, productively, and efficiently.

3.1. Categorization/Classification of DSS

We have previously observed the order of DSS based on innovations utilized in the set of experiences area. One should now take a categorization at the order based on the description of processes (Minhas, Majeed et al. 2011):

- *File Drawer System (FDS):* As the name propose, an FD-DSS network gives us useful data or information to settle on a particular task. It works like a file drawer where various kinds of data are put away under various names or classifications.
- *Data Analysis Systems (DAS):* These decision systems (DSS) networks depend on a procedure; and subsequently, are utilized to mark a comparative and proportional study. These utilize basic information from processing software, tools, for example, stock investigation, and inventory analysis.
- *Information Analysis System (IAS):* This sort of DSS network examines the numerous arrangements of information to produce the educational informational intelligence that can be utilized to evaluate a circumstance for formulating a decision process.

- *Accounting and Financial Support System (AFSS):* This kind of system depends to monitor money and stock inventory system in an organization or a company.
- *Representation or Solver Model:* This kind of system perform or speak to represent in a specific domain or for a particular issue. It ascertains, computes, and looks at the results of various decisions path. The leader can direct a what if examination besides settling in an educated choice premise on the results produced.
- *Optimization Model (OS)***:** These DSS depend upon the artificially simulated model, significantly giving rules, guidelines to the activities that are performed by the executives for the operational business management. The emphasis is on giving ideal optimal arrangements on employment booking, job scheduling, product mix, and material mix decision making process choices.

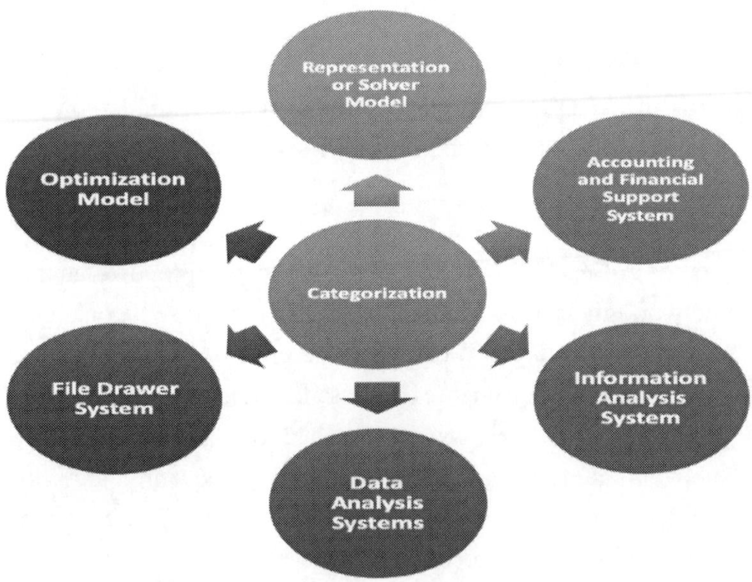

Figure 3. Categorization of a DSS.

4. Limitation and Disadvantages of Decision Support System

4.1. Limitations of Decision Support Systems (DSS)

DSS networks are fused in organizations to help human intelligence since a long time. In any case, these frameworks are not perfect. Although DSS prevents a leader, manager from advancing an inclination or bias, these systems just guide the decision-makers by offering helpful experiences into efficiently consumable help. The thinking is to extant all considerable, substantial information related to data in the kinds of diagrams, outlines, pictures, graphs, or text, so you can't neglect the reality. Unforeseen a ton upon a DSS organization and placing a lot of trust in its anything besides a sound sign (Arnott and Pervan 2008; Bright, Wong et al. 2012; Power 2013). A lot of vulnerabilities are identified with the DSS, for instance:

- *Difficulty in Quantifying the Data:* A DSS network fundamentally relies upon quantifiable informational data. Thus, it's difficult to dissect immaterial or indescribable information, data. Few qualities can't specifically be confined and considered in numbers. Even though a DSS may measure a portion of these angles, aspects, the final product should be appropriately considered by the leaders. They ought to utilize their own decision when settling on a final decision
- *Unaware of Assumptions:* As a decision-maker, you may not be careful of the suspicions that a DSS network has considered while exploring the data for a specific issue. Settling on choice without considering the uncontrolled factors may end up being dangerous. A leader should understand that an automated DSS is just a supporting tool. One have to think about an unstructured or intermediate, partially organized instance inside and out to investigate the constraints and suppositions.

- *System Design Failure:* Decision support systems (DSS) network remains intended for the particular requirements of a decision-maker. You don't have an idea what process you want a DSS to organize or how it would assist you, it will be hard to plan, design a system that meets decision-makers' requirements. Also, when you utilize an obscure DSS, the results delivered are not what you re looking for. Such occurrences may arise as a result of system design failures.
- *Difficulty in Collecting All the Required Data:* As a decision-maker, one should understand that its impractical to capture, gather, and store the entirety of the connected information precisely. Though some information is hard to store in the form of documentation, some can't be recorded using any means. Along these lines, the worth value introduced by a DSS may not be 100% valid.
- *Lack of Technology and the Technical Knowledge in DSS Users:* Although decision support system networks have gotten a lot more straightforward throughout the long term, numerous leaders think that it's hard to utilize. The absence of innovative information stays an issue.

4.2. Disadvantages of Decision Support Systems

Other than restrictions, DSS networks likewise have a few obstructions, for example, (Lambin, Van Stiphout et al. 2013):

- *Information Overload in the DSS system:* At some points mechanized, and computerized decision-making may bring data information overload. Since it investigates, analyzes all parts of the problem, it leaves the user in a dilemma about what to consider and what not to consider. Not each portion of data is important in decision making. However, when it is contemporary, a decision-maker thinks that it's difficult to disregard the interrelated information that doesn't need significance.

- *Dependence on DSS:* The facts demonstrate that DSS networks are coordinated into organizations to settle on a consistent decision. Some leaders build up a propensity to rely a lot upon modernized decision making and don't have any desire to apply their minds. There is a move in concentration and managers may not sharpen their abilities further in light of unnecessary reliance on DSS.
- *Depreciation of Subjectivity leads to devaluation:* A good DSS network advances discerning the relational decisions by recommending options and suggestions to premise objectivity. While limited judiciousness or confined roles assume a basic part/role in the process of decision, subjectivity cannot and ought not to be dismissed or rejected. A DSS advance objectivity and consigns subjectivity, which can have a genuine effect on a business.
- *Over prominence on Decision Making:* Obviously, the focal point of mechanized computerized decision building is thinking about all parts of an issue constantly, which may not be needed in a significant number of circumstances. It is fundamentally basic to set up the customers to ensure and guarantee the effective and ideal use, utilization of DSS.
- *Expenditure of Development Cost*: The expense of dynamic DSS once a support system is introduced. Yet, the advancement and usage of a DSS need enormous money related to speculation investment. Personalization may attract higher charge costs. In case you're on a strict budget, you probably won't get a modified DSS explicit to your needs.

5. Analyzing a Business Decision Making Process

Continuous analysis of authoritative, dynamic DSS is fundamental to the high caliber and straightforward transparent decisions. In any case, a trade runs with a predisposition: the idea that it is acceptable at settling on making decisions, regardless of whether it is not. Also, most likely this is the reason both, decision-makers and the DSS examiners attempt to get significant comprehension information of the association, organization-wide decisions range to construct a highly profound personalized DSS software framework. This implies a ton of attempts into the arrangement, planning, and implementation of a DSS network (Weygandt, Kimmel et al. 2020). Decision making is significant and complex as well. However, its extension is wide. It's not confined to a specific degree of progression; rather employees at all levels across all offices or departments decide and make decisions, dependent upon the positions they are working and conditions they face the problem of decision making. Some of the decision choices are identified with an assessment of ventures, investments, dispensing assets allocation, evaluating consolidations, and securing recommendations. Some are connected to introducing new things, examining their time period of practical convenience, upgrading producing effectiveness contemplating their timeframe of realistic usability for improving the manufacturing and accumulating effectiveness (Ferrell and Fraedrich 2015). There are, furthermore, ordinary decisions that are legitimate for a state of time. Commonly, more objective decisions are made at lower levels of the hierarchy, which can be evaluated. More significant levels of progressive system management deal with an unstructured or poorly organized system, which is abstract, subjective in nature, while targeted objective choices may not need imagination, emotional, subjective decisions. Like choices made in every division at each level are unique, also a decision support system network analyst should consider the kind of choices and recognized variables impacting dynamic before going to the planning phase and planning the engineering designing the architecture. Understanding the setting in which decisions are made is a significant thought in building a DSS (Edelenbos and Klijn 2007; Vercellis 2009; Murphy 2016). Allow us to investigate the elements that a DSS examiner should consider.

5.1. Types of Managerial Decisions

As said before, decisions are made at all levels of hierarchy. Along these lines, it's imperative to comprehend that what kind of decisions will be supported by DSS managerial decisions (Mullakhmetov 2016).

- *Strategic decisions:* As essential choices are not identified with the general working of organization and association. These are non-monotonous and need a great deal of time to be shown arrived up at. For the most part, decision taken by the highest level of hierarchy of importance, strategic decisions include a careful analysis of the circumstance and consequences. A few instances of strategic decisions: assessment of a speculation proposition, choices identified with consolidations and acquisitions, asset assignments, resource allocation, and so on, etc. (Lovallo and Sibony 2006).
- *Operational decisions:* These sorts of decisions fall under two classes. The first class is the choices related to plant area location, production volume, allocation of a channel, and strategies are taken by top administration management. These are long-haul choices that straightforwardly sway the working of a business. The second classification of decisions is identified with everyday working, which is taken by centre and lower-level directors, managers, supervisors (Puig, Marques et al. 2009).
- *Managerial decisions:* These choices relate to asset assignment, the ability of the executives, innovative work, and new product introduction, pull out, or redo old items. These are consolidated decisions taken by top and upper center administration, management. Each sort of choice requires a diverse degree of help. A decision support analyst needs to investigate and analyse, what sort of decisions should be upheld; who is associated with the decision cycle; and whether alternative courses of activities are needed to appear (Velychko and Liudmyla 2017).

- *Nature of Problems:* Decision-making is straightforward or complex relying on the nature of the problem. It could be monotonous or non-repetitive, organized, or unstructured. Also, every difficult type requires diverse methodology, problem-solving technique procedures, and subjectivity. We should comprehend this in detail:
  - Non-structured based problems
  - Structured/Organized problems
  - Non-repetitive problems
  - Recurring/Repetitive problems
- *Participation of Clients:* A DSS analyst should consider individuals engaged with a decision-making process. There is a bunch of choices that are taken by a group of people. In such a case, a DSS should empower individuals required to interface, impart, share records, files, and information with one another.
- *Decision Environment:* Managers can take the help of DSS network experts in understanding these inward and outer elements of decision-making. The outer variable like innovation, technology, distributors, wholesalers, competitors, and customers. Inner elements include individuals and their insights, capacities, recurrence of decisions, kind of choices they take, office where a DSS is to be actualized, and authoritative elements systems, cycles, financial plan, change the board management (Argent, Perraud et al. 2009).
- *Determine the extent or the scope of the Support System:* For conventional issues, a DSS can offer total help, yet for a not well-organized issue, it can just show all conceivable elective courses of activities with their upsides and downsides, leaving the end choice for client. Contingent on a decision-maker setting, a DSS examiner can believe objectives to be accomplished, inspect other important options, attract a cycle to rank other options, foresee choice climate inward and outer elements influencing choices and distinguish the attributes of decision-makers (Burstein and Holsapple 2008).

6. Developpent of a Decision Support System

6.1. Role of Decision Support System in the Management Information System (MIS)

DSS network remains an exceptional class of organization framework that encourages decision making. As in an association, at every single point and time, decisions need to be independent of decision-maker's temperament or nature. Few decisions are frequent practice or programmed and non-customized choices. In any case, one thing is sure that decision is done at all degrees of the executives or managerial level. DSS network includes a programmed package which assists the management, managers with taking the right and convenient choices. Decision support system networks use information, available data from the overall administration databases, and they are utilized by a manager or a leader to take decisions (Asemi, Safari et al. 2011). The fundamental characteristic of choice based DSS network is that it depends on some software tool, technique, or available organization's standard models. These available systems are utilized here and there for testing new alternative options, training, and learning. They are likewise utilized for exploring the different, new boundaries of a model. The MIS creator needs to search for every single such circumstance and design, develop the DSS network for combination in the system. The administration database management system would turn out to be more helpful if the decision making is made individual free and executed with an all-around planned and well-designed DSS network. All such implanted system frameworks cover the ordinary assortment of different decision circumstances. On the off chance that anything outside the considered assortment manifests, the DSS network will bring to the notification of the chiefs that activity is called for in the circumstance. The system assumes a prevailing party in the management information system administration data framework as help to decide in the organization (Asemi, Safari et al. 2011; Tripathi 2011).

6.2. Designing, Building, and Implementation of an Ideal Decision Support System

A portion goes into planning, designing, and making an ideal DSS network. It functions as an intelligent system network simply after it is taken care of by knowledge during the turn of its development. Building up a DSS is a complex cycle process and took a long time. It goes repeatedly throughout three phases - sources of input activities, output during each period of the system development lifecycle (SDLC). You give an input, carried out the desired, ideal action, and degree the output (Berner 2007; Bonczek, Holsapple et al. 2014).

A DSS system plan and development experiences these different stages:

- *Intelligence:* On that level of a support system the goal, objectives are to look for the problems/situations/conditions that we need a decision-based system to build up.

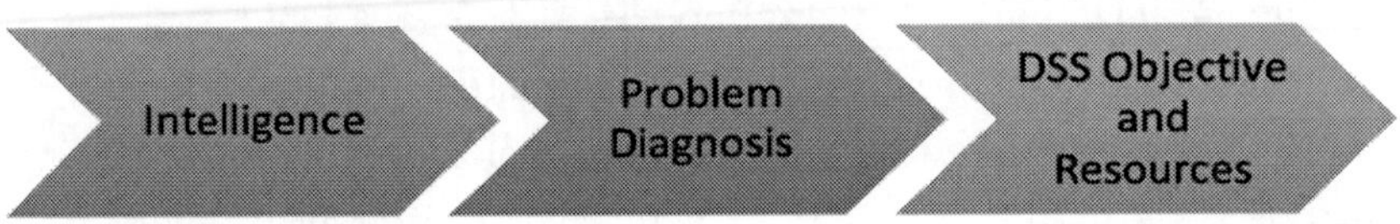

Figure 4. The process involved in intelligence.

As a businessman, you are relied on and estimated, expected upon to recognize and characterize the issues set for which solution, encouragement is needed. You should characterize and define the goals which are accessible, with the goal that the results produced to meet up to your expectations.

- *Design of an ideal DSS:* This phase deal with analyzing down every conceivable, possible activity, alongside the determination of organization plan and system development.

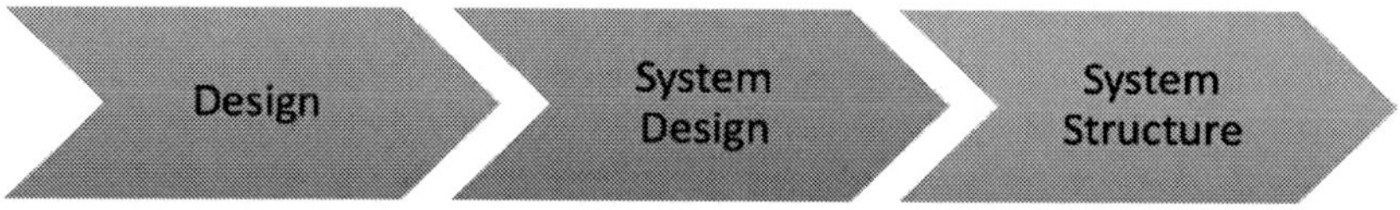

Figure 5. The process involved in the design of Ideal DSS.

- *System design* includes and incorporates the declaration of components, platform, working libraries, and special programming language.
- *System structure* is connected to picking up the model philosophy and methodology. This stage also incorporates the identification of hardware requirements. The advancement and development in the DSS start from here.
- *Implementation of a DSS network:* This is the last stage of a support system where testing, assessment, evaluation, adjustment changes, and the deployment of DSS takes place. Nevertheless, this is the final result however it can be changed, refined, upgraded premise your exercises activities, prerequisites and based on end-user requirements.

When building up a custom DSS, these are significant elements that should be considered and kept in mind:

- Data management functions in the DSS
- Available hardware platforms that support the system
- User interface the system uses
- Compatibility with other applications in the organization
- Overall cost

6.3. Gaining Competitive Advantage with Decision Support Systems

Over the last fifty years, Decision Support Systems (DSS) has progressed significantly. They have changed from an automated system to rearranging/simplifying the calculations into profoundly sophisticated arrangements plans consolidating the hardware, programming-based software, tools, and the human intelligence for taking care of enormous volumes of information or data sets, examining various results/outcomes, recognizing new chances, opportunities via implementing the methodological strategies successfully. Old DSS appears to have overwhelmed human intelligence (Noe, Hollenbeck et al. 2017).

DSS comes as a significant tool that can rapidly measure all the boundaries, parameters, complete inside in-depth analysis, and out an examination, predict future patterns, trends and suggest potential blueprints, course of action. This implies that a cutting edge DSS is fit for visualizing and forecasting, envisaging future patterns in a given territory/areas, offering helpful insights of knowledge to organizations. In this way, it makes an upper hand for a business. Besides, the advancements in computers, mobile phones, and web advances/internet have intensely affected the plan, design of a DSS, and its abilities. We should examine what can be foreseen anticipated from DSS in the future (Trkman, McCormack et al. 2010).

6.4. Technology Trends in DSS

The Support Systems are continuously developing. There are innovations, emergence of new technologies, methodologies and steadily changing business needs that are subject to their constant advancement, evolutions. Development has had the critical and highest effect on their turn and on their development. Experts recognize new key developments or examples, a pattern that you may discover in this class of programming systems frameworks, software systems in a not so distant future. These include:

- GIS (Geographical Information System) will accept a critical part in a borderless global business world in the near future. It's a system designed intended to oversee, manage, and analyze geological data information, helping the decision-makers in arranging area-based services or area-based manufacturing. GIS innovation additionally facilitates with scopes of latitudes and altitudes to locale to decide its reasonableness for supply chain management for their plant and assembling/manufacturing unit. Also, when combined with GPS, it will permit decision-makers to change their thing creation network, depend upon the direction of customers in a particular district, region, area, or state (Mbilinyi, Tumbo et al. 2007).

- The part of OR (Operational Research) techniques, methods will increment in building DSS, to give a more realistic picture in offered situations to the leader or decision-makers. Web innovation, internet technology strongly affects nearly everything that we do. The next-generation DSS, no doubt will meet web search engine to quickly look and address a particular issue which arises in the organization (Simpson and Hancock 2009).
- A future DSS may have the alternative to choose the nearby correct, right timespans for the ease of use of a product. It is very smart well enough to comprehend the psychological and emotional factors engaged with the purchasing choices, decisions. A future DSS may have an alternative to utilize scholarly intellectual features, seriously utilizing visualization, highlights, memory, thinking, consideration, attention, and appreciation or comprehension (Charles and Chemelle 2012).

6.5. Designing and Developing Decision Support Systems

The business intelligence (BI) empowered software or DSS help dynamic decision making in an association, corporation. A viable DSS furnishes you with unbiased, impartial data analysis, ongoing real-time system monitoring, and rich detailing in the system, supporting you to make an informed choice at all possible periods (Turban, Sharda et al. 2010). A prudently planned DSS uses scientific, scientific-analytical models, diverse real and econometric instruments, human-based information knowledge model, intelligence, and experiences to help in decision making (Bonczek, Holsapple et al. 2014). This demonstrates the significance of innovation, prominence of technology, philosophy, methodology, and approach behind designing, planning, and improvement of a DSS. As a decision-maker, you should be very cautious in choosing the DSS innovation and formative technique. You need to get the fundamental rights to get a dependable right tool, software to help a different kind of data and perform decision-making techniques (Turban, Sharda et al. 2010). Since planning, designing, developing and improvement of a DSS network is an intricate critical process, you may go up against different issues, for example:

- *Incompatibility and misalliance between the perceptions of the programmer and decision-maker:* On one hand decision-makers have no information about the need to plan and build up a DSS network. On the other hand, a programmer or software designer probably won't have a sensible considered or probably can't consider rationally that how the business dynamic has become unpredictable in today's highly variable time. Innovation, technology purpose may appear to be perplexing and ambiguous to the decision-maker while the inclinations, necessities, and desires for the decision-maker may not fit the system design of framework plan and advancement. This will match among points of view prompts difficulties. And yet, this improves the likelihood probability of production of a powerful and able DSS.
- *Identification of unambiguous, specific requirements of clients:* The greater part of the occasion, that even decision-makers have no idea about what's inside data is stored to form a decision support system network. This is especially the circumstance when managements, executive, the director needs an instrument to help in settling of ineffectively coordinated or unstructured issues. It's not hard to pick what is helpful in DSS should have when issues are routine and organized. Administrators, managers can look for

help from their partners and direct meetings to produce novel thoughts, outline the capacities and advantages of a decision support system (Kremic, Tukel et al. 2006).

- *Technology selection:* At the present exceptionally serious professional business environment, you need an intelligent and responsive DSS network that boosts your presentation, performance. In such a situation, the determination of innovation assumes an urgent job. Notwithstanding, it's not generally important to utilize the most recent form of version at a specific stage. It relies upon the targets, objectives you wish to accomplish. A DSS advancement organization may push you for the most recent innovation, which will add to your costs. The general guideline is to request value cites from various organizations (Lakhno 2017).
- *The approach followed to system software development and design:* As discussed before, there is no standard methodology or philosophy to plan, design the best DSS network. There are three principal ways to deal with framework plan and improvement: 1) the traditional System development life cycle (SDLC) approach; 2) Rapid prototyping and 3) The end-user approach. You might need to pick one methodology system that guarantees that the eventual outcome achieves your destinations, objectives. Yet, each approach has its advantages and disadvantages, making it hard to pick the best one (Ali 2017).
- *Feasibility Study Analysis and Pre-Design Diagnosis of a DSS:* What is the way to make sure about the privileged DSS formative strategy, methodology. Indeed, a pre-plan design diagnosis of a dynamic decision-making process and attainability feasible study of a DSS idea can help you pick up and gaining clarity. Conclusion, diagnosis, and possible testing are two distinct cycles yet are entwined with each other. Contingent on how decisions are made in an association, organization, a software engineer, and programmer complete the plausibility testing of all the possible

thought on which a DSS is to be created (Doufene, Sakhrani et al. 2020).

- *Decision-Making Process Diagnosis:* There is one demonstrative diagnostic, analytical study of DSS. In an association DSS help pick up clearness on various points, *for example*, the Problem Identification process, what is the information, data collection procedures and techniques, How the decision was made, What kind of people from the administration are associated in decision making, and the Norms relating to decision making in an association, organization?

6.6. Choosing a System Development Approach

As referenced above, picking a system development approach is a basic issue. This is because there is no single cycle that can be named as best. What advancement approach on which you rely on the consequences of plausibility, feasibility study, and a share mutual arrangement between decision-maker and developer. You should pick a formative software development methodology, when you choose to settle on a custom DSS network. On the off chance that you choose to purchase a bundled package arrangement, solutions, you just advise the master to pick an appropriate programming framework, and execute it. It is more affordable than making a good support system network. However, in case you're not convinced with the usefulness of a bundled arrangement, deals to make it furnish with all the capacities and highlights that you require (Sommerville 2004). Here are three ways to deal with framework system improvement, a growth that you might need to find out about:

- *System Development Life Cycle Approach(SDLC):* The official SDLC is a consecutive sequential cyclic process that starts with distinguishing the system framework primarily objective, client requirements (necessities of end-user, clients), and experiences at different stages, including, System design (architecture), System plan (design), Coding (programming), Testing (finding error and bug fixing), Implementation of DSS (execution in the association), end-users clients utilizing DSS for evaluation and to check the functional capacities and capabilities where modification required. Usually, it's the most utilized and most inflexible rigid system framework development approach. In complex circumstances, it gets hard to utilize this methodology, as the requirements of the end-users, clients are continually evolving. It doesn't advance the repeating improvement, development, design, and testing (Jirava 2004; Sommerville 2004; Radack 2009).

- *Rapid Prototyping Approach (RAD model):* As the name proposes, rapid prototyping stands as a technique that advances quick framework, software, system improvement, development. Also, it's the consolidated exertion of decision-makers and system analysts. A DSS expert works intimately with a decision-maker, to graph out the specific requirements. Although a leader utilizes general terms, experts use the DMS (data management system) to help quick advancement of the application. Rapid prototyping experiences include as identification of objectives to be achieved, client necessities, requirement, Development of the first principal model, Evaluation of the main model, recognize the changes required, modification, testing the developed DSS interface, return to assessment and alteration. In rapid prototyping the necessary implementation in DSS is consistently open, assessment and adjustment occur at a quick movement. This is the reason it's viewed as a preferable methodology over SDLC in complex circumstances and viewed as a better solution in the development of a support system in less time interval (Jones and Richey 2000; Sommerville 2004).
- *End-User DSS Development Approach:* End-users DSS advancement approach advance the planning, improvement of a system software relying on the particular individual for decision-making. It resembles like as modify your personal computer. As an administrator utilize different applications, they may need a

framework, software that coordinates all the dimensions they require. In addition to this side of the methodology is a manager makes his DSS all alone. The negative side is that the person may wind up picking the unfortunate programming language or software. Besides, they may settle on mistake accidentally when building up a DSS as a result of the absence of specialized, technical skills. This methodology is once in a while utilized (Sommerville 2004; Miah 2009).

6.7. User Interface (UI) platform for Designing a Decision Support System (DSS) an Approach

The adequacy of an automated method framework or a product stage relies upon its UI plan design. Being it's a standard software package or a top of the DSS network, the client's interaction with the UI framework should be as straightforward as simple, successful, and hassle-free as could be expected under any circumstances (Dellermann, Lipusch et al. 2019). It is anything but miserable that incredible on DSS networks have fine UI plans. These are designed to give a prevalent client experience. Planning a UI include accomplishing the total comprehension of client needs and how they decide to make the decisions. All in all, the inquiries emerge - whatever goes into their arrangement and how to plan a decent good client user interface? We will result in these present circumstances. Before that, we dive into the refinements in UI. We should initially attempt to comprehend what UI implies on DSS. What is a good interface and what it contains? In software engineering, computer science, boundary implies that piece of a modernized computerized framework that permits its clients to collaborate, interact through it. This is the main thing that clients see and then use the developed product. UI is significant yet it encourages, facilitates the collaboration and interaction between the client and the product framework without causing a lot of consideration to itself. It is that concealed part of a PC program that reinforces its convenience and usability. A good user interface contains commands, menus, graphics, icons (Smethers 2004).

Features of a Good User Interface (or A Good interface should have the following features): Following are the most significant highlights of an ideal UI:

- Its stimulus how clients, users' interface with the DSS.
- Stabilities the details, usefulness of the system framework, and user mindset toward UI client's perspective.
- Provide a picture-oriented visual approach to clients to connect with the software UI.
- Create a perfect correspondence announcement and collaboration between the client and the support system network.
- Decrease mistakes, errors, speed up, underpins great dynamic.
- Logical and instinctive simultaneously

6.7.1. User Interface Styles

Probably we are aware that UI is there, where collaboration between humans and-machine occurs. This chooses, how the client inputs the data and how the system framework presents the result. There are various approaches to collaborate with automated computerized decision-making software. Regardless, which UI style is to be used, should be picked before the advances, the development process begins. Before the advanced development process begins, it should be decided which UI style is to be used. There are no firm standard rules about which is the best UI style. A Decision Support System might practice one interface style or a blended mix of two styles, user interface at any rate. A DSS designer can give a few control successions to oversee or run a product program, contingent on client needs (Ho 2000). Here are six prevailing dominant UI styles that can be utilized to make good decision-making system software.

- Command-Line Interface (CLI)
- Menu-based GUI interface:

- Graphical based interface (Icons, Emoji):
- Question-and-Answer interface:
- Voice-based command user interface:
- Touch user interface:

Rules that you should follow when planning the user interface for the DSS:

- *Consistency in DSS design, Architecture:* A DSS network programming-based software should look, feel, and act comparable all through. The colour combination, themes of the tools, menus in software, and other visuals should be reliable and consistent. It makes a DSS look coordinated and thoroughly examined.
- *Information Overload should be less:* The fundamental goal of a support system network is to reduce the database information over-burden and streamline things to the degree of extent of possibility. Likely, this is the reason most associations utilize modernized frameworks to help dynamic decision making. Where appropriate, the designed plans should be limited and orders should be shown as the group of activities should be abbreviated and shortened.
- *Create Aesthetically Appealing yet Minimal Interface Design:* The interface should be engaging. In any case, you need to show your creative side to design and UI. It should be adjusted balanced, calming, intelligent, interactive, and responsive.
- *Feedback based system should be informative:* Clients anticipate enlightening informative input feedback about the order they have given or activity they have performed. Minor orders may offer modest unassuming input feedback, while solid criticism should be offered for infrequent actions.
- *Interactions between the different designs:* Each collaboration ought to have a succession or a request at the starting, centre, and the end. This keeps track of the progression of the exchange. The design tries to make user interaction much more intuitive and easier to interact with the DSS system. It should be easy to operate.

- *Anticipate Errors:* You need to envision potential mistakes that a client can make when utilizing the supportive system network. At certain places, the framework should make clients mindful of what mistakes they will make by pressing a system command.
- *Users Control of the System in the Support System:* Individuals utilizing a choice based DSS network need to control every part of the system framework. Powerlessness to control make them on the edge and unconfident. Give them control of the framework and let them investigate it as much as they need.
- *Provides Acceleration to the organization in the development of their business processes:* As a manager or executives a DSS all the more much of the time, they would prefer not to offer the same data or information is needed each time in the system as they sign into the framework. Furnish them with quickening agents to abbreviate the cooperation's and increment the speed.
- *Provide Documentation and Help Capabilities:* A DSS even though isn't fragmented on the off chance that it doesn't give documentation abilities however to clients it might appear to be inadequate and incomplete. A compelling effective UI makes a framework simpler to utilize. It eliminates out uneasiness and fear of innovation and advances its utilization. A DSS support designer should keep all the above rules when planning an intuitive user interface.

6.7.2. Elements Influencing User Interface Design Success

There is a lot of components that impact and influence the accomplishment of a UI plan, design. A DSS creator is required to perceive and consider these elements when planning and designing a UI for a DSS network (Al-Maskari and Sanderson 2010).

- *Execution Time:* For what reason an executive uses a computerized system framework to help in decision making. Clearly, to decrease execution time! As a DSS designer, you should attempt and try to reduce the execution time for an order given and the activity action performed. The speed of execution should be maximum to limit the wastage of time.

- *Versatility:* An intelligence supportive system network should be sufficiently clever enough to play out the decision-maker task assignments that an executive to perform when settling on a decision utilizing DSS. Besides, it should be sufficiently adaptable to incorporate new tasks at whatever point needs to emerge.
- *Adaptability:* A decision support system should be sufficiently intelligent to adjust as per the most conspicuous prominent habits for its client. This implies it should act naturally fitting or customizing in itself. It might appear to be unreasonable, yet actually, it isn't. Or maybe this is the thing that is normal for a smart DSS framework network.
- *Learning Time:* A DSS UI should be adequately straightforward to reduce the learning time for their clients, with the goal that they can utilize it to its full limit when possible.
- *Uniformity of Command:* As said before, a DSS UI should have a uniform subject all through. It should offer a similar look and belief and command all through as the previous DSS system work.
- *Quality of Help:* At the point when an executive is a client (sometimes executive or client both) use a DSS developed by you, the person expects complete offline help from your side. The achievement of a DSS relies on the nature of help provided by the company or developer. Perceive what the client may do on/with the DSS and offer self-improvement manuals both on the web and offline. There must be a help section in the support system through which one can read and troubleshoot their problems.
- *Memory Load:* An individual has impediments limitation with regards to recollecting or remembering the numbers. The thought isn't to barrage the client with an excessive number of factual or mathematical numerical information data interpret all at once. A decent UI configuration takes the memory load off the client's mind and executes it on less memory. Load balancing should be in

the system at the time of full load testing or in the actual environment.

- *Ease of Recall:* When a client returns to DSS after a long, it should help him/her review what was done previously history. It causes them to accomplish a similar speed within a short period.
- *Fatigue:* Mental exhaustion happens as a result of the complexity of the plan and design. Keep things simple and straightforward. Keep the command visual with the goal that the client does not need to recall that anything when they frequently use the system.
- *Errors:* Envision of errors that a client, the executive may perform when utilizing a decision supportive network system. Give them the control to turn around the activity and help to manage them what to do straightaway next. Designing a DSS network UI is the hardest piece of the improvement system development cycle.

6.8. Networking and Security Related Issues in DSS Architecture

Organizations are based on decision-driven. The rate of success and the failure of every decision with an organization's system directly or indirectly affect the growth and the support system which decides the strategies for the organization. If in hierarchical organization decision is lined up with the man-made artificial intelligence-based software program, probabilities are that the exhibition, performance of the association, the organization will improve by and large. DSS networks have picked up gigantic popularity in different areas, including armed, security, medication, manufacturing, designing, engineering, and business. These containers uphold the decision making in circumstances where accuracy is important. Also, they give admittance to pertinent information by incorporating different structures of relevant knowledge and wellsprings integrating various forms of data, supporting human intellectuals. Whereas the DSS utilizes AI to address issues, you shouldn't overemphasize its significance. It's a method to get near figures to premise a few or a mix of some conventional procedures. The end decision for decision making remains at the parts with your end (Seaman 2020).

In some organization, a DSS is used in an implicit and incompetent way. The development design process is abbreviated and is completed in a quick approach. While this is justifiable in light of the relentless competition, always changing business strategies and economically unstable setting. Yet organizations need more opportunity to get together to look into inventive data sources, work on the plan, design, foundation, and development of a DSS, alongside DSS analyst and software engineers recognize possible security features, systems administration issues. This will help in building a solid, more appropriate, and exceptionally compelling DSS network. Except if every segment of a DSS is carefully planned, created, and designed. It is very difficult to make an independent framework to help in the decision making. This requires equivalent inclusion of decision-makers and DSS analysts, planners, designers, and developers. Everyone in DSS design segments requires a careful approach and resolutely uphold from all the gatherings in an organization who use the system (Subashini and Kavitha 2011).

6.8.1. How Are the DSS Based Architecture, Network, and Security Is Interdependent?

DSS network is used in engineering, organization, and security is interconnected with each other. Investigation of DSS design includes getting out thinking of how a user will collaborate, interact with the software framework, and how data will move starting with one point then onto the next. DSS network is worried about how equipment is connected, in this way the information is transferred all through the system framework, how DSS segments are related, and whether the information is taken care of and got to utilizing over the website, extranet, or intranet. While DSS engineering is worried about the origination of the structure, model, and conduct of a software framework that is to be created. Organizing is about the association between the different parts of software, programming, and computer hardware. Security is integral to any computer programming framework and a DSS is no exemption from the standard. A malicious virus attack, hacking endeavour, leakage, or data leakage within the organization can make harm the software framework just as the association, company, or organization. As a DSS is a network that contains secret encrypted data, it should be 100% free, safe and secure. It's likewise fundamental for defending safeguard for representative and client information. Let's take a close look at these components (Holsapple 2008).

There are four central segments of DSS based engineering and architecture:

1. The type of user interface that a DSS have
2. Type of database is used
3. Model for the contextual or situation representation in system software
4. Knowledge about the DSS system working

- *The type of user interface that a DSS has:* In the previous article, we learn what to plan and design a powerful UI plan. Meanwhile, it's an obvious topic of study. We acquired prerequisites of a good user interface, at the essentials of a respectable, decent UI setup, concerns identifying with discourse dialogue advancement, adaptableness, strategy for dealing with information, interface design rules, and the factors impacting the achievement of a UI idea.
- *Type of database is used:* Afterwards, approaches comes on the type of database used for information. It serves and provides as the storeroom of information. It comprises personal data details are gathered from inside the association, organization, representatives, employees, and clients. It influences, incorporates thoughts, ideas, your own experiences, encounters, and bits of knowledge. External data information, data gathered from outside sources, similar to independent researchers, web, internet, government organization, associations, and so on.
- *Model for the contextual or situation representation in system software:* This part of the DSS project deals with the DSS model

and DSS model management system. A prototypical made a critical fragment of DSS design plan since it grants you to finish a particular specific kind of data that you're required for a specific type of decision making.

- *Knowledge:* In this constituent of DSS design, the architecture gives data about the relationship among information, which is disproportionately too complex for understanding. It deals with the information and gives executives, managers a solution of arrangements of a particular problem. It additionally sends signs to managers when there is any problem that needs to be a concern.

7. Decision Support System Models

As the name itself clarifies, a model-driven DSS network uses a model to tackle issues or help in decision making. A prototypical model can provide the statistical, numerical, financial, arithmetical solution for the optimization problem. A DSS model may utilize a single based model, a mix of at least two models or more than two models, contingent on the particular requirements, specification of its clients. Simply the models give essential, basic usefulness while the fusion of at least two models allows clients to analyze complex information. Commonly Model-driven DSS does not contain serious information or maybe they use boundaries-based parameters to enter by leaders in the assessment when analysing the situations. They produce ideal explanations that are steady, reliable, and dependable with time and asset limitations or restrictions. The possibility of the model-driven DSS is immense and can be additionally upgraded by integrating the web-based online applications. Making a DSS driven model necessitates an extensive degree of expertise. Decision-makers and DSS analysts need to work close to build up a productive and efficient system framework, which is adaptable, scalable flexible, simple to coordinate, integrate, and utilize with the other systems also (Kuik and Diong 2019). DSS driven model can be utilized to help in dynamic decision making and diversity of assortment and circumstances. It can help administrators in the creation of the following: -

- Credit-based and advancing conclusions for the customers
- Product demand forecasting in weather
- Budgeting decisions for future trends
- Marketing decisions in companies
- Production forecasting decisions in the manufacturing unit
- Resource allocation decisions in the organization
- Investment decisions for the investors, stock market investors

7.1. Building a Model-Driven based DSS (MDSS)

The main part of a model driven DSS is the model it utilizes for dynamic decision making. This implies that the determination of a model is the most significant and crucial step in the advances of building an MDSS (Kuik and Diong 2019). All in all, how you go about it? How about we comprehend let's look into it now:

- *Modelling:* Displaying modelling is the way toward identifying a proper model for a model-driven DSS network. It experiences the following stages in an ordered way, starting after problematic identification proof. Once the modelling is done, it's essential to choose the authorized model, to guarantee that its functions are working well and create suitable outcomes in taking up the decisions.
- *Expectations & Predictions:* Assumptions are expectations or best estimates. Each model has certain suspicions about the time and risk included with a specific circumstance. These outcomes are tried through affectability for what-if analysis. Assumption plays a significant part in characterizing an issue, distinguishing and managing of vulnerability.

- *Static Analysis:* This kind of system doesn't think about the drawn-out reaction of a system framework. The static investigation is done when a circumstance in which the organization settles on a choice is static in nature.
- *Active Analysis:* Active analysis is involved in the testing of a database, software, or product-based software framework in the actual time. This technique considers that the circumstance transformations over time, because of any explanation, for example, cost, rules and guidelines, time, and so on. What type of study should need to be led relies on the circumstance. Leaders and DSS investigators should recognize whether it is proper to accept confidence, vulnerability, risk in a situation in the company.

7.2. Model Types

As declared before (discuss earlier or mentioned above), a piece model-driven DSS deals with some sort of model or a mixed arrangement of models. Consequently, thinking about different models is paying off. A DSS conveys one or a blend of beneath the models:

- *Explanatory/Descriptive Model:* Depicts besides clarifies approximately, what is it and why, how it functions, and the working.
- *Contemplative Model:* Figures consequences or results that might be delivered since a particular arrangement of boundaries and parameters.
- *Algebraic Model:* A significantly high-level demonstrating modelling system framework for resolving the multifaceted conditions. It is utilized to streamline, optimized a variable or condition, comparison. Best of all, it can deal with numerous conditions at a time.
- *Accounting and Financial Models:* These model-driven choice DSS networks help in decision making in different circumstances

identified with bookkeeping, accounting, and Financially management. The models incorporate many other things related to finance.

- *Budget Financial Model:* DSS with the planning budget model is normally an enterprise-wide presentation. Numerous organizations utilize such frameworks for expenditure arranging, preparation, and estimating, predicting their decisions.
- *Pro Forma Financial Statements:* A DSS with this model sums up the foreseen monetary outcomes for a particular time-frame in the future. Expenses are assessed dependent on past information, net deals are anticipated and benefit then determined on these connections.
- *Ratio Analysis:* These aides a commercial in assessing its economic summaries. Proportion investigation makes monetary information more significant, by indicating coherent connections between information.
- *Decision Analysis Models:* The fundamental occupation of DSS is to distinguish, classify, and assess the options with their separate upsides and downsides. The decision-makers at that point evaluate all the other options and pick the one that they believe is the best. The point of choice analysis procedures is to perform the tasks.
- *Simulation Models:* DSS with reproduction models lead tests to distinguish conditions or circumstances that imprecise from the real conditions. These models are used to take care of various issues, including, manpower arranging and task, Inventory control, Reliability and replacement, Sequencing and planning, Stock-in and stock-out, Queuing and blockage in the decision systems.

7.3. The Following Are Different Sorts of Decision Analysis Processes in DSS Models

- *Analytical Hierarchy Process (AHP):* It's a multi-standards decision technique, a strategy that consolidates quantitative and subjective variables while assessing the different options. The insightful hierarchy process begins and measures that start with building up a progressive portrayal of an issue. With the general goal on the top the decision options at the base, applicable properties, and determination models in the middle. After you compose decision alternatives at the base, you need to analyze the options by creating social information(Das 2019).

- *Decision Trees:* As the name recommends, a decision tree utilizes a tree-like flowchart of decisions, draw from left to right, with additional branches clarifying their results. The point is to distinguish the most suitable procedure to arrive at an objective. A decision tree has three sorts of centres. The hubs, nodes and decision rules, principles are the basic foundation structure of DSS. The decision trees are easy to comprehend, offer important bits of knowledge, decide the best and most noticeably terrible situations, and can be joined effectively with other choice strategies (Hu, Rudin et al. 2019).
- *Multi-Attribute Utility Analysis (MAUA):* Multi-attribute utility exploration provides a lot of significance to attribute weights. The data is given about every kind and a decision on each attribute is determined. A decision-maker at that point sees the utility of handiness of a decision option regarding its attributes. This technique is commonly utilized when the properties of an option are sure.
- *Forecasting Models:* Forecasting models structure a fundamental piece of an enormous number of DSS networks. Their fundamental occupation is to anticipate the estimation of interrelated factors, variables eventually of interval in the future. The two fundamental kinds of figures are:
  - *Short and long-run forecasts:* Where the forecast will be utilized whenever/long time before long predominantly in deterministic models.
- *Regression and Econometric Models:* These kinds of anticipating models utilize straight and multiple regressions to build up

circumstances and effect relationships. These strategies are viewed as more remarkable than time-arrangement yet besides complex. Simultaneously they are complex because they utilize the refined models and incorporate more factors. The outcomes acquired are more exact.

- *Network and Optimization Models:* Organization then network improvement models remain incorporated into a DSS. When the decision is concerning about resource allotment, venture control, area, planning, transportation, dispersion, size, shortage, worldwide income, stock administration, cash flow management, and broadcasting organization network should be completed. For instance: The best area for an activity or manufacturing, the resources expected to complete the tasks, most appropriate airplane course to ship items. Organizational network and optimization models ordinarily utilize the linear regression technique procedure, which comes in the category of mathematical numerical programming in available device, tools.
- *Judgment Based Methods:* The expectations or determining the forecast depends upon the insights and assessments, thoughts of specialists rather on hard the information. It's an abstract subjective evaluation, utilized since quite long-run figures forecast where the external variable plays a critical role. The outcomes are not exact they are just the approximation.
- *Time Series Extrapolation:* This technique considers the financial-economic variable factors that are estimated at the continuous period of interval. It is accepted that the information on past conduct of the variable at successive periods will help comprehend the conduct of the behaviour of the factors in the better future.

7.4. Data Mining and Creating Knowledge

Previously, information-based data mining system frameworks came into reality and the organizations had business analysts examining the information. They would take data, the information associated with detailed theory to do a test to the hypothesis, as a result, carries approval or rejection. Be that as it may, an information-based data mining programming software doesn't have to set up speculation to be approved or rejected. Maybe it works in revelation mode, discovery mode, and searches for patterns in the data. There are two sorts of information mining models that can be deployed to develop the DSS model (Zhu and Davidson 2007).

- *Predictive Model:* This information-based data mining model predicts which possibilities are probable to react to a specific upgrade. It estimates clear outcomes results dependent on examples distinguished from identified consequences. It considers those individuals who have just reacted to a comparative or same improvement.
- *Descriptive Model:* This model depicts designs in existing information to make critical socioeconomics, demographics subgroups, which would then be able to be utilized for target advertising with the help of data mining DSS.

7.4.1. Data Mining Tools and Techniques

There are a countless large number of available tools and methods, techniques used to extract/mine information. Which procedure is to be utilized relies upon the sort of information to be extricated (Kaur and Chopra 2016)?

- *Case-based Reasoning:* Case-based reasoning apparatuses are utilized to decide the distance between or association amongst different segments, components. An issue settled utilizing these data mining tools experience five different phases.
  - *Presentation:* The problem is designated, analyzed, and submitted to the data mining system.
  - *Retrieval:* The system competitions the current data, system through the cases deposited in the organizational software.

  - *Adaptation:* The system coordinates the recovered nearest coordinating case and the issue to produce an answer.
  - *Validation:* The arrangement at that point experiences a validity test and is supported if the client gives positive inputs and feedbacks.
  - *Update*: The substantial arrangement is accepted and added to the case base in the system framework.
- *Fuzzy Query and Analysis:* Fuzzy query and analysis are information-based data mining techniques that follow the numerical idea for fuzzy logic the logic of indecision, vulnerability to decide results that are near a specific basis. Clients would then be able to pick one, depending on their arrangement.
- *Data Visualization:* As the name suggests, this assists the analysts with imagining, visualize complex connections in multi-dimensional data information. The advantage is that this apparatus graphically speaks to connections among parts from alternate points of view. Measurable statistical tools such as regression, classification, or clustering-based analysis are part of these data mining tools.
- *Genetic Algorithms:* By way of the name proposes, this assists the analysts with imagining, visualize complex connections in multi-dimensional data information. The advantage is that this apparatus graphically speaks to connections among parts from alternate points of view. Measurable statistical tools such as regression, classification, or clustering-based analysis are part of these data mining tools.

7.5. Development of Inter-Organizational Decision Support Systems and web-based interconnected W-DSS

Critical thinking and information the executives go inseparably. Together they have gotten one of the main parts of hierarchical in decision making. Directors around the globe understand that a lot of their organizations worth relies upon their capacity to accumulate, break down, oversee information and use it to resolve problems. To accelerate the way toward changing data into information and operating it to determine, resolve the issues, companies use properties in human insight. These resources assist them with finding and designs patterns, distinguish text where these examples work and dissect elective, analyze the alternative solution. A computer-based mechanized DSS network accomplishes all the work and helps directors in settling on to make the correct decision. With the appearance of the web in present-days correspondence the modern communication, advancements in support system, the organizational DSS networks sends electronic-based web-technology in taking decisions (Kim and Eom 2016). The novel knowledge of the common meeting and allocating the data to the system adds productivity to DSS, eventually assisting the executives with settling on the more suitable and reliable decisions. Best among all, the web-based DSS networks can be information-driven, interchange the communication, model data-driven, or could be hybrid. Web advancements can coordinate with any DSS network. Since the internet-based web advances are powerful, faster, and more secure in data transfer, the electronic-based web DSS can be utilized across the association, companies, and by at least two associations where there is a requirement for data sharing (Kasie, Bright et al. 2017).

7.5.1. Designing and Developing Web-Based DSS

Most organizations incorporate an internet web browser on their current support systems networks, for upgrading, sending, and deploying an electronic-based web DSS. The outcomes, in all likelihood, are inadmissible, unsatisfactory, and questionable. This is because the web innovations are incorporated without conveying a possibility, feasibility analysis. At the point when a DSS is at first planned, it centres and focuses around is the current necessities of its different users. In a perfect world, managers shouldn't anticipate that it should be productive in different areas. All in all, the inquiry remains - what goes into planning and building up a web-based DSS network. Here is the bit by bit process to measure clarifying how an electronic-based web system framework is planned and created. This is a standard cycle and any of the underneath referenced advances can be eliminated during system framework development, contingent upon the agreement and preferences of designers, developers, testers, analysts, end-users' clients (Alvandi, Sadodin et al. 2019). The steps involved in the development of the web-based decision support system includes are as follows:

- *Problem Identification:* This is generally in light of the fact that without understanding what you need an online DSS to do and perform tasks for you. It is difficult and impossible to push forward not to mention getting things right. Conceptualize with your colleagues to distinguish the issues you need to determine resolving with the help of using a DSS.
- *Conceptualization:* Following the next stage is to conceptualize the ideas on which your DSS will be based on. This process needs the gathering of more information related to problem identification and formalizes the basic requirement before feasibility analysis.
- *Feasibility Analysis:* When you have an away from a prospective DSS network, you should evaluate it. An attempt to reveal, its qualities, strength, limitations, opportunities, and threats resources needed to assemble, build the DSS analysis system for progress. Moreover, an attainability examination, feasibility analysis reveals insight into a venture's operational, conservative, economic, innovative, booking, legitimate feasibility, and viability.
- *System Development:* When the probable system framework has gone through your feasibility assessment-based test analysis, you can start with system framework advance. Recollect that system framework for improvement doesn't simply require the need for specialized technical expertise; rather it's a community orient effort of managers, decision-makers, DSS analysts, engineers, and financial experts. The emphasis essential be on:
    - *UI Development:* Building up a UI remnant the most essential part of any computer-based framework. Furthermore, it turns out to be more significant when a forthcoming framework will

be utilized by people of different degrees of refinement and specialized skill. Control, memory helps in suggestions that are dependent on the client's set of experiences are a significant part of a UI, with regards to an electronic web-based system framework.

- *DSS Architecture:* UI remains only a piece of DSS design and architecture isn't isolated from it. However, we referred to it independently because UI resembles an agent that makes the communication between the system framework and the client or users. It's the main part of DSS design. Typically, an online DSS is based on three or four-tier engineering architecture. One, the client sends a request through an internet browser utilizing HTTP over to a network-based web protocol. Second, the web worker at that point utilizes a program or content to deal with the web request. Three, the script may establish a connection to a model, measures information from the database, or format a document. Four, the internet browser where the client sent a request shows results generally fit the query.
- *Tool Selection:* HTML is (HyperText Mark-up Language) the utmost normally utilized language used for creating electronic based web DSS. HTML isn't a programming language, however can be utilized for front-end development and DSS which are developed in Java or JavaScript. HTML takes essentially intended to specify the reasonable association of reports with hypertext augmentations.: XML (Extensible Mark-up Language), CGI (Common Gateway Interface Scripts), JavaScript codes in HTML web pages, Java applets, and ActiveX are different programming software/tools that can be utilized to create electronic web DSS. To measure your alternatives, you should advise your designer then decide on improvement expenses.
- *System Implementation:* When the framework is created, the following stage is to implement, deploy the developed DSS.

Various tools are accessible that represent considerable authority in the execution, implementation of DSS. These are ColdFusion and dB Probe commonly used for the implementation.

7.6. Managing Web-Based and Inter-Organizational Decision Support System

Management of electronic besides inter-organizational based DSS networks can overwhelming. This remains because these frameworks are utilized by numerous people for settling on shared choices. Regardless of noticing an outrageous, problem when building up a system framework, some genuine issues will undoubtedly emerge. Reengineering the business cycle can be truly testing and a challenge also. It is anything but simple to restructure or re-engineer a business decision process once it includes countless no of different clients. Supervisors, managers in the associated organizations should contemplate the following issues to guarantee successful execution, the accomplishment of an electronic-based DSS. The primary significant subject is who will utilize the system framework by administrators, suppliers, providers, clients, or all. At the point when you answer this inquiry, you'll recognize the related inquiries. Regardless of whether there will be a requirement to reclassify, re-define the measures, how you are going to prepare the clients to work with a DSS, what are the chances of its prosperity and achievement. If the responses to these inquiries are ambiguous, your DSS is bound to fail. The subsequent significant issue is the accessibility of specialized technical ability to build up an electronic web-based DSS. Specialists need to decide on the equipment, programming, and labour needed to build a system framework. In this way, managers need to inquire as to whether they have in-house capacities to work and evolving up the system framework for the DSS. Assuming nowhere are they going to discover the use of appropriate technology, programming language. The third significant issue is the legitimateness of the material is dispersed through DSS to outer gatherings and outside stakeholders. Reflect, on the off chance that you are probably going to face any copyright or security issues (Shu, Pang et al. 2020).

8. Machine Learning/Deep Learning-Based Approach, Algorithm and Case Studies for a Decision Support System

As the human starts understanding the things that start happening around him, he tries to make the everyday process done with little or much more effort. In this case, the rise of technology takes place. As the industrial development took place in the 18th century and the invention of electricity things are going so much faster speed. During the late 19th century human tries to automate things with the help and invention of the computer, information technology. In this scenario advancement took place and in the digital era more automation took place and emergence of new technology like Artificial Intelligence, Machine Learning, and Deep Learning comes into play to solve problem. The term Artificial Intelligence was first coined by *"Herbert Simon and Allen Newell"* in "1955". Artificial intelligence uses some logic to learn the processes done by the machine with the help of some algorithms. The first breakthrough in the field of AI was done at MIT in the field of image processing with the project called the *"Summer Vision Project."* Soon *Newel* and *Simson* had worked on some mathematical problems and they solve them with the help of AI. During the second world war, German forces send some code to their military forces to decode these code Britishers had developed one machine termed the "ENIGMA MACHINE" which decodes the messages sent by the German forces, and as time passes there are different advances in the AI captures almost every field like as in medicine the program called MYCIN (Medical Diagnosis Application) had developed, then program called DENDRAL developed for chemical structure analysis. In 1977 we see that the program Deep Blue developed by IBM has defeated the world champ in chess which uses the Brute force algorithm to find the best answer and this was a breakthrough in the field of artificial intelligence.

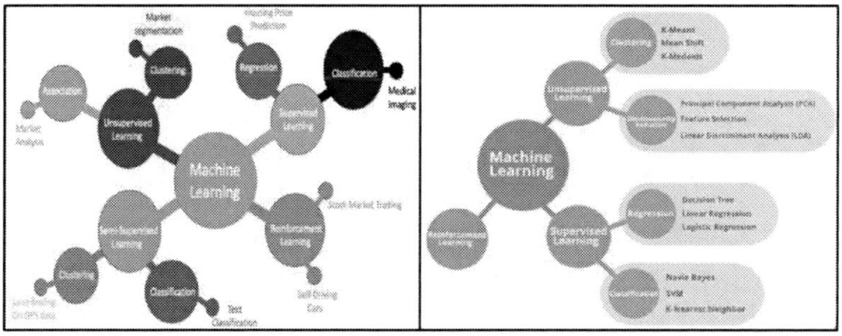

Figure 6. Different machine learning classification and machine learning algorithms.

With the advancement in technology Machine Learning came into play which is again a subset of AI, where AI deals with the generalized problem mostly the use the what-if statements, machine learning uses some of the advanced techniques like Neural Network, Random Forest, Support Vector Machine based classifications to automate the things. An ML-based program uses some sort of data on which we built our model and train on the existing data sets. ML is an interdisciplinary field that uses various things like the algorithmic mathematical procedure and some other technique to make an automated model on the pre-existing data set. Machine learning uses the feature-based learning technique where different kinds of features were extracted from the available data set and based on these data set, we developed our model. Basically, ML models were classified into different categories like Supervised Machine learning, Unsupervised Machine Learning, and Semi-Supervised Machine Learning, and Reinforcement based learning. In a nutshell supervised machine learning-based approach uses the pre-labelled data for the model development where an unsupervised learning uses the unlabelled data for the model building, hence in this case we don't know how our model will behave based on the data set. In other cases, like semi-supervised used mix kind of approach and reinforcement technique use the brute force mechanism to search out the result from the thousands of possible combinations in the data set. The supervised learning model is again further divided into the classification-based model and regression-based model. The classification is like binary classification which has only two labels and in the case of multi-classification has multiple labels to predict, regression-based classification uses the linear regression and logistic regression between the data points in the given data sets. The figure demonstrates the different types of ML-based classification and learning algorithms.

8.1. Case Studies Involved Which Uses the Machine Learning and Deep Learning

8.1.1. Case Study 1. DSS and ML Method for the Big Data Mining

As in the above section, the author has discussed the data mining techniques, as time passes there is the explosion of the data rapidly. People are uploading videos, photos, images, tweets, posts, and other kinds of data. Hence it is very difficult to handle this kind of multidimensional data which has diversity in terms of Velocity, Volume, Variety, Value, and Veracity in the given data. Hence the researchers have developed a technique to support the DSS based model for data mining used the machine learning-based technique to solve the problem. In this model what has been done is first of all the data set is selected and then the analyst has done some kind of analysis on the given data which includes the data cleaning and removal of the outliers. After that, they have selected some kind of targeted variables. Based on the selected preferences developer has decided that what kind of task to be performed on the available data. Here the model is trained on the given data set and results were visualized based on the trained model(Shailaja, Seetharamulu et al. 2018; Rudnichenko, Vychuzhanin et al. 2020).

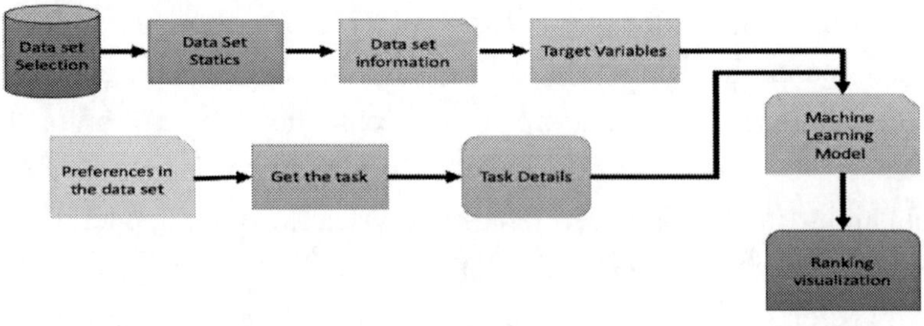

Figure 7. DSS and ML process for the data mining.

This concept is based on the following steps:

- First, the data is imported
- Formation of the metadata information from the downloaded data information
- Data mining methods and the task performed to perform the task
- Assessment of the machine learning-based quality for developed model.
- ML model for the evaluation and creation of the specified data set.
- Result visualization and the ranking of methods list which gives the appropriate solution in the DSS.

8.1.2. Case Study 2: Credit Card Detection, Scoring Based Machine Learning Approach

Money is the most important part of the human being's life and to run the economy it is very essential to a smooth-running circulation of money. People generally use the money either digital payment or in terms of cash for buying the good to spend a healthy conferrable life. To this sometimes people/customers buy expensive things and took credit from the banks and payback in terms of instalments or other payment schemes provided by the banks. Sometimes customers are not able to pay back the credit taken from the banks thus it is a challenge to provide to credit only those customers who willing to pay back to bank credit. In that case, banks have to make a decision support system that is powered by the machine learning techniques through which the model provide the scoring function to each customer based on their banking activities, the bank provides the credit for that. In this case study, a similar kind of system is developed which scores the performance of customers for a particular bank, and based on that score bank provides the credit loan. For the credit scoring, they have used many features like contract value time, the balance of a customer, collateral values, client size, seniority basics, time or duration, etc. In this credit card scoring system the system has obtained great accuracy to avoid the faulty customer stay away to provide the bank credit(Matsatsinis 2002; Teles, Rodrigues et al. 2019).

8.1.3. Case Study 3: Decision Support System In Case of a Health Care System

Health is wealth as the prove says, a healthy body attracts everyone, since the advancement in medical science going on new techniques were develop to diagnose the disease. Before diagnosis, it is really important to detect the disease first next steps come the treatment and diagnosis. The biomedical field has done a great advancement and new instruments were developed with the combination of information technology. New decision support systems were developed across the globe like an automated diagnosis of Alzheimer etc. (Salehi, Baglat et al. 2020). Hence a deep learning-based approach has tried to solve most of the problems in the field of biomedical as heart disease detection, Alzheimer's, medical retinopathy, etc. There are several examples where deep learning has done a great job. This is possible because of the data availability and increase in computing power, development of new algorithm like CNN based classifiers which automated diagnose the disease and predicts the results. In this COVID-19 pandemic, no. of tools were developed to find out the diagnosis or to take care of health records of different countries as no. of patients defected, diagnosis or dead from this COVID pandemic(Salehi, Baglat et al. 2020). Online clinical assessment with the help of a Deep Neural network has been done, in this case, one online-based assessment system is developed which provides the solution to the patients via online interaction. Thus, these types of Decision support systems will help in the improvement of the systems in the field of health care and automated diagnosis(Farhadian, Shokouhi et al. 2020; Pandey, Ma et al. 2020; Wu, Yang et al. 2020).

8.1.4. Case Study 4: Decision Support System in the Field of Sports, Manufacturing

Machine learning takes the sports and manufacturing industry up to a new set of standards. Deployment of electronic sensors and other imaging devices in the playground provides real-time data analysis based on this system that can predict the results. Like in the case of cricket the developed system provides the Real-time data analysis of the match predicted score, player previous record, timestamps of bowling, other umpire-related decisions, etc. This is possible due to the making of an automated decision support system. All other activities were monitored and captured by the sensors or cameras and the DSS system automatically monitor these and give us the result. The same happens in football also, the football players were constantly tracked during the match to check their playing behaviour or to get any other records. This will help in the pre or post-match data analysis. Here the researchers have developed some sort of algorithm which helps the coach and the selection committee through the analytics methods where the players' performance is evaluated, measured, and based on that decisions are framed. Hence a good decision support system will help in the all the context of sports industry including the manufacturing process also which include the requirement of the player need other the equipment they need play, company where the distribution will take place, etc. (Kröckel 2016; Peterson and Evans 2019).

Hence here we see that the decision support system will use in almost every field ranging from health care to sports, and banking, etc. Today almost every organization is developing their own DSS and dependent upon their systems.

FINAL THOUGHTS/CONCLUSION

A decision support system is not a new technology. We observe it everywhere. In today's world most of the things we see are related to a sort of support system. There is one support system that is responsible for most of the things that are happening around us. Hence the development and research will be remained to continue as the technology get advanced and the process gets changed in an organization. Support systems powered by artificial intelligence and the deep learning-based algorithm will provide a great solution for problems in manufacturing, development, handling the daily resources, and other chat bots-based support system. Hence while designing this book chapter, the author tries to touch every aspect related to the support system so that the reader will get a touch, understanding about DSS and do not have to rush to any other resources. Special take care should be opted so that a layman can understand the basic concepts of the decision support systems and enhancer their knowledge.

ACKNOWLEDGMENTS

I would like to dedicate this book chapter to the anonymous reviewers who are going to spend to review this book chapter and able to highlights the correction and make it happens. I would like to thanks my friends, Rohit Shukla and Shashi Kala for helping me to make a draft of this book chapter. I would like to thank Dr. Gaurav Gupta who provides me this opportunity to write and contribute to one book chapter.

REFERENCES

Abdullah, W. M., K. L. Kabir, et al. (2015). Development of a smart learning analytics system using Bangla word recognition and an improved document driven DSS. *2015 International Conference on Computer and Information Engineering* (ICCIE), IEEE.

Accorsi, R., R. Manzini, et al. (2014). "A decision-support system for the design and management of warehousing systems." *Computers in Industry* 65(1): 175-186.

Al-Maskari, A. and M. Sanderson (2010). "A review of factors influencing user satisfaction in information retrieval." *Journal of the American Society for Information Science and Technology* 61(5): 859-868.

Alavi, M. and J. C. Henderson (1981). "An evolutionary strategy for implementing a decision support system." *Management Science* 27(11): 1309-1323.

Ali, K. (2017). "A Study of Software Development Life Cycle Process Models." *International Journal of Advanced Research in Computer Science* 8(1).

Alvandi, E., A. Sadodin, et al. (2019). "Designing and developing a web-based decision support system in order to improve water quantity and quality in the Bonekooh Watershed." *Iranian Journal of Ecohydrology* 6(4): 849-863.

Argent, R. M., J.-M. Perraud, et al. (2009). "A new approach to water quality modelling and environmental decision support systems." *Environmental Modelling & Software* 24(7): 809-818.

Arnott, D. and G. Pervan (2008). "Eight key issues for the decision support systems discipline." *Decision Support Systems* 44(3): 657-672.

Asemi, A., A. Safari, et al. (2011). "The role of management information system (MIS) and Decision support system (DSS) for manager's decision making process." *International Journal of Business and Management* 6(7): 164-173.

Baumeister, J. and A. Striffler (2015). "Knowledge-driven systems for episodic decision support." *Knowledge-Based Systems* 88: 45-56.

Beheshti, H. M. (2010). "A decision support system for improving performance of inventory management in a supply chain network." *International Journal of Productivity and Performance Management.*

Berner, E. S. (2007). *Clinical decision support systems*, Springer.

Bonczek, R. H., C. W. Holsapple, et al. (2014). *Foundations of decision support systems*, Academic Press.

Boza, A., M. Alemany, et al. (2014). "A model-driven DSS architecture for delivery management in collaborative supply chains with lack of homogeneity in products." *Production Planning & Control* 25(8): 650-661.

Bright, T. J., A. Wong, et al. (2012). "Effect of clinical decision-support systems: a systematic review." *Annals of internal medicine* 157(1): 29-43.

Burstein, F. and C. W. Holsapple (2008). *Handbook on decision support systems 2: variations*, Springer Science & Business Media.

Campion Jr, T. R., L. R. Waitman, et al. (2010). "Social, organizational, and contextual characteristics of clinical decision support systems for intensive insulin therapy: a literature review and case study." *International journal of medical informatics* 79(1): 31-43.

Charles, J. and P. Chemelle (2012). "The history of duplex developments, nowadays DSS properties and duplex market future trends." *World Iron & Steel* 1: 46-57.

Chen, Z. and H. Dong (2010). The effects of documents lineage on use of explanation in document-driven DSS. *2010 Second International Conference on Intelligent Human-Machine Systems and Cybernetics, IEEE.*

Das, S. (2019). "Comparison among influencing factor, frequency ratio, and analytical hierarchy process techniques for groundwater potential zonation in Vaitarna basin, Maharashtra, India." *Groundwater for Sustainable Development* 8: 617-629.

Dellermann, D., N. Lipusch, et al. (2019). "Design principles for a hybrid intelligence decision support system for business model validation." *Electronic markets* 29(3): 423-441.

Doufene, A., V. Sakhrani, et al. (2020). "*Model Based System Design to Support Variability and Flexibility, and Early Bidding Phase of New Procurement.*"

Edelenbos, J. and E.-H. Klijn (2007). "Trust in complex decision-making networks: A theoretical and empirical exploration." *Administration & Society* 39(1): 25-50.

Eom, S. and E. Kim (2006). "A survey of decision support system applications (1995–2001)." *Journal of the Operational Research Society* 57(11): 1264-1278.

Eom, S. B., S. M. Lee, et al. (1998). "A survey of decision support system applications (1988–1994)." *Journal of the Operational Research Society* 49(2): 109-120.

Farhadian, M., P. Shokouhi, et al. (2020). "A decision support system based on support vector machine for diagnosis of periodontal disease." *BMC Research Notes* 13(1): 1-6.

Ferrell, O. C. and J. Fraedrich (2015). *Business ethics: Ethical decision making & cases*, Nelson Education.

Galimore, S. E. (2011). *Educational decision support system and associated methods*, Google Patents.

Gudigantala, N., J. Song, et al. (2011). "User satisfaction with Web-based DSS: The role of cognitive antecedents." *International Journal of Information Management* 31(4): 327-338.

Ho, S. B. (2000). *Computer user interface system and method having book image features*, Google Patents.

Holsapple, C. W. (2008). DSS architecture and types. *Handbook on Decision Support Systems 1*, Springer: 163-189.

Hoogenboom, G., J. Jones, et al. (2004). "*Decision support system for agrotechnology transfer version 4.0.*" University of Hawaii, Honolulu, HI (CD-ROM).

Hu, X., C. Rudin, et al. (2019). Optimal sparse decision trees. *Advances in Neural Information Processing Systems*.

Jirava, P. (2004). "System development life cycle." Scientific papers of the University of Pardubice. *Series D Faculty of Economics and Administration*. 9 (2004).

Jones, T. S. and R. C. Richey (2000). "Rapid prototyping methodology in action: A developmental study." *Educational Technology Research and Development* 48(2): 63-80.

Juan, Y.-K., P. Gao, et al. (2010). "A hybrid decision support system for sustainable office building renovation and energy performance improvement." *Energy and buildings* 42(3): 290-297.

Kasie, F. M., G. Bright, et al. (2017). "Decision support systems in manufacturing: a survey and future trends." *Journal of Modelling in Management.*

Kaur, A. and D. Chopra (2016). *Comparison of text mining tools*. 2016 5th International Conference on Reliability, Infocom Technologies and Optimization (Trends and Future Directions)(ICRITO), IEEE.

Kim, E. B. and S. B. Eom (2016). "Decision Support Systems Application Development Trends (2002–2012)." *International Journal of Information Systems in the Service Sector* (IJISSS) 8(2): 1-13.

Kremic, T., O. I. Tukel, et al. (2006). "Outsourcing decision support: a survey of benefits, risks, and decision factors." *Supply Chain Management: an International Journal.*

Kröckel, P. (2016). Decision support enhancement for player substitution in football: A design science approach. *International Conference on Business Information Systems*, Springer.

Kuik, S. and L. Diong (2019). "Building model-driven decision support system in product redesign plan." *Designs* 3(1): 18.

Lakhno, V. (2017). "Development of a support system for managing the cyber security." *Радіоелектроніка, інформатика, управління*(2): 109-116.

Lambin, P., R. G. Van Stiphout, et al. (2013). "Predicting outcomes in radiation oncology—multifactorial decision support systems." *Nature reviews Clinical oncology* 10(1): 27-40.

Lovallo, D. P. and O. Sibony (2006). "Distortions and deceptions in strategic decisions." *McKinsey Quarterly* 1: 18.

Matsatsinis, N. F. (2002). "CCAS: An intelligent decision support system for credit card assessment." *Journal of Multi-Criteria Decision Analysis* 11(4-5): 213-235.

Mbilinyi, B., S. Tumbo, et al. (2007). "GIS-based decision support system for identifying potential sites for rainwater harvesting." *Physics and Chemistry of the Earth, Parts A/B/C* 32(15-18): 1074-1081.

Miah, S. J. (2009). "End user as application developer for decision support." *AMCIS 2009 Proceedings*: 142.

Minhas, N. M., S. Majeed, et al. (2011). Controlled vocabulary based software requirements classification. *2011 Malaysian Conference in Software Engineering, IEEE.*

Mullakhmetov, K. (2016). "Control in the system of managerial decisions procedures: A conceptual view." *Problems and Perspectives in Management* 14(3): 64-76.

Murphy, C. (2016). *Competitive intelligence: Gathering, analysing and putting it to work*, CRC Press.

Neustadt, R. E. (2011). *Thinking in time: The uses of history for decision makers*, Simon and Schuster.

Noe, R. A., J. R. Hollenbeck, et al. (2017). *Human resource management: Gaining a competitive advantage*, McGraw-Hill Education New York, NY.

Pandey, S. R., J. Ma, et al. (2020). "A supervised machine learning approach to generate the auto rule for clinical decision support system." *Trends in Medicine* 20(3): 1-9.

Peterson, K. and L. Evans (2019). "Decision Support System for Mitigating Athletic Injuries." *International Journal of Computer Science in Sport* 18(1): 45-63.

Power, D. J. (2007). "*A brief history of decision support systems*." DSSResources. com 3.

Power, D. J. (2013). "Mobile decision support and business intelligence: An overview." *Journal of Decision Systems* 22(1): 4-9.

Puig, F., H. Marques, et al. (2009). "Globalization and its impact on operational decisions." *International Journal of Operations & Production Management.*

Radack, S. (2009). *The system development life cycle* (sdlc), National Institute of Standards and Technology.

Rudnichenko, N., V. Vychuzhanin, et al. (2020). *Decision support system for the machine learning methods selection in big data mining*. CMIS.

Salehi, A. W., P. Baglat, et al. (2020). "*Review on machine and deep learning models for the detection and prediction of Coronavirus*." Materials Today: Proceedings.

Salehi, A. W., P. Baglat, et al. (2020). A CNN Model: Earlier Diagnosis and Classification of Alzheimer Disease using MRI. *2020 International Conference on Smart Electronics and Communication (ICOSEC), IEEE.*

Seaman, J. (2020). The Evolution of PCI DSS. PCI DSS, Springer: 29-60.

Seidling, H. M., S. Phansalkar, et al. (2011). "Factors influencing alert acceptance: a novel approach for predicting the success of clinical decision support." *Journal of the American Medical Informatics Association* 18(4): 479-484.

Shailaja, K., B. Seetharamulu, et al. (2018). Machine Learning in Healthcare: A Review. *2018 Second International Conference on Electronics, Communication and Aerospace Technology (ICECA), IEEE.*

Shu, W., S. Pang, et al. (2020). "Achieving structured knowledge management with a novel online group decision support system." *Information Development*: 0266666920969842.

Simpson, N. and P. Hancock (2009). "Fifty years of operational research and emergency response." *Journal of the Operational Research Society* 60(1): S126-S139.

Smethers, P. (2004). *Graphical user interface features of a browser in a hand-held wireless communication device*, Google Patents.

Sommerville, I. (2004). *Software engineering*, Pearson Education India.

Stanek, S., S. Drosio, et al. (2014). *Experiences with Building Modern Communication-Driven Decision Support*. DSS.

Subashini, S. and V. Kavitha (2011). "A survey on security issues in service delivery models of cloud computing." *Journal of network and computer applications* 34(1): 1-11.

Teles, G., J. J. Rodrigues, et al. (2019). "Machine learning and decision support system on credit scoring." *Neural Computing and Applications:* 1-18.

Tripathi, K. (2011). "Decision support system is a tool for making better decisions in the organization." *Indian Journal of Computer Science and Engineering (IJCSE)* 2(1): 112-117.

Trkman, P., K. McCormack, et al. (2010). "The impact of business analytics on supply chain performance." *Decision Support Systems* 49(3): 318-327.

Turban, E., R. Sharda, et al. (2010). "*Decision support and business intelligence systems (required).*" Google Scholar.

Velychko, O. and V. Liudmyla (2017). "*Logistical modelling of managerial decisions in social and marketing business systems.*"

Vercellis, C. (2009). *Business intelligence: data mining and optimization for decision making*, Wiley Online Library.

Weygandt, J. J., P. D. Kimmel, et al. (2020). *Managerial Accounting: Tools for Business Decision-Making*, John Wiley & Sons.

Wikström, P., L. Edenius, et al. (2011). "*The Heureka forestry decision support system: an overview.*"

Wu, G., P. Yang, et al. (2020). "Development of a clinical decision support system for severity risk prediction and triage of COVID-19 patients at hospital admission: an international multicentre study." *European Respiratory Journal* 56(2).

Zada, F., S. K. Guirguis, et al. (2012). "Development of a Dynamic Model for Data-Driven DSS." *Journal of emerging trends in computing and information sciences* 3(2): 255-261.

Zhang, D., X. Chen, et al. (2015). "Development of a prototype web-based decision support system for watershed management." *Water* 7(2): 780-793.

Zhu, X. and I. Davidson (2007). *Knowledge discovery and data mining: challenges and realities*, Information Science Reference Hershey.

In: Mobile Health
Editors: G. Gupta, N. Kumar et al.
ISBN: 978-1-53619-420-3

Chapter 4

INNOVATION INSIGHT FOR HEALTHCARE PROVIDER DIGITAL TWINS: A REVIEW

Chitresh Sharma[1,]* and Gaurav Gupta[2]
[1]Scientific Data Acquisition Competence Centre Leader,
L'Oréal Paris, Paris, France
[2]Yogananda School of AI Computers and Data Science,
Shoolini University, Solan, Himachal Pradesh, India

ABSTRACT

Digital twins are evolving into a required next-generation capability for healthcare process simulation modeling. As healthcare delivery organizations gear for digital transformation, IT must meet the increased demands to deliver accurate digital twins assistance in reducing human intervention in almost every domain. In simple terms, a digital twin is a virtual copy of a tangible entity (such as vehicle engines or people) or an intangible system (like manufacturing processes or marketing systems) that can be analyzed independently of its real-world counterpart in order to make informed decisions. NASA employed a similar concept. It had physical replicas of its spacecrafts on Earth while the actual ones were in

* Corresponding Author's Email: schitreshsolanhp@gmail.com.

outer space. This proved crucial in the Apollo 13 mission where engineers on Earth could determine the issue and find a solution with the same assets as the astronauts. Such undertakings eventually gave way to fully digital simulations applied in various sectors. Siemens, the German engineering giant, has employed such a twin for its Amberg factory, which produces industrial computer-control systems. "This digital twin is identical in every respect and is used to design the control units, test them, simulate how to make them and program production machines. Once everything is humming along nicely, the digital twin hands over to the physical factory to begin making things for real," writes The Economist. With the increasing prevalence in the use of wearables, social media, smart living, and personalized recommender systems for consumer health, it becomes imperative to converge these technologies to provide personalized, context driven, proactive, and preventive care in real time. Digital Twins are a convergence technology and involve making a digital replica of any living or nonliving entity. At present, Digital Twins are extensively used in Industry 4.0 where Digital Twins help in optimizing the performance of machines by proactive and predictive maintenance. This chapter gives an overview of the existing literature and aims to provide an overview of existing literature on Digital Twins for personal health and well-being—key terminologies, key applications, and key gaps.

Keywords: digital twins, medical science, healthcare, sensors, data mining, prediction, AI, well being, blockchain

1. Introduction

Digital twins have the potential to transform and accelerate decision making, reduce clinical risk, improve operational efficiencies and lower cost of care, resulting in better competitive advantage for HDOs. However, digital twins will only be as valuable as the quality of the data utilized to create them. The digital twin of a real-world entity is a method to create relevance for descriptive data about its modeled entity. How that digital twin is built and used can lead to better-informed care pathways and organizational decisions, but it can also lead clinicians and executives down a path of frustration if they get the source data wrong. The underlying systems that gather and process data are key to the success for digital twin creation. Get those systems right and digital twins can accelerate care delivery and operational efficiencies.

A digital twin is a digital representation of a real-world entity or system. The implementation of a digital twin is a model that mirrors a unique physical object, process, organization, person or other abstraction. For healthcare providers, digital twins provide an abstraction of the healthcare ecosystem's component characteristics and behaviors. These are used in combination with other real-time health system (RTHS) capabilities to provide real-time monitoring, process simulation for efficiency improvements, population health and long-term, cross-functional statistical analyses.

1.1. Digital Twins in Healthcare Delivery

The fact is that HDOs have been using digital twins for years. Although rudimentary in function, digital representations of patients, workflow processes and hospital operations have already been applied by caregivers and administrators across the HDO. For example, a physician uses a digital medical record to develop a treatment plan for a patient. The information in the medical record (a rudimentary digital twin) along with the physician's experience, training and education combine to provide a diagnostic or treatment plan. Any gaps in information must be compensated through additional data gathering, trial-and-error treatments, intuitive leaps informed through experience or simply guessing. The CIO's task now is to remove as many of those gaps as possible using available technology to give the physician the greatest opportunity to return their patients to wellness in the most efficient possible manner.

Today, one way to close those gaps is to create the technology-based mechanisms to collect accurate data for the various decision contexts within the HDO. These contexts are numerous and include decisioning perspectives for every functional unit within the enterprise. The more accurate the data collected on a specific topic, the higher the value of the downstream digital twin to each decision maker (see Figure 1).

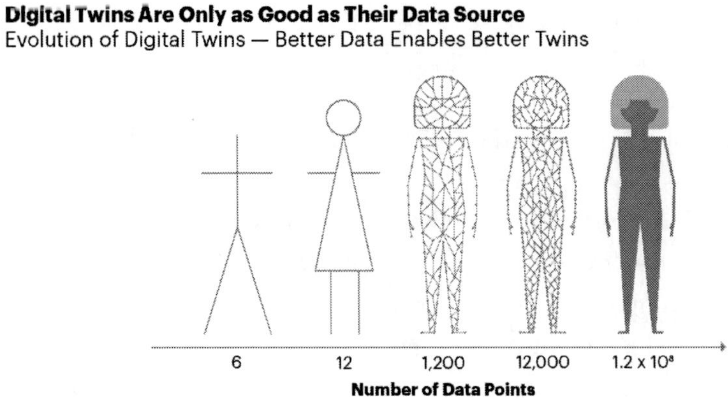

Source: Gartner.

Figure 1. Digital twins are only as good as their data source.

HDO CIOs and other leaders that base decisions on poor-quality digital twins increase organizational risk and potential patient care risk. Alternatively, high-quality digital twins will accelerate digital business and patient care effectiveness by providing decision makers the best information in the correct context, in the right moment and at the right place — hallmarks of the RTHS. Now imagine applying this concept to medicine: a virtual representation of the human body and its organs where the effects of drugs can be studied. This sounds like what in silico trials and organs-on-a-chip aim to achieve.

But imagine a virtual representation of individual people on whom every known drug for that person's condition can be tried. This will allow the deduction of the optimal treatment. It can even monitor that virtual "being" and alert before a medical condition arises. Thus, the real person can undergo preventive measures. This is what the digital twin model in healthcare, which delves into the realm of personalized medicine, promises.

1.2. Digital Twin Types in Healthcare Delivery

Current practices for digital twins take two basic forms: discrete digital twins and composite digital twins. Discrete digital twins are the type that most people think about when approaching the topic. These digital twins are one-dimensional, created from a single set or source of data. An MRI study of a lung, for example, is used to create a digital representation of a patient that can be used by trained analytics processes to detect the subtle image variations that indicate a cancerous tumor. The model of the patient's lung is a discrete digital twin. There are numerous other examples of discrete digital twins across healthcare delivery, each example tied to data collection technologies for specific clinical diagnostic purposes. Some of these data sources include vitals monitors, imaging technologies for specific conditions, sensors for electroencephalography (EEG) and electrocardiogram (ECG). All these technologies deliver discrete data describing one (or very few) aspects of a patient's condition.

When these discrete sources are combined for the patient, a multilayered set of data is created that can describe a group of physiological systems in one model. This is a composite digital twin — and this is where digital twins begin to show their true power. By combining related data from multiple sources, the composite twin exposes the measurable effect of one biological system on another, thus providing a more detailed and quantitative view of a patient. And by combining multiple composite digital twins together, users can create a digital twin of organizations (DTO). In the patient example above, the organization is the group of related human biological systems — think cardiovascular, respiratory, lymphatic — that layer on top of each other to provide a clearer, more informed model of the patient.

The examples used have been clinical and centered on a patient, but digital twins provide value for any entity or system within the HDO. Any characteristic of activity or process that is occurring within the organization that has collectible digital data is a candidate for a digital twin. The facilities themselves have discrete digital twins available for HVAC, physical security, energy consumption, lighting, elevators and many more. These individual twins can be layered to form a composite facility twin that can create the correct level of situational awareness to enable a new level of decision-making capability. The same can be said for the supply chain process, emergency department, operating room, medical/surgical units and others. The combination of these various composite twins can layer together to form a true DTO, in this case of the HDO.

Situational awareness is at the heart of HDO digital twins. They are the culmination of information gathered from IoT and other sources to create an informed, accurate digital model of the real-world healthcare organization. Situational awareness is the engine behind various "hospital of the future," "digital hospital" and "smart patient room" initiatives. It is at the core of the RTHS.

Digital twins, when applied through the RTHS, positively impact these organizational areas (with associated technology examples — the technologies all use one or more types of digital twins to fulfill their capability):

Care delivery:

- Clinical communication and collaboration
- Next-generation nurse call
- Alarms and notifications
- Crisis/emergency management

Patient engagement:

- Experiential wayfinding
- Integrated patient room
- Interactive patient care

Facilities and operations:

- Patient throughput and capacity management
- Real-time operational dashboards
- RTHS supply chain

Management and administration:

- Real-time costing
- Healthcare information exchange
- Healthcare interoperability
- Revenue cycle management

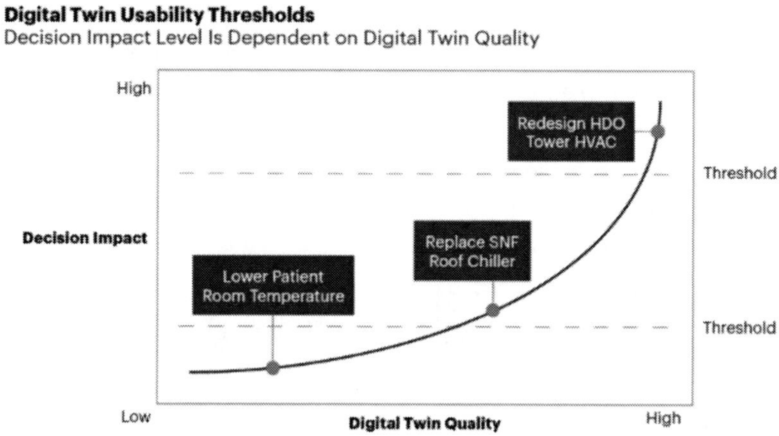

Figure 2. Digital twin usability thresholds.

1.3. Digital Twin Usability Risks

Some Digital twin risk is tied directly to usability. Digital twin usability is another way of looking at the issue created by poor data quality or low data point counts used to create the twins. Decision making is a process that is reliant on inputs from relevant information sources combined with education, experience, risk assessment, defined requirements, criteria and opportunities to reach a plausible conclusion. There is a boundary or threshold that must be reached for each of these inputs before a person or system can derive a decision.

For example, the amount of information about a patient room required to decide if the space is too hot or cold is low (due to a single temperature reading from a wall-mounted thermostat). In addition, the accuracy or quality of that data can be low (that is, a few degrees off) and still be effective for deciding to raise or lower the room temperature. To decide if the chiller on the roof of that patient wing needs to be replaced, the decision maker needs much more information. That data may represent all thermostat readings in the wing over a long period of time with some level of verification on temperature accuracy. The data may also include energy load information over the same period consumed by the associated chiller.

If viewed in terms of a digital twin, the complexity level and accuracy level of the source data must pass an accuracy threshold that allows users to form accurate decisions. There are multiple thresholds for each digital twin — based on twin quality — whether that twin is a patient, a revenue cycle workflow or hospital wing. These thresholds create a limit of decision impact; the lower the twin quality the less important the available decision for the real-world entity the twin represents.

Trusting Digital Twins for HDOs - The concept of a limit of detail required to make certain decisions raises certain questions. First, "how does a decision maker know they have enough detail in their digital twin to take action based on what the model is describing about its real-world counterpart?" The answer lies in measurement and monitoring of specific aspects of a digital twin, whether it be a discrete twin, composite twin or organization twin.

Users must understand the inputs required for decisions and where twins will provide one or more of the components of that input. They need to examine the required decision criteria in order to reach the appropriate level of expected outcome from the decision itself. These feed into the measurements that users will have to monitor for each twin. These criteria will be unique to each twin. Composite twins will have unique measurements that may be independent from the underlying discrete twin measurement.

The monitoring of these key twin characteristics must be as current as the target twin's data flow or update process. Digital twins that are updated once can have a single measurement to gauge its appropriateness for decisioning. A twin that is updated every second based on event stream data must be measured continuously.

The trap the user of a digital twin can fall into is trusting a twin to provide accurate input for a decision that is based on past successful results with that trust remaining, even as the twin changes over time. Perhaps the changes reflect an unnoticed degradation in data input quality, reducing the usability of the twin. Additionally, it may leave the decision maker unaware that they are taking action based on a twin that is no longer worthy of that level of decision.

This trap is the same for all digital twins regardless of context. The difference is in the potential impact. A facilities decision that leads to cooler-than-desired temperatures in the hallways pales in comparison to a faulty clinical diagnosis that leads to unnecessary testing or negative patient outcomes.

All it takes is a single instance of a digital twin used beyond its means with negative results for trust to disappear — erasing the significant investments in time and effort it took to create the twin. That is why it is imperative that twins be considered a technology product that requires constant process improvement. From the IoT edge where data is collected to the data ingestion and analytics processes that consume and mold the data to the digital twin creation routines, all must be under continuous pressure for improvement.

Obviously, for such a concept to materialize many factors will come into play. These range from financial resources determining which healthcare center or even which patient will be able to afford the technology, to the very technological advances required to make sensors that people can wear without disrupting their daily routine.

The sheer computing power required to run simulations of the human body or even organs can also be intimidating. For the Blue Brain Project, modelling of an individual neuron leads to some 20,000 ordinary differential equations. For entire brain regions, we're looking at 100 billion equations that have to be solved concurrently.

1.4. Digital Twin Process Improvement Cycles

The process improvement cycle for digital twins is more complex than typical due to the variety of systems and workflows in play. At a macro level, the process mimics the archetype with create, test, identify and update steps. Each one of these steps represents a cycle of their own with specific digital-twin-related inputs and outputs that cross the physical and the virtual (see Figure 3).

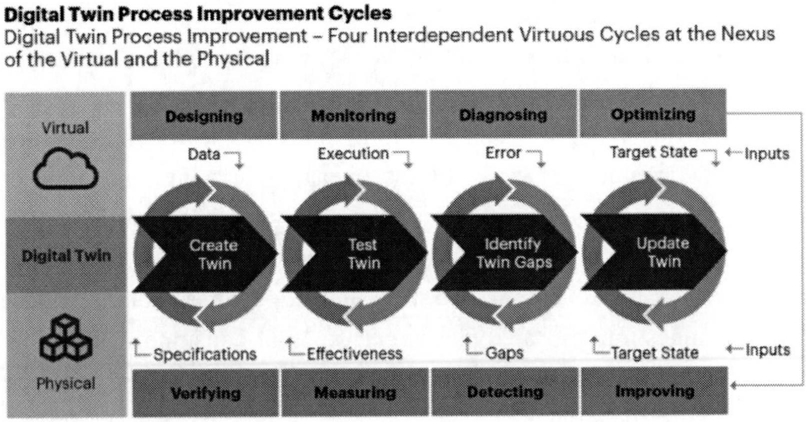

Source: Gartner.

Figure 3. Digital twin process improvement cycles.

The four cycles are:

- Create Twin Cycle — Twins start with an identified need to model a component of the HDO, which could be anything from a process, workflow, department, a role (such as patient, nurse, physician, housekeeper). The twin creators define specifications that describe the requisite data for the model and where to acquire that data. Based on feedback about the availability, quality and applicability of the data to the model, the designers will enter a change cycle until the data and the design conform to the twin requirements.

- Test Twin Cycle — The new model is then tested to make sure it will meet the modeling needs. This cycle combines monitoring output from the digital twin with measured outcomes of the twin's effectiveness in the physical world. If the dependent actions in the real world do not enable the intended positive change for the users, the testing methodology must be reviewed until validated. Once the test process is reliable, the output of the testing feeds into the next cycle.
- Identify Twin Gaps Cycle — Based on testing output, twin designers perform a gap analysis by detecting gaps between the expected outcomes detected and the test results. Those gaps inform the diagnosis of errors within the digital twin that are remediated in the next cycle.
- Update Twin Cycle — In this cycle, the twin is updated with improvements based on the previous cycle outputs with the twin optimized with a better understanding of the target state. This is done not just for the twin itself, but also for the physical counterpart that is the target for the twin.

2. Recommendations for Digital Twin Strategy

2.1. Include a Concise Digital Twin Vision within the HDO Digital Transformation Strategy

Digital twins are one of the foundational constructs supporting digital transformation efforts by HDO CIOs. They are digital representations of the real-world entities targeted by organizations that benefit from the advances and efficiencies technologies bring to healthcare delivery. Those technology advances and efficiencies will only be delivered successfully if the underlying data and associated digital twins have the appropriate level of precision to sustain the transformation initiatives.

To ensure this attention to digital twin worthiness, it is imperative that HDO CIOs include a digital twin vision as part of their organization's digital transformation strategy. Binding the two within the strategy will reinforce the important role digital twins play in achieving the desired outcomes with all participating stakeholders.

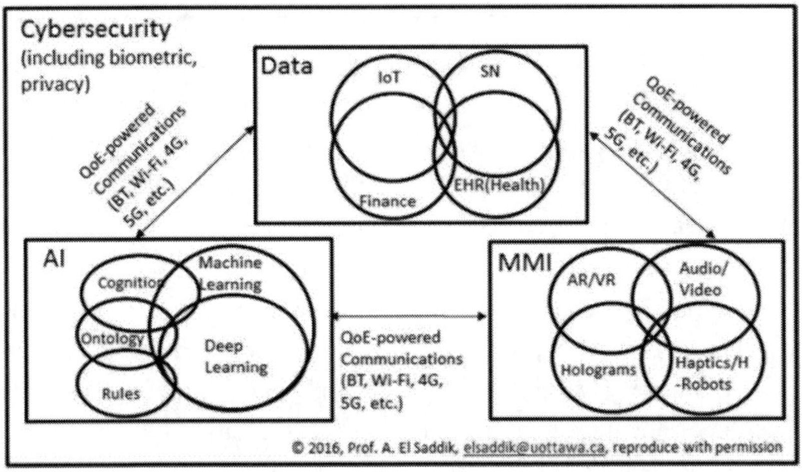

Figure 4. Digital Twins multimedia ecosystem for health and well-being.

Some key action areas that are common to digital transformation strategies are listed below and should be used by the CIO as touchpoints for creating linkage points to the digital twin vision.

- Laying the foundation - The enterprise must have the infrastructure, architecture, governance and other basics to support the digital platform.
- Building new capabilities - APIs, artificial intelligence (AI) and other new technologies enable the connections and automation that the platform provides.
- Leveraging existing systems - Legacy systems that an HDO already owns can be adapted and connected to form part of its digital platform.

- Applying the platform to the industry - Digital platforms must support specific use cases, and those use cases will reflect the needs of patients, employees and other consumers.

2.2. Educate Business and Clinical Units About Digital Twins

Educate business and clinical units to inform them about the benefits of digital twins and how they fit in with departmental and organizational goals. This begins the process of identifying the right data to create highly effective digital twins along with establishing a collaborative environment for the initiative among stakeholders. Accurate data collection is core to the success of digital twins and that accuracy in many cases lies in the hands of individuals within the HDO.

Laying the groundwork to justify why digital twins are important to the organization is vital to helping all stakeholders connect the value proposition of digital twins to their daily workflows. The technologies involved are part of transformative innovations and may seem daunting or unobtainable by working units within the HDO. It is your task to influence the department and unit leads to accept digital twins into their daily operation. To get started with the education process:

- Create an educational program to inform employees about digital twins and their importance to your existing digital transformation program. These can take the form of computer-based training, classroom sessions and external training. If you have existing training materials that support your overall transformation effort, consider added digital twin information where appropriate.
- Segment the training by the various levels of digital twins: discrete, composite and organizational. Different parts of the organization will find connection and meaning to the type of twin that most impacts their daily task load. A lab technician will have tangible touchpoints with discrete twins, a department lead will use many composite twins and management will take the most

advantage from organizational twins. Ensure that the right roles are attending the correct level of training.

Identify department-level key performance indicators (KPIs) that monitor value delivery or work efficiency. Those KPIs are based on specific measurements that tie directly to the most important workflows within a department. Those measurements are key to data that will eventually form a digital twin of that department. Show the department how better data collection and better analysis of the data will lead to less variance for their KPIs, allowing them to perform their jobs easily and more efficiently.

2.3. Create a Digital Twin Pilot Program

Like other advanced technology ideas, a digital twin program is best started as a simple project that can act as a starting point for maturity over time. Begin this by selecting a simple model of a patient, a department or other entity tied to a specific desired business or clinical outcome. The goal is to understand the challenges your organization will face when implementing digital twins.

The target for the digital twin should be discrete and easily managed. For example, a digital twin of a blood bank storage facility is a contained entity with a limited number of measurement points, such as temperature, humidity and door activity. The digital twin could be used to simulate the impact of door open time on temperature and humidity within the storage facility. The idea is to pick a project that allows your team to concentrate on data collection and twin creation processes rather than get tied up in specific details of the modeled object.

- Begin by analyzing the underlying source data required to compose the digital twin, with the understanding that the usability of the twins is directly correlated to its data's quality. Understand the full data pathway from the IoT devices through to where that data is stored. Think through the data collection type needed for the twin, is discrete data or real-time data required? How much data is needed to form the twin accurately? How accurate is the data generated by the IoT devices?

- Create a simulation environment to exercise the digital twin through its paces against known operational variables. The twin's value is tied to how the underlying data represents the response of the modeled entity against external input. Keep this simple to start with — concentrate on the IT mechanisms that create and execute the twin and the simulation environment.
- Monitor and measure the performance of the digital twin. Use the virtuous cycle to create a constant improvement process for the sample twin. Experience gained through this simple project will create many lessons learned and best practices to follow for complex digital twins that will follow.

2.4. From Evolution to Revolution

Several companies have developed digital twin models of human organs. Partnering with Ecole Polytechnique Fédérale de Lausannes (EPFL) on its Blue Brain Project, Hewlett Packard Enterprise deployed its supercomputer to create digital models of the brain for research purposes. Siemens Healthineers has a Digital Twin model and Philips has its own version of a virtual heart. At a glance, these models might seem like the natural evolution to radiological imaging and diagnosis – detailed depictions of patients organs – but in fact they snowballed a revolution.

A.I. helps in the design of digital twins to weave together organs' physiological data to output a 3D image. The latter can then be modeled to a specific patient from their specific parameters. Siemens Healthineers trains its algorithms on a huge database with over 250 million annotated images, reports and operational data. This enables them to design digital heart models based on patients data with the same parameters of the given patient (size, ejection fraction, muscle contraction). In this way, the operator is able to test therapies on the model and look at the outcome. Eventually, one can select the best therapy for this specific patient.

Dorin Comaniciu, Vice President of Artificial Intelligence at Siemens Healthineers, said that they've used this method in projects with hospitals Europe to assess cardiovascular risks. The company is also developing models for other organs such as the lungs and liver.

However, it is clear that the concept is still evolving, with only organ twins demonstrated. While organizations like the Swedish Digital Twin Consortium push for the idea, we are still far from a completely digitized version of ourselves. However, we might already digital versions of our organs that could serve as templates for the future of personalized care.

2.5. Future Perspectives

The way digital twins work in the manufacturing industry is as follows. The physical object in need of a digital twin, like an engine, is equipped with sensors which relay real-time status information. The data and parameters from those sensors then feed the software mapping the digital twin. It is thus able to get insights about its performance and predict when the object (the engine) needs maintenance. As such, operators don't need regular checkups of this particular engine but only when indicated by the digital twin.

Now, are there any sensors for the human body? Well, there's plenty thanks to the advent of digital health. Health trackers now allow us to measure a gazillion of data. There's literally a device to measure your health parameters from head to toe; the Philips SmartSleep headband will track your sleep, the Polar H10 chest strap will measure your heart rate in detail while the Fitbit Ionic will keep track of your steps and running routine. All of these devices output data that allows you to make informed decisions. In fact, they already offer a disconnected picture of your digital self.

The next step in personalized medicine will be to link those insights to 3D- models of your organs. Wearable sensors, as tiny as the BioSticker, will feed real-time data to a remote server maintaining your digital twin. Both you and your GP will receive regular notifications regarding specific tests/procedures that need to be done as preventive measures.

"Imagine that in the future, we have a patient with all their organ functions, all their cellular functions, and we are able to simulate this complexity," explained Benjamin Meder, a cardiologist at Heidelberg University Hospital in Germany who is testing Siemens Healthineers' digital heart software. "We would be able to predict weeks or months in advance which patients will get ill, how a particular patient will react to a certain therapy, which patients will benefit the most. That could revolutionize medicine."

3. Case Studies

3.1. DT for Heart Care

Most heart-related diseases can be avoided only by leading a healthy life. There are risk factors associated with these diseases, alcohol consumption, obesity, smoking, sedentary lifestyle, and poor diet are the main factors. By reducing these risk factors or even suppressing them, the individual can significantly reduce the chances of being affected by any of these diseases. With Digital Twins you can promote a healthy lifestyle as a strategy to prevent heart diseases. Digital Twins collects data from different BAN type of sensors, for example, an accelerometer, GPS, or a smartwatch that monitors heart rate and galvanic response. The AI module can use machine learning to estimate the level of physical activity for the real twin on a daily basis. From this estimation, the real twin receives recommendations on different activities outdoors or indoors to participate according to personal preferences or physical condition in the real twin. Digital Twins knows everything about its real counterpart, based on caloric consumption, weight, clinical data, and/or biological signals obtained from different sensors, it can also detect situations related to obesity, alcohol, or tobacco consumption for which it can help the real twin to reduce or suppress effectively based on your personal preferences. This is how Digital Twins can also act as a persuasive system that supports the user to reduce or even eliminate the risk factors associated with heart disease and ultimately, prevent them. Take obesity, for example, since the Digital Twins knows about food consumption preferences, what the real twin likes or dislikes it can recommend the best meal plan that is best suited for the real twin along with a set of exercises and activities that are more adequate to the physical state of the real twin.

3.2. DT & Emotions

Digital Twins is the enabling technology that facilitates the means to monitor, understand, and provides continuous feedback to improve quality of life and wellbeing. Thus, a Digital Twins can consider a solution to enhance mood to enhance the quality of life and emotional well-being. The Digital Twins for emotional wellbeing system is a closed loop feedback system in which information taken from the human body is translated into a language perceivable by any of the human senses. The loop begins with human sensory information from the body. The physiological signals are then interpreted and converted to a recognizable emotion state. Feedback is provided to the individual through recommendations while monitoring the user behavior and action tendency. If the quality of service is not satisfied, then the system will loop back to the matching process to recalculate the feedback. Once the biofeedback information is consumed by the human brain, a change in the mental state will occur, which will cause a change in the human physiological state. The cycle then starts again. The primary goal of Digital Twins system for emotional well-being should include tracking, assist, remind, intervene, and reinforce learning. A biofeedback loop can allow users to see their bodily reactions in real time, and assist users in finding both the positive and the negative stressful patterns in their behavior. While opportune moment detection helps provide just-in-time interventions as needed. Then, reinforce learning helps to learn the user preferences.

3.3. DT & Sports

The Digital Twins has many applications related to health and well-being, among which is sport. Indeed, Digital Twins can help improve tremendously the quality of sport both by giving the athletes access to automated training as well as by giving them the benefit of personalized feedback during and after the training. Indeed, the DT can allow athletes to work out even in the absence of the coach but following his/her recommendations. We suggest here an application of the DT in sport, where we show that how athletes can benefit from it. We used sensors as the DT data source and actuators as DT representation to give feedback to the real twin who is here the athlete. The DT replaces temporarily the coach by helping the athlete follow his/her recommendations without the coach's presence. We studied the case of training for soccer sprinting. As sensors, we used the smart insoles [24] in order to collect pressure point data and send it to the DT storage. The DT was configured by the coach for each athlete following their level, then the DT sends notifications to the athletes to inform them of the availability of a new training set for them. The athlete can start their sprint training at their own preferred time, during which the DT accompanies them with tracking and feedback. The feedback is delivered through haptic armbands that signal to the athlete when to start sprinting and when to switch to periods of recovery for the duration recommended by the coach. After the training is completed, the DT makes it available to the coach (and the athlete) by means of visualizations in the form of graphs and feet heatmaps showing the results of the training that the coach can analyze and provide the next training recommendation based on the athlete performance. We performed a pilot study with three soccer athletes who reported that the DT for sport proved very useful for them. They rated it at an efficiency of eight out of ten and declared that they would adopt it to facilitate their sprint training. The Digital Twins system can also automate the performance analysis using artificial intelligence, and act as a coach assistant, providing him/her with suggested athlete recommendations and waiting for the coach's approval before notifying the athlete of the training outcome and next steps.

3.4. Digitizing the Human Body Using Virtual Simulations

Digital Twins have not yet developed sufficiently to analyze the human body in its entirety, but progressions have been made. An example comes from software company 'Dassault' who released 'Living Heart', which is the first realistic virtual model of a human organ accounting for blood flow, mechanics and electricity. The software is capable of turning a 2D scan of a human into an accurate full dimensional model of an individual's heart. Capturing the human body will have multiple benefits for doctors such as; discovering undeveloped illnesses, experimenting with treatments, and improving preparation for surgeries. Body parts such as the brain, however, are far more complex than the heart. France based start-up 'Sim&Cure' have made advances in assisting medical researchers' treatment of brains while developing a digital patient for treating aneurysms.

4. Empowering DT with Blockchain

4.1. Blockchain as a Powerful Antidote

In the first part of this chapter, we have extensively discussed about the futuristic and fabulous implications of the digital twin paradigm across industry verticals. The perpetual and perplexing question is that if data breaches happen here. As we all know, wrong or corrupted data leads to wrong decisions. Thus, securing digital data and twins gains.

Data is extremely essential for the intended success of the digital twin paradigm. New data streams in the connected world typically comprise the participating physical objects' attributes, the interaction data with other physical objects, and future states. The data interchange happens between the physical and digital worlds. While digital twin instances (DTIs) are mirroring a physical entity and activity, the digital twin aggregates (DTA) is a composite of individual DTIs to achieve bigger and better things. With this combination and collaboration, a breach of a DTI will compromise one product. A breach of DTA will expose a set of participating products.

The emerging blockchain technology has the innate potential to surmount the safety and security lacunae to put digital twin projects on the track. As blockchain technology is blessed with the decentralization and immutability attributes, digital twins projects can innovate better and faster through the shrewd usage of blockchain.

The cryptographic characteristics of blockchain ensure safe and secure data transfer. By having a robust authentication of users and data sources, data immutability along with the safety of digital twins promises a lot for the digital world. As explained in the previous chapters, through one or other consensus mechanism incorporated in the blockchain technology, multiple stakeholders, collaborators and users, can be brought under one umbrella. The stakeholders have become the gate-keepers enforcing transparency and accountability. Thus, confidential, customer, and corporate information gets transmitted without any fear.

Through the astute combination of DTAs and blockchain, we can unquestionably expect the blockchain-enabled and path-breaking digital twins. From there, every business domain can visualize next-generation products, processes, operational models, etc.

Blockchain technology is a decentralized ledger with public records of all physical products and their transactions. The data can be viewed and verified publicly. However, modifications to it can be made only by authorized executives, and the ledger retains a history of every modification. In the previous chapters, we have discussed about the power of blockchain in surmounting many current problems and in laying down a breakthrough platform for envisaging and implementing newer use cases. Having understood the impacts, every noteworthy business domain is fast experimenting and evolving a strategic and sustainable blockchain plan. The blockchain technology is being empowered through a smart integration with other pioneering technologies such as the IoT, digital twin, AI, etc. On other hand, these technologies are being succulently and solidly empowered through the sagacious synchronization with blockchain. There are white papers, case studies, research publications, and best practices authored by technical experts, evangelists, and exponents clearly accentuating and eulogizing how the technology combination works wonders for several perpetual problems. In this and subsequent sections, we are to expound and espouse how different popular industry domains are tremendously benefiting out of this unique combination.

4.1.1. Eliminating Counterfeits

On the supply chain side, now by combining digital twin and blockchain, businesses, and brands can easily protect their products from being wilfully counterfeited and increase the revenue remarkably. As widely known, one of the biggest concerns for worldwide businesses these days is skilled counterfeiting of their products. With the arrival of advanced technologies and tools, fraudsters can quickly create replicas for various expensive products and sell them to unsuspecting people at a cheaper price. This dangerous situation not only damages the brand name but also causes huge financial losses. Digital twin in conjunction with blockchain can bring forth a competent solution to thwart such frauds. They together guarantee the authenticity of products. As articulated above, digital twins facilitate the digitization of physical artifacts. As explained in the previous chapters, blockchain with its decentralization capability will bring in the much-needed transparency. This strengthen the security of any digital data.

4.2. Combination of Digital Twins and Blockchain

The advent of the Blockchain technology has redefined the progress of digital twins. At macro level, blockchain enables the storage of information in a decentralized manner with no single point of control. Fresh transactions can be added, but the existing ones cannot be changed or corrupted. This clearly ensures transparency and data integrity.

Creating a digital twin on blockchain would mean that all information regarding a physical product can be saved immutably. Furthermore, the product's transaction records can be saved. This means prospective buyers can get all the information of the product from its origin and also the journey it took off. This will help create proofs of authenticity and identity.

4.2.1. Consider a Premium Watch

There exist countless replicas of this costly watch. Fake watches can be made along with fake documents for proving their authenticity. However, creating digital twins on blockchain decimates such fake products and documentations. Digital twins, in a way, act as digital certificates for the digital age. Digital certificates stored and issued with the help of Blockchain will ensure that these certificates can't be stolen, modified, and used wrongly.

Blockchain is becoming a popular digital technology that allows every transaction to be tracked in an inviolable way. The blockchain technology is gaining the inherent capability to redefine the concept of digital twins. It could turn out to be an indispensable tool to skilfully aid the application of digital twins in the ensuing IoT era. Sectors such as manufacturing, healthcare, and retail are set to benefit immeasurably from these technologies interlinking with one another. There is a tight coupling between the physical world and the digital world.

A digital twin built with traditional technologies must need a central intermediary for stocking digital data and for doing data analytics. Now, with the booming blockchain technology, the aspect of digital twins is bound to go through strategically sound transformation. The security and immutability being guaranteed by blockchain are to take digital twin to the next level in the days to come.

Keeping a digital twin (more specifically digital certificate) on blockchain helps businesses to retain information about their products perpetually and securely. Further on, the data regarding transactions for these products also can be saved in the blockchain database. This allows any perspective buyer to get the complete details including the real manufacturer, who are the other owners of the product, etc., about the product during purchase. Precisely speaking, it helps establish the authenticity and provenance of the product. It is possible to craft a fake document to prove its authenticity. By creating digital twins/certificates on the blockchain, fake products can be eliminated from the sordid market. An immutable and tamper-proof digital certificate for each of the products is the way forward to nullify any kind of fraud.

Blockchain actually stores digital certificates that embed all the relevant data regarding the products registered by businesses. Blockchain ensures that the data embedded in the digital certificates cannot be copied, modified, and even deleted by others. Businesses can register their items on blockchain platforms. As enunciated above, every concrete product has its corresponding digital twin and in this case, it is digital certificate. The digital certificate gets updated at every stage of the product cycle right from the manufacturing stage. When the product is shipped, the information regarding the place, mode, and shipping destination can be updated with timestamps. When customers buy the product, they can verify the authenticity of the item by verifying the digital twin of the product on the blockchain. After the item is purchased, the ownership gets transferred to the new owner by the authorized salesperson. All the previous data stored is maintained as such. No modification is possible.

Without an iota of doubt, blockchain brings the much-needed reliability and credibility to businesses. Clearly, blockchain is being touted as an anticounterfeiting and antitheft technology. If businesses across the world implement this with a proper care, then the evil things of faking and falsification can be easily surmounted. The confidence of people on various products gets a strong boost. Buyers get all the right information about any product instantaneously. Unverified ownership will become a thing of the past and people get to know the complete details about every product. This inspiring combination is penetrating into every industry vertical ranging from manufacturing, healthcare, advertisement, and logistics.

4.2.2. Digital Twin and Blockchain in Logistics

Supply chain processes can be unequivocally streamlined and secured using digital twin and blockchain together. Shipping containers embedded with a number of IoT sensors are connected to the blockchain platform in order to ensure a complete transparency in the complex logistics process.

The products empowered through multiple sensors can have their own digital twins, which land on blockchain. This powerful entitlement helps to track and trace the products. This helps the stakeholders to have complete information about the product and the transportation process. The documentation for the products also can be stocked in blockchain database eliminating any kind of modification and forgery. The documents with product and payment details can be tracked digitally. The transparency aspect of the logistics sector can be fulfilled through blockchain and digital twin combination.

4.2.3. Digital Twin and Blockchain in Utilities

Digital twin and blockchain can be used in the utility sector to help utility operators in efficiently fulfilling their consumers' requirements. As we know, the production and consumption of power energy varies sharply based on consumer behavior. Nowadays, electricity meters in our homes are being attached with IoT sensors to be transitioned into smart electricity meters. These connected meters can directly communicate the consumption data every few minutes to the smart energy grid. The energy consumption details of every individual consumer can be digitally updated on the blockchain to guarantee transparency. The corresponding digital twin for the smart energy grid can receive and analyze the energy consumption data to extricate actionable intelligence. This gives energy service providers (energy generation, transmission, and distribution) a clear understanding about the consumer behavior. Accordingly, power producers and suppliers can do everything in an optimal manner. On the other hand, consumers based on peak energy costs could adjust the power usage time to time to reduce expenditure on energy.

4.2.4. Digital Twin and Blockchain in Healthcare

The use of digital twin and blockchain together can bring in drastic changes for the healthcare industry. As the whole world is severely stricken with Covid 19 virus, the smart combination of multiple technologies is the way forward to comprehensively overcome the grave challenges especially in curtailing the growing fatalities.

For a prime example, the digital twin of a patient's heart can be realized through the digital version of a pacemaker. This digital twin can specially empower cardiologists, who are carrying out cardiac resynchronization therapy, in precisely identifying the position of leads on the specific patient. All the lead placement positions pinpointed through the digital twin can be tried virtually to determine the best suitable position. This happens well before the real surgery begins. The best suitable position enables the surgeons to complete the operation with all the intended success. Blockchain can safely hold records of the medical history of the patient. The trustworthy and timely data can be accessed anytime by healthcare providers and professionals to ponder about the next course of action in case the person develops any untoward complications in the future.

Thus, digital twins and blockchain can blend together to bring in a bevy of transformational effects across industry verticals. By merging digital twin with blockchain technology, a secure and decentralized digital ecosystem can be formed and sustained. This solemnly assures businesses and end-users the authenticity of the products and services.

4.2.5. Aircraft Industry

The manufacturers of different components of aircrafts are being strictly governed by unambiguously written technical standards. The ultimate aim is to certify and monitor the component production process. Further on, this industry domain increasingly uses additive manufacturing technologies to accomplish rapid prototyping of product components. Aided by highly optimized supply chain, the time to market comes down sharply while not compromising on the product quality. There are recommendations for producing and sustaining digital twins for additive manufacturing. It is recognized that the fusing of digital twin and blockchain can be a trend-setter for many industry sectors.

4.3. Usage of IBM Watson & Blockchain Approach to Digital Twins

IBM Watson IoT, a cognitive system that learns from and infuses intelligence into the physical world, is fervently expanding its scope further by creating digital twins by using blockchain. Also, IBM is implementing blockchain to existing digital twins. It is believed that blockchain can substantially increase the cost-effectiveness of digital twins. Utilizing blockchain with digital twins facilitates digital identity and data tracking through blockchain traceability.

With a greater understanding, enterprises are keenly experimenting with the blockchain paradigm, which is fast penetrating and participating beneficially in many business domains. As we all know, Internet is the world's largest information superhighway. However, data transmission through the Internet, which is the most affordable and global-scale communication infrastructure, is battling a few security and privacy challenges. Blockchain is being projected as the promising savior here. Further on, blockchain-based infrastructure is being pronounced as the next-generation phenomenon for the secure exchange of value.

4.4. Blockchain and Digital Twins for Enhanced Digital Value

With blockchain in place, the concept of digital value transfer will be implemented in a completely decentralized way. Crypto chips, which can be easily and quickly implanted on any physical asset, are enabling scores of physical assets getting directly linked to a blockchain platform of choice. The asset can be anything ranging from credit cards, personal devices, consumer electronics, drones, robots, and appliances, medical instruments, to industry machineries. The metadata of physical assets are being stored in blockchain databases. This guarantees that transactional and operational data actually originate from highly trustworthy sources and spread across with proven integrity. Private keys never leave the crypto chip and hence transaction data is fully encrypted while in transit until it gets formally recorded in an immutable ledger system.

Digital twins are increasingly stored on blockchains. Therefore, digital twins, while gaining the much-needed trust, are used efficiently to regulate business transactions involving multiple participants and parties. With trust enshrined through blockchain, we can safely expect that here will be many more innovations in the flourishing field of digital twin.

Digital twins for sharing economy - The realization of industrial IoT (IIoT) has led to smart manufacturing. The industry 4.0 vision gets accelerated through the astute usage of the IIoT competencies. Factory floors are skilfully automated through a variety of IoT sensors and actuators. IoT data, which is typically big in size, is being meticulously analyzed in order to get the useful insights in order to plan and execute appropriate tasks in order to steer businesses in the right direction. Industry machineries are not only connected but also made smart in their actions and reactions. IIoT in consonance with transformative technologies such as AI, blockchain, digital twin, etc., can be a fulsome hallmark for the future of our business powerhouses. However, industry players' efforts to monetize their industry IoT devices, which they own or use for production were without any grand success thus far. The rise of the sharing economy and its supporting technologies represents a paradigm shift in the access and consumption of IoT systems and services.

In traditional transactions, the transfer of ownership of a product to a buyer is the end of the story for the manufacturer or vendor in the value-creation process. In the new sharing economy, either the asset is a shared entity or the device/asset's output is portable. For example, a car is a physically portable asset that can be collaboratively consumed. But in the case of a windmill, it is the asset's output (wind energy) that gets shared across.

The dual concepts of digital twins and machine-to-blockchain networks are portrayed as key technology facilitators for intrinsically empowering industrial IoT devices to participate in the fast-evolving sharing economy. These concepts can support and sustain the distinct ideals of the sharing economy. As the digital era evolves, newer business models are emerging. One promising model is a service-based business model. This can be deftly applied to individual IoT devices, and this can result in gaining an auxiliary revenue stream based on usage or outcomes. This new paradigm brings two important things. The first one is digital twins, which can virtually articulate the unique capabilities of the IoT device to any prospective buyer. The second is machine-to-blockchain, which facilitates smart and secure monetary transactions.

CONCLUSION

Digital Twins bring about the promise to help improve the health and well-being of individuals, provided they are able to get their trust and provide data privacy. Some challenges exist among which delivering a high degree of personalization, which is context aware, culturally apt, matching user's lifestyle, and preferences. Our current interest is the study of role of incentives to self-health behaviors and links them to create a well-being economy or to initiate dialogue for a well-being economy. In the end, we need consumer evangelism and participation in use and scale of digital technologies for personal health and well-being. With the flourish of interactive IoT devices, a massive amount of multistructured data gets generated, transmitted, and stored in local and remote storage systems. There are powerful AI algorithms and integrated data analytics platforms for processing IoT data using batch and real-time processing methods to extract actionable insights. On the other hand, there are digital twins being built for IoT devices in order to deeply understand and articulate their structural properties and behaviors in different contexts. Existing and emerging IoT devices and their constant interactions with others in the vicinity and with remotely held applications and data sources/stores are being decisively investigated through their digital counterparts individually and collectively. Digital twins even simulate the working of physical products according to changing situations and hence a lot of useful knowledge gets delineated before the said products are physically manufactured. Thus, the scope of usage and benefits of digital twins are consistently on the rise. However, IoT devices can be remotely pierced through by brilliant hackers damaging the device networks to do irreparable damages to the IoT systems and applications. Similarly, IoT device data, when in transit and rest, can be breached to steal confidential information. Further on, digital twins can be made inaccessible, or corrupted data can be submitted to digital twins to make wrong decisions, etc.

With the faster maturity and stability of blockchain, the IT experts are exploring the possibility of establishing a linkage between digital twins and blockchain in order to ward off the security threats. The combination of these two technologies presents a positive future for the business and IT domains. How the blending of these two path-breaking digital technologies could bring forth a number of digital innovations and disruptions gets detailed in this chapter. The combined entity has laid down a strategically sound platform for envisaging and implementing a number of business, technology, and user cases.

Digital twins are also being continuously updated and upgraded by incorporating the cutting-edge technologies such as machine and deep learning (ML/DL) algorithms, computer vision (CV), and natural language processing (NLP) methods. Thus, with the cool synchronization with blockchain, the digital twin domain is to flourish in the years to come.

References

Badawi, H., F. Laamarti, F. Arafsha, A. El Saddik, Standardizing a shoe insole based on ISO/IEEE 11073 personal health device (X73-PHD) standards, in *Proceedings of the International Conference on Information Technology & Systems (ICIT)* (2019).

Demiris, G., Consumer health informatics: past, present, and future of a rapidly evolvingdomain. *Yearb. Med. Inform. Suppl* 1, S42–S47 (2016). https://doi.org/10.15265/IYS-2016-s005.

El Saddik, A., Digital twins: the convergence of multimedia technologies. *IEEE MultiMedia* 25(2), 87–92 (2018). https://doi.org/10.1109/MMUL.2018.023121167.

Ferguson Report (1999), http://www.fergusonreport.com/articles/tfr07-03.htm.

Fleerackers, T., M. Meyvis, Web 1.0 vs Web 2.0 vs Web 3.0 vs Web 4.0 vs Web 5.0 – *A Bird's Eye on the Evolution and Definition*, https://flatworldbusiness.wordpress.com/flat-education/previously/web-1-0-vs-web-2-0-vs-web-3-0-a-bird-eye-on-the-definition/.

Hermann, M., T. Pentek, B. Otto, *Design principles for Industrie 4.0 scenarios*, in 2016 49th Hawaii International Conference on System Sciences (HICSS) (IEEE), pp. 3928–3937. https://doi.org/10.1109/HICSS.2016.488.

Last, J. M., J. H. Abramson, International Epidemiological Association, *A Dictionary of Epidemiology* (Oxford University Press, 1995).

Libbrecht, M. W. and W. S. Noble (2015). "Machine learning applications in genetics and genomics." *Nature Reviews Genetics* 16(6): 321-332.

Loftus, T. J., P. J. Tighe, et al. (2020). "Opportunities for machine learning to improve surgical ward safety." *The American Journal of Surgery.*

Ottawa Charter for Health Promotion, https://www.who.int/health promotion/conferences/previous/ottawa/en/.

Parrott, A., L. Warshaw, No Title, (2017), https://www2.deloitte.com/insights/us/en/focus/industry-4-0/digital-twin-technology-smart-factory.html.

Roser, C., *Illustration of Industry 4.0, Showing the Four "Industrial Revolutions" with a Brief English Description*, AllAboutLean.com.

Shajahaan, S. S., S. Shanthi, et al. (2013). "Application of data mining techniques to model breast cancer data." *International Journal of Emerging Technology and Advanced Engineering* 3(11): 362-369.

Stokes, J., J. Noren, S. Shindell, *Constitution of the World Health Organization* (1982), https://www.who.int/governance/eb/who_constitution_en.pdf.

Stokes, J., J. Noren, S. Shindell, Definition of terms and concepts applicable to clinical preventive medicine. *J. Community Health* 8(1), 33–41 (1928). http://www.ncbi.nlm.nih.gov/pubmed/676.

Suwalka, I., A. Sanadhya, et al. (2012). *Identify malaria parasite using pattern recognition technique*. 2012 International Conference on Computing, Communication and Applications, IEEE.

Suzuki, K. (2017). "Overview of deep learning in medical imaging." *Radiological physics and technology* 10(3): 257-273.

The Ferguson Report: The Newsletter of Consumer Health Informatics and Online Health.

Thuemmler, C., *The Case for Health 4.0, in Health 4.0: How Virtualization and Big Data are Revolutionizing Healthcare*, (Springer International Publishing, Cham, 2017), pp. 1–22.

World Health Organization. Regional Office for Europe, *Health Promotion: A Discussion Document on the Concept and Principles*. Summary report of the Working Group on Concept and Principles of Health Promotion, Copenhagen, 9–13 July 1984 (WHO Regional Office for Europe, Copenhagen, 1984), http://www.who.int/iris/handle/10665/107835. http://apps.who.int/iris/bitstream/handle/10665/107835/E90607.pdf?sequence=1&isAllowed=y.

In: Mobile Health
Editors: G. Gupta, N. Kumar et al.
ISBN: 978-1-53619-420-3

Chapter 5

LASIK INNOVATION TECHNOLOGY FOR DISEASE IDENTIFICATION DURING LACTATION

G. S. Pradeep Ghantasala[1,*] ***and Anuradha Reddy***
[1]Department of Computer Science and Engineering
Chitkara University Institute of Engineering and Technology,
Punjab, India
[2]Malla Reddy Institute of Technology and Science,
Hyderabad, Telangana, India

ABSTRACT

During pregnancy, alterations in keratometric standards and refractions can take place. Therefore, it is not advised to adjust the refractive recommendation of a patient or undergo corneal refractive surgical treatment during pregnancy. Though, it is not as well recognized to what degree these corneal alterations occur for the duration of lactation. Pregnancy and lactation cause hormonal alterations that influence the construction of the cornea. LASIK or other forms of

* Corresponding Author's Email: ggspradeep@gmail.com.

refractive surgical treatment are not suggested until all the subsequent necessities are satisfied: ending of lactation, re-establishment to regular menstruation, and restitution to pregnancy refraction. Besides, patients must be advised that if they are pregnant within one year of LASIK, refractive deterioration can take place. PLO is a special kind of osteoporosis distinguished by enlarged bone desorption and abridged BMD, like VCFs. Phosphorylation therapy in the PLO organization was well endured and triumphant but had to be further tested in a randomized proscribed examination. Through pregnancy and lactation, calcium demands increase, and an intricate sequence of hormonal alterations attains this. The improvements in tissue bone structure and the whole bone level detected at some point in pregnancy and lactation tend to cure in great assess over time. The severity of the changes observed during lactation can be related to the breastfeeding volume and length and return to regular menses. Research investigating the long- term effects of pregnancy and lactation indicates that bone density has mild, site-specific benefits and that bone structure may also be affected. Osteoporosis (PLO) caused by lactation and pregnancy is an infrequent stipulation for which the pathos's physiological origin is not yet fully understood. Lactation-associated osteoporosis (PLO) and Pregnancy is an infrequent, extreme, premature type for osteoporosis in adolescent females in attendance for the period of late pregnancy or lactation with fractures, typically multiple vertebral fractures. We in pre-menopausal women registered 80 Females with small trauma fractures and with 40 safe tests in idiopathic osteoporosis (IOP) studies, all about it regular Menses and no other reason for Loss to the bone. During late pregnancy, fractures had occurred, or lactation in 15 females exaggerated the PLO subgroup. We speculated the physiological, Structural skeleton, and metabolic distinctiveness of people with PLO and others with IOP and controls (Non-PLO) would vary. Everything has been estimated > a postpartum of 12 months when systemic and changing distinctiveness is unspecified to reproduce the premenopausal baseline category rather than transitory postpartum modifications.

Keywords: breastfeeding, LASIK, lactation, premenopausal osteoporosis, pregnancy and lactation-associated osteoporosis

1. Introduction

Human milk is a species-specific and the entire replacement milk provision for feeding vary manifestly commencing it, generating the outstandingly advanced human milk for child feeding [1]. The milk of human beings isn't a standardized body liquefied, although a composition changing Secretion of the gland in the breast. Foremilk varies as of hind milk, and intermediate and mature milk is strikingly distinct from colostrums. During the process of lactation, milk varies with time of day and. Nutrients like as trace, minerals, lipids, vitamins, carbohydrates and proteins rudiments are part of human milk., which are important for meeting the dietary requests of adolescent tot and for maintaining regular enlargement and improvement [2].

For infant feeding, human milk is exceptionally greater and is the prime Examples of pediatric individualization. The milk of human beings is not a standardized body fluid, but a composition-changing Breast gland secretion. Foremilk varies from hind milk, and transitional and mature milk varies markedly from colostrums. During the process of lactation, milk varies with time of day and. The clinical, nutritional, immunological, the social, psychological, environmental and economic repayments of human milk for growth have been demonstrated by comprehensive studies. In both the developed and developing world, breastfeeding results in better child and maternal health outcomes.

Some particular issues resolve to converse, like as the deterrent impact of human milk on diseases, plumpness, diabetes and obesity, malignant disease, neurodevelopment effects, narcotic enter colitis diminution, etc. For mothers, significant health advantages, often, breastfeeding and lactation are identified. Lastly, breastfeeding contraindications and breastfed baby supplementation are discussed. Interventions are relatively easy and inexpensive to facilitate breastfeeding. There should not be baby feeding seen as a preference of existence, but moderately as a fundamental issue of physical condition.

Changes in values and keratometric during pregnancy, refraction may occur. For this one, therefore, it is not advised to alter A refractive prescription or a patients undergo During breastfeeding, corneal refractive surgery. The degree these corneal improvements to continue all through lactation, however, it's not all that known. Pregnancy and lactation contribute to changes in hormones which influence the constitution of the cornea. Until any of the following requirements are met, LASIK, or added forms of refractive surgery, Recommended it isn't: cessation of lactation, restoration of normal menstruation, and restoration to refraction for prepregnancy. Also, the patients need to be warned if they get pregnant after one year of LASIK, refractive regression may occur.

During pregnancy, the female body undergoes several dramatic changes. While some of these improvements are evident, for both observers and patients, others are harder to spot. Corneal modifications come into the above group. Although LASIK is contraindicated during pregnancy, our goal is to fix corneal modifications that begin and continue during lactation in pregnancy and to include guidelines for refractive postpartum corneal surgery.

Although hormone levels can differ in pregnancy, based on based on the personality, here is substantial growing progesterone and many types of progesterone, estrogen, together with estrone and estradiol [3-5]. The concentrations of oestrogen and progesterone within a couple of days of birth, return to pregnancy values [6]. This drop in the echelon of oestrogen and progesterone disinhibits prolactin such that lactation takes place shortly thereafter [7]. Oxytocin also manages the milk let-down]. If there is inadequate milk removal, the amount release of an enzyme lowers the pro-lactation hormone [8-10].

If a female does not breastfeed once birth, the return of menstruation typically takes about 6 weeks [11]; nonetheless, if a female breastfeeds, she's not going to see the revisit of menstruation for 6-9 months, on normal [12]. The cornea of humans has estrogen, progesterone, and androgen sex-hormone receptors [13-15]. The function is suspected that these receptors induce hormone-mediated corneal changes from menstruation [16] to pregnancy and menopause [17-19] during periods of hormonal fluctuation.

During breastfeeding, corneal thickness changes [20]. It is postulated that this impact of thickening is secondary to the retention of dampening. There is contradictory data, however, stating no substantial change in at some point in pregnancy or lactation, corneal thickness. There is evidence that when oestrogen and progesterone levels are incredibly high, a shift

Corneal thickness arises throughout the third trimester, but this increase in the postpartum period does not continue.

Less overall protein in human milk 8-10 g/l compared to bovine milk, this is of greater biological importance, however, and human milk proteins consists of the correct combination of caseins and whey proteins that cover nutritional and handy needs represented by a clear postprandial retort. The optimum Ratio of long shackle polyunsaturated fatty acids n-3 and n-6 also characterize the person milk of strong mothers. These are triglyceride and phospholipids constituents that form complex structures that are essential for metabolism and brain growth. Throughout lactation, these lipids differ [21-23]. The disaccharide lactose is the main carbohydrate in human milk.

Many Immune-related apparatuses like as interferon-γ, lactoferrin, lysozyme, sIgA leukocytes, cytokines, nucleotides, and others are also found in human milk. In the digestive system and the superior respiratory tract to some extent, some of these compounds provide passive defense, preventing pathogens from adhering to the mucosa and thereby shielding breastfed infants from all-encompassing infectivity. Human milk also consisting of indispensable hormones, fatty acids, polyamines, carbohydrates, intensification factors, [24-25] and further geologically vigorous compounds that can cooperate a significant position in the healthiness settlement of breastfeeding.

2. Breastfeeding Along with Operation for the LASIK Ogle

Several breastfeeding mothers have been advised that LASIK ogle surgery should not be conducted before their child is weaned; it is often suggested that the mother wait 3-6 months or longer until considering this procedure after breastfeeding has ended. The belief that breastfeeding can induce improvements in the corneal [26] curve that will endure as long as breastfeeding continues is based on these guidelines. The problem with getting LASIK surgery during lactation is that if the vision of the mother improves after weaning, the surgery will need to be resumed later. Breastfeeding should not be affected by general anesthesia. When you are awake and conscious enough to carry your infant, you can comfortably nurse. At that time, the level of drugs in your bloodstream is minimal enough that it will not be relevant to the levels in your milk. After general anesthesia, the point at which you wake up is the point where enough of the medication has left your system that it no longer affects. Furthermore, pediatric operations need, and that is more intense than mom's milk exposure. Mom may want to nurse in case she's out for a while or too groggy to work normally for a while just before the operation.

While a few women experience changes in eyesight during lactation, I did not locate substantiation to sustain the belief The reality that all mothers will undergo changes in vision or with the intention of changes in vision that transpire will necessarily continue all through lactation. Some believe that once their cycles have returned and are routine, a mother's eyes will be back to their "natural" state. Many mothers enter this state well before weaning.

If her eyesight has improved, a mother would most likely realize, as will her ophthalmologist [27] or optometrist. LASIK surgery should be delayed until her vision has been stable for some time if her vision has changed (because she will need to have the surgery reworked if her vision changes again). Of course, one of the regular LASIK surgery guidelines is that the prescription of the glasses has not improved in the last year, so this alone should preclude any women who have changes in vision during pregnancy and breastfeeding. It was previously assumed that refractive surgery would not be acceptable for breastfeeding patients the hormonal changes that transpire throughout pregnancy are due to and the possible risk of drugs that may pass through breast milk to infants. Researchers recently confirmed that at least not for LASIK and photorefractive keratectomy, this is not the case; both have been found safe and successful in women who are breastfeeding.

Pregnancy can also, for better or for worse, bring about improvements in existing eye conditions. If you have diabetes, see an ophthalmologist to check for damage to the blood vessels in your retina before you become pregnant and again in early pregnancy. This disorder, called diabetic retinopathy, sometimes worsens during pregnancy, so when you are pregnant and in the postpartum period, you will need more regular eye examinations.

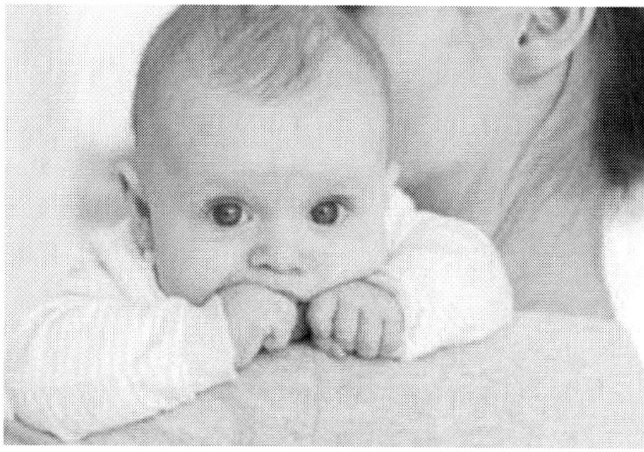

Figure 1. LASIK Ogle representation.

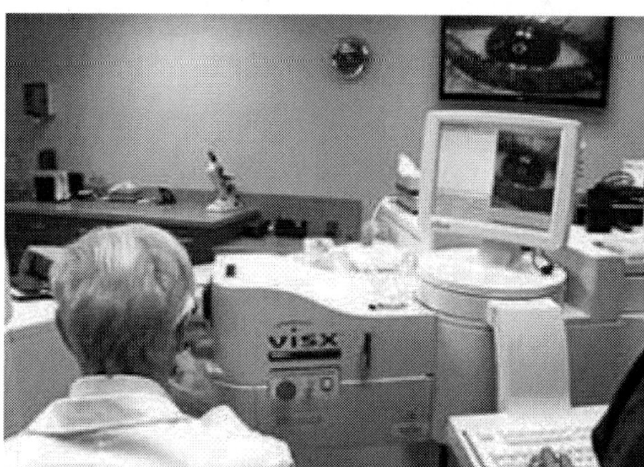

Figure 2. Test for LASIK surgery.

3. Basics of LASIK

You could think about surgery to fix your vision if you wear glasses or contact lenses. In a LASIK operation, a laser is used to remake your cornea, the translucent, circular arena at the facade of your eye, to enhance the means your eye concentrates luminosity rays on your retina. For laser-assisted keratomileusis in situ, LASIK is shorthand. LASIK is an operation on a very sensitive part of the eye that cannot be reversed. There are risks and potential complications, as with any operation. LASIK has been used by millions of people, many quite successfully, but it is not for all. You might not be granted full hallucination by LASIK. The American Academy of Ophthalmology (AAO) estimates that somewhere between 20/20 and 20/40 vision is attained by nine out of 10 patients, but for convinced work or relaxation actions, the 20/40 vision may not be sharp enough. And 20/20 doesn't for eternity connote full vision. Detailed, right vision might be vaguely affected. In your mid-40s, you would still need to read glasses Also in regulate to accurate your distance vision with LASIK. LASIK surgery, the lack of age-related concentrating ability to see near objects, does not fix or avoid Presbyopic [28]. If you are myopic and don't necessitate to read bifocals yet, getting LASIK can signify that you necessitate reading bifocals sooner than stipulation you didn't have the procedure.

3.1. Are You a Successful LASIK Contender?

- LASIK isn't for all people,
- You ought to be 18 years of age (21 for certain lasers) at least. The hallucination of individuals younger than 18 is also evolving.
- You're not supposed to be expectant or a nurse. It may alter the eye's calculated refraction.
- Some prescription medications, Accutane or oral prednisone, for instance, should not be taken by you.
- Your eyes need to be safe and your medicine stable. LASIK should be postponed until the refraction is finished normalized if you are myopic. In some patients, Myopia will continue to grow until the middle then to late 20s.

- Your healthiness in general ought to be fine. Glaucoma, Rheumatoid arthritis, lupus,
- herpes eye infectivity, cataracts, corneal disorders and retinal disease are seen in patients with diabetes, LASIK may not be prescribed. Discuss with your surgeon your general health condition.
- The narration of "desiccated eye" can issue. If you have desiccated eye issues, contact lens wear, some drugs, or some other cause

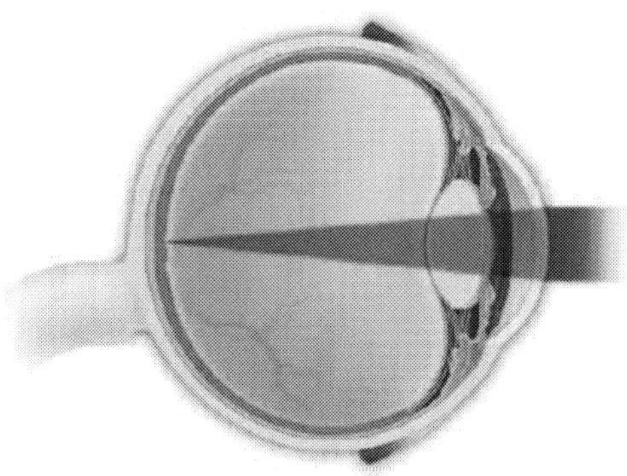

Figure 3. With natural vision, light rays are specifically centered on the retina.

3.2. The Eyes Understanding

In order, the cornea along with the lens have to curvature or refract light rays to see clearly, so that the spotlight on the retina, a stratum of light-sensing cells lining the backside of the eye. The retina turns light rays addicted to the brain's impulses, where they are remembered as images. The photo you see is fuzzy if the rays of light do not settle on to the retina. This is considered a mistake of refraction. By creating rays of light concentrate on the retina. These inaccuracies are minimized by glasses, contact lenses, and refractive surgery [29]. Refractive inaccuracy arises the origin by a defectively fashioned eyeball, lens, or cornea, or by a lens that, in the case of Presbyopia, does not amend figure adequate to focus on surrounding things, and are of these particular forms. A further term for shortsightedness is myopia, where merely surrounding objects are visible or separate. Hyperopia is a different term for forethought, where simple or distinct astigmatism is just things far away when details are distorted, irrespective It is a condition that normally happens between the ages of 40 and 50 and makes it more difficult to see very closely if they are close to or distant Presbyopia, or "ageing eye," It may be fixed among reading glasses or bifocals, but LASIK or some other refractive surgery is commonly used cannot fix it.

3.3. Additional Considerations

- The threats and bonuses. You may want to forgo the surgery if you're able to wear contacts or glasses.
- Your surgical preferences. Realistic, are they? In broad-spectrum, having exceedingly pitiable perception decreases the probability of accomplishment with LASIK and augments the likelihood of retreat.
- Requisites and routine practices for the workplace. To make sure LASIK is safe for you, discuss work, sports, and leisure with your physician.
- If you are a contender for monovision, one eye corrects for remote vision with the further eye corrects for near vision. LASIK does not remedy Presbyopic, one eye can see both close and far. Nevertheless, it can be used to the acceptable distance for one eye and close vision for the other. If you are able to amend to this transition, the need for reading glasses can be removed or decreased. Monovision, however, has threats of its own:
- The two eyes no longer function together after mono-vision. This triggers a vision of lower quality and a decline in the perception of depth. In conditions of low lighting and when conducting tasks involving very clear vision, these effects are most apparent.
- As a result, when the stage visually challenging activities, alike driving at nighttime, operating hazardous paraphernalia, or

performing professional duties require very spiky, close vision, you might should bear glasses or contact lenses for distance or close vision.

3.4. Complications and Threats

Before the procedure, the surgeon must Explain the risks and potential complications of getting one or both eyes done on the same day, including the pros and cons. This is the "informed consent arrangement" procedure.

- *Menace* Blindness and the sight is permanently damaged. In rare cases, Irreversible eye injury, including constant blindness, may be caused by errors during surgery (such as laser system malfunction) or complications following surgery (such as inflammation). In other cases, with further surgery or other procedures, the symptoms may be fixed.
- *Loss of vision.* Although with glasses or contacts, after the operation, you may not see as well, as you did before with glasses or contacts the procedure. Or, to see as clearly as you did before surgery, you may need glasses or contacts.
- *Extreme difficulties with night vision.* You can the development of painful visual symptoms that can have a significant effect on night vision, particularly glare, halos, and/or double visualization.
- *"Dwindle in contrast compassion," "moistness," or "serration."* In nature, objects might be fuzzy or grayish. Also, On the eye map with a clear vision, you cannot notice well in low contrast circumstances after treatment compared to before, such as at night or in fog.
- *Extreme syndrome of dry eyes.* As a consequence of the surgery, your eye might Not be able to fabricate sufficient tears to remain it clammy and relaxed. Not just that does dry eye cause soreness, but because of intermittent blurring and other visual symptoms, it can

reduce visual quality. This disease could be lifelong. It can require extensive Usage of plugs or other treatments and drop therapy.

3.4.1. Inconvenience

- *The contagion of the corneas or inflammation.* Supplementary surgery or further treatments may require certain tribulations.
- *Problems with the post-operative corneal flail.* These involve abnormal or imperfect flaps, cell growth beneath the flap that will have to be replaced by surgery, and abnormal curative that results in a blurred cornea that can solitary be resolved by transplantation of the cornea.

3.5. Why Is LASIK Not Made Up of Women Who Are Pregnant or Breastfeeding?

If you would like to see better and your reliance on corrective lenses (i.e., glasses, contacts), LASIK is a great choice to consider. For people suffering from refractive errors, it's a great choice to consider, which you might know better with the following names:

- Myopia
- Hyperopia
- Astigmatism

Although many individuals can be treated by laser eye surgery, some individuals are not good candidates for treatment. Right now, we would like to take a few moments to discuss why pregnant or nursing women are not considered suitable contestants for surgery.

4. Regarding LASIK Surgery

Next, going over some of the ground rules of LASIK surgery is a good idea. The use of a laser to reshape the cornea, the transparent, frontal/outer portion of the eye, requires LASIK surgery. Light will correctly focus on the retina, the Tissue with light-sensitivity situated at the backside of the eye, by correcting the corneal shape. Under local anesthetic, which is administered by eye drops, LASIK is carried out. In general, overall surgical healing is swift and free of significant complications.

4.1. Surgery and Breastfeeding in LASIK: The Whole Thing You Should Be Familiar With

The verdict to start a family is enormous and one that can only be taken if it feels right. There are some things that you should know first if you are starting your family but have been thinking of getting LASIK. Before attempting laser eye surgery while pregnant or breastfeeding, we've gathered all the details we think women should know.

4.2. LASIK Pregnancy Before, During and After

As you most probably know, a lot of major changes in the carcass are caused by pregnancy. There are also signs of pregnancy that people don't know about. You hear about morning sickness, mood swings, swelling, and the coveted glow of pregnancy, but you rarely hear anyone speak about how your eyes can be affected by pregnancy. Here at New York Eye Specialists, as part of our diverse patient base, we respect women. Therefore, when consulting and caring for them, we take into account their distinct needs.

4.3. How Your Vision Is Affected by Pregnancy and Breastfeeding?

Their bodies experience major hormonal changes when a woman becomes pregnant, or is breastfeeding. Throughout the body, these changes will cause a great deal of swelling. It involves the eyes! Your corneas can swell and change shape when you become pregnant. This could make your vision fuzzy. While this issue ends after pregnancy for many women, for others, it may last until after they stop breastfeeding.

4.4. LASIK before Pregnancy Surgery

When you are planning to start a family but are not pregnant, if you want LASIK pre-baby, there are some things you should remember. Many physicians suggest waiting at least six months to become pregnant following LASIK surgery. When some women did not wait long enough after LASIK, they experienced vision regression. After pregnancy, your vision can return to normal, but you risk requiring LASIK improvement to achieve the vision you had after your first process. The safest solution for vision correction during pregnancy or breastfeeding is the use of corrective lenses, such as glasses or contacts. This helps to ensure good vision and the baby's health.

4.5. During Pregnancy, LASIK

A successful LASIK surgeon won't perform laser eye surgery on a pregnant woman knowingly. For a few factors, this is inadvisable. The main factor, and one that we have already touched on, is that her vision is likely to regress and that after pregnancy she will need a second operation. Another reason is the added vulnerability of pregnant women to post-LASIK dry eye syndrome [30]. The beginning of irritating dry eye symptoms may be reason by pregnancy alone. A common side effect of surgery with LASIK is dry eye. Together, both may significantly worsen the problem throughout pregnancy. So, we suggest waiting until after pregnancy to undergo LASIK surgery to prevent a lot of needless annoyance and discomfort. There's a moistened cheek. To prevent the moving eye and the cornea in the eye right position, a suction ring is placed. A special system cuts the outer layer of the cornea of the eyeball [31-33] with a hinged flap of thin corneal tissue and the dither is raised Out of the Course. The corneal tissue that underlies is reshaped by the laser, and the surgeon removes the flap, adhering to the eyeball rapidly. No stitches are required. To cover the flap, a mask, either transparent the eye is placed over plastic or perforated metal.

4.6. LASIK Following Pregnancy

Although not inherently harmful during the nursing process, LASIK may still produce some of the above-mentioned negative effects. Many physicians suggest waiting to undergo LASIK eye surgery six months after you finish breastfeeding. This is not intended to unnecessarily make vision correction difficult for nursing women, but to keep them protected from side effects that they would not otherwise encounter. Healing is reasonably quick, but after the procedure, you may want to take a few days off from work. Stop Athletics for three days after surgery; for four weeks, contact sports or related practices. Be mindful of the fact that:

- After surgery, you can feel a slight burn or impression for a few hours. Don't itch your eyes. If you need one, your doctor will prescribe a painkiller to relieve some discomfort.
- On the day of surgery, your vision will still be blurry, but when you return for a follow-up, it should boost considerably by the next day examination.
- Aggravating or irregular side impacts should be reported to the doctor instantaneously.

- If your vision has changed adequately to do so comfortably, you should not drive until
- Swimming, hot tubs, and whirlpools should be avoided for two weeks after the procedure.

4.7. Why Pregnant Women Are Not Successful LASIK Candidates

Although LASIK is a safe and efficient treatment choice, surgeons will not perform the procedure on pregnant women. This goes for all pregnancy stages. The explanation for this is that the consistency of a woman's vision can be affected by hormonal changes that arise during pregnancy. Also, as part of the LASIK procedure and LASIK aftercare, there are anesthetic eye drops and other drugs that are given, all of which can have adverse effects on a developing fetus. It is desirable for surgeons to behave conservatively and postpone the surgery until a few weeks after the woman has had the child to ensure proper vision correction and to protect the health of the infant.

4.8. Why Nursing Women Are Not Successful LASIK Candidates

For females who are also breastfeeding, the same limitation on LASIK applies. The reasoning for this is the same as the rationale for not allowing pregnant women to undergo LASIK. A woman's hormones [34-35] can take time after pregnancy to return to normal levels, and thus their vision will take time to meet its prescription for pre-pregnancy. Also, surgery-related eye drops and drugs may find their way into breast milk.

4.9. Candidacy during Pregnancy and Breastfeeding for LASIK

The candidacy of a woman for LASIK after pregnancy and breastfeeding will be decided on a case by case basis by eye doctors. It will be necessary to even out the hormones of a woman and to finish breastfeeding. As a general rule, after giving birth, LASIK is considered viable for a woman for around two menstrual cycles.

5. Is It Possible to Take LASIK Surgery for a Pregnant?

A prevalent dream expressed by numerous individuals those who suffer from myopia, Hypothermia or astigmatism is LASIK surgery. This surgery, done through an ophthalmologist, uses a laser to recast the cornea to correct vision, enhancing optical acuity, which is the clarity and serration of images. LASIK surgery is a comparatively harmless, austerely invasive surgery that greatly enhances the life of patients who are normally capable to avoid using eyeglasses and contact lenses. However, there are some important considerations for a woman who is pregnant or breastfeeding a baby that ought to be in use into account before deciding to continue with this process.

5.1. Corporal Eyesight Improves Appropriate to Pregnancy

Pregnancy is a moment of transition in the body of a female. Eyes and eyesight are included with some of these improvements. Some are temporary only, although others may be permanent. Many females experience changes in vision due to variations in hormone levels, Such as nearsightedness, farsightedness or astigmatism at new or increased levels. It may alter the form and the cornea thickness, and it may also swell due to fluid retention. The progression of diabetes and hypertension, which be able to occur throughout pregnancy, can also cause changes in eyesight. Another common problem is dry eyes. These corporal changes in the body of a pregnant woman compose her a bad contender for LASIK surgery, as the adjustment obtained might not be precise if, after the birth of the baby, the eyes change again.

5.2. Issues of Protection during Pregnancy

There are several adjustments in the eyes of a pregnant woman that justify waiting for LASIK surgery, but there are also some safety concerns. During and after surgery, LASIK surgery patients are administered drugs that can reach the bloodstream via mucous membranes. Many of these drugs have not been checked and cannot be assumed to be safe for the fetus in pregnant women. Before surgery, the doctor must dilate the eyes, and medications, such as Valium [36-38], are also provided for relief during the operation. Upon surgery, there could Antibiotics and eye drops containing steroids. All of these will penetrate the stream of blood and the pose possible hazards to the infant. The lasers themselves may have a slight risk of radiation. To any pregnant woman, these protection issues are warning flags that this is not the right moment to investigate LASIK surgery.

5.3. The Nursing Mother's Considerations

A pregnant woman can wait to undergo surgery with LASIK until after her birth. There are issues, conversely, As well as for the pregnant mother. And after birth, she will undergo hormonal changes. These may hurt post-operation healing. It is also possible for breastfeeding to cause corneal changes that may not be resolved until after weaning. The risk of drugs finding their way into breast milk is also increased. Even in limited quantities, post-operative drugs, Steroid eye drops and antibiotics both enter the breast milk. These drugs are not checked for children, so nearby is no undertaking of protection, and they may be probably harmful to a breastfeeding child. The months of pregnancy and breastfeeding are not the time for LASIK surgery to be considered. The physical changes in the eyes of a woman, as well as the safety concerns associated with some forms of drugs, will not be fully addressed until after the breastfeeding phase has ended. Most physicians suggest that after the baby is weaned, women wait for the treatment for about two or three menstrual cycles for the best results. So, being polite, following the orders of the doctor and waiting for the correct period of the moment are the correct approaches to guarantee the best possible operation for LASIK outcomes.

6. Consider Correction of LASER Vision

Have you considered LASIK laser vision correction, but continue to come up with excuses to avoid treatment? Not alone are you. Many individuals have been weighing the decision for years. A number of our patients, however, have admitted that they would like to have LASIK earlier. Make 2016 the year that you eventually experience better vision and independence from contact lenses and glasses. The team at King LASIK shares the top five reasons for getting LASIK in 2016 in this article.

6.1. Clearer Vision Comfort

There is life-changing independence from reliance on glasses and contacts. With better vision, without searching for your glasses or putting in contacts, you can perform basic tasks, like looking at the alarm clock or testing a medicine bottle. You will fly with ease and avoid thinking about packing your lenses or cleaning solutions or forgetting them. LASIK makes living an active lifestyle simpler. Without thinking about your glasses slipping off or fogging up, you can take a long jog outside. At a moment's notice, you can leap into a tub. Without thinking about breaking your glasses, you can play contact sports.

6.2. Investment of Wise

LASIK makes sense financially. Over time, by not having to purchase contact lenses, glass lenses, frames and associated products, you can save thousands of dollars. You may also be able to pay with a flexible spending account (FSA) provided by your employer for your LASIK operation, or by special patient funding services offered by the doctor.

6.3. Almost-Instant Results

Usually, a lengthy, drawn-out recovery does not require LASIK. Almost right away, enjoy your performance! Many of our LASIK patients wake up with significantly better vision the day after surgery. During the next few days, the findings appear to change. It is highly unlikely to encounter severe side effects.

6.4. Reduction in Signs of Allergy

A reduction in painful allergy symptoms such as itchiness, red eyes and burning has been noticed by some of our LASIK patients, so they no longer need to wear contact lenses. After LASIK, patients who have experienced chronic headaches or sinus issues [39-40] due to wearing glasses will find relief.

6.5. Raise the Quotient of Your Style

You'll love your appearance after LASIK if you don't like the way you look with glasses but can't handle contacts. All the time, you should go bare-faced and show off your lovely skin. Without exchanging the lenses for prescription-strength lenses, pick your favorite sunglasses.

6.6. Recognizing the LASIK Patient Ideal

In determining the ideal LASIK patient, there are two viewpoints to consider: the scientific basis of expertise and the empirical so-called soft skills of an accomplished surgeon. The considerations to be considered when deciding If an individual is a good candidate for treatment, this refractive surgical procedure is discussed in this expose.

7. Issues of Corneal

Refractive surgeons are well aware that candidates with LASIK should have a minimum corneal thickness of 500μm. This cap should be respected when a LASIK procedure is scheduled. In certain nations, disregarding it is considered a matter of iatrogenic inability. When assessing a patient's candidacy for LASIK, corneal steepness should also be considered. After treatment, the cornea should not become too smooth, because the flatter the cornea is, the more optical problems can occur. The suggested corneal flatness limit is 36.00 to 38.00 D. The corneal steepness, on the other hand, should not exceed 50.00 D, as greater steepness could lead to nutritional problems and instability of the tear film. As a rule of thumb, to approximate the result in terms of corneal curvature, refraction may be applied to the steepness. Ideally, a myopic patient should have a 48.00 D keratometric (K) reading and refraction of -5.00 D; after treatment, this patient should end up with a K reading of around 43.00 D. On topography and 4.00 D of Hyperopia, the ideal hyperopic patient will have a K reading of 39.00 D. It will also be expected that this patient would have a K reading of 43.00 D after treatment.

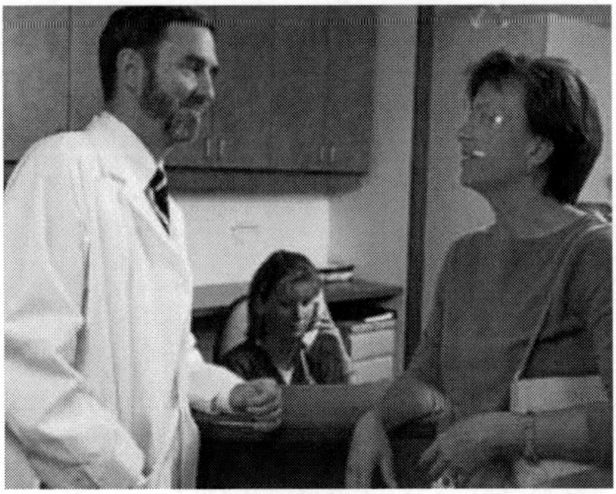

Figure 4. The mask of the eye worn behind LASIK.

8. Astigmatism

Similarly, the preparation of astigmatic ametropia is determined, and the same limits should be observed. To define lentogenic astigmatism, that is, astigmatism caused by the lens rather than the cornea, the estimated treatment should take into account the cylinder axis. Only corneal astigmatism should be seen in the ideal LASIK candidate. If lentogenic astigmatism is remarkable, one should be aware of the fact that corneal astigmatism is caused by the expected LASIK procedure. Therefore, the surgeon would be responsible for the continuity and proper alignment of both ametropia over time and the fact that, after lens detachment, the patient would be left with extreme iatrogenic astigmatism. You should discuss this detail with the patient. Correction by implantation of a toric IOL is the ideal treatment in eyes with lentogenic astigmatism.

9. Criteria Exclusion

When deciding whether a patient is a candidate for LASIK, exclusion criteria resulting from other diseases should be taken into account. It is important to classify patients with rheumatoid arthritis or other collage nous. Cataract patients should undergo lens extraction first. To distinguish patients with keratoconus, in particular the not-so-evident early cases and types of agitation, great care should be taken. Visualization of the back surface of the cornea is extremely useful, so having a corneal topography system with this skill is advantageous for the refractive surgeon. Since there is an increased risk of epithelial development in these cases, patients with diabetes are usually not suitable candidates for LASIK. This should be clarified to the patient, and it is important to address the PRK alternative. Measurement of refraction can also be troublesome in patients with diabetes; the measurement will overestimate myopic values under elevated blood sugar conditions, and vice versa. The best time for the refractive measurement to be measured is when the blood sugar levels of the patient are normal. It is therefore desirable to test the blood sugar of the patient first, and then to test his or her refraction when the reading is fine.

9.10. Motivation and Comprehension of Patients

There are two important aspects to remember in terms of soft skills: (1) the patient's confidence, and (2) the capacity of the patient to understand refractive therapy. To assess if the patient has unreasonable expectations, it is beneficial to explore the patient's motivation for undertaking LASIK during the visit before the surgery. Additionally, poor motivation, especially in times of pain, can lead to problems during the healing process. Freedom from glasses and contact lenses is defined by most patients as their key reason to undergo LASIK. Maybe because of dry eyes, they do not wear contact lenses or cannot regulate their use. Some patients may choose to save the money they have historically spent on contact lenses or glasses. Regardless of the motivation of the patient, to recognize any latent issues that might arise postoperatively, it is necessary to know his or her exact objective. A patient who is active in martial arts, for example, is not an ideal candidate for LASIK, as a punch could reach the cornea and loosen the flap. The specifications of a driver's or pilot's license, which may not be met for some time after LASIK, maybe another concern. Divers should be prepared for around 2 months after the operation to avoid these practices. If the patient's ultimate reason for LASIK is physical appearance, one should brace him or her to feel potential discomfort from facial wrinkles that are more noticeable without glasses. All patients, particularly hyperopic patients who undergo surgery later in life and are reaching the age at which presbyopia occurs, should be educated about the eventual onset of presbyopia.

9.11. Patients Presbyopic

Those with presbyopia are a category of patients that deserves special attention. If a Presbyopic patient is given correction for long vision by the surgeon, he or she must be told of the continued need to read glasses after surgery. The patient must be prepared for issues with enhancement operations and visual impairments caused by multifocal effects, including loss of glare and contrast sensitivity if a multifocal corneal pattern is used. If monovision is provided, the patient with glasses or contact lenses should be shown the procedure. It is crucial that the patient fully understands the treatment with monovision. He or she needs to be told that there will be only one focal plane for each eye, so there are two distances to use, far and close. In this sense, the patient needs to be told about the depth of field in his or her close-vision eye. Patients should realize that only one focal length is close, but it can be broadened by maximizing the lighting of the workplace.

9.12. LASIK's Medical Alternatives

You may want to explore with your eye doctor some surgical alternatives to LASIK. These operations are usually comparatively innovative and are carried out less repeatedly than conventional LASIK surgery.

- *Photorefractive keratectomy (PRK)* In surgery using PRK, like Epi-LASIK and LASEK, surgeons exploit lasers to allow "surface ablations" on the cornea exclusive of building a corneal flap. As these operations cut only the very top (epithelial) stratum of the cornea, the possibility of convinced complications allied with LASIK surgery can be condensed.
- *Keratoplasty Conductive (CK)* This is a thermal surgery that refracts technique used in people over the age of 40 to correct mild to moderate farsightedness (Hyperopia) by using a small prod that liberates regulated quantities for Radiofrequency (RF) energy for heat transfer to the peripheral part of the cornea instead of a laser. Farsightedness, over time, can return.
- *Phobic Intraocular Lens (IOL)* An IOL is a variety of contact lens inserted surgically within the eye in the facade of the lens. Such implants are used to fix vision tribulations grounds by cataracts and other refractory tribulations that are too serious to be fixed with refractive surgery based on the cornea. In addition to improving distance vision, some types of IOLs, like multifocal lenses or accommodative lenses, can also remove the need for reading glasses.

10. Laser Surgery Drawbacks

There is only one thing that comes up with our min, LASIK when we think about correcting the vision. As technology progresses day by day, so are LASIK's hopes and aspirations. But there are still cases where it cannot be achieved, even with LASIK's new techniques. The following are some cases in which it is not possible to perform LASIK eye surgery:

10.1. Limitations on Age

- *18 Years Minimum Age* by 18 years, in most individuals, the strength of glasses appears to become constant. There can be no hard and fast rules in a human environment, however. It means that the number may also become stable by 16 years in some individuals, while in some it may not be stable even at 22 years. LASIK should not be done at this point, even if the number is 16 years stable, since it is difficult to foresee the future, and if the number increases later, it can merely direct to regret. As a general observation, it is shown that even before 18 years of age, low numbers like -1.0 to -3.0 appear to become stable. Numbers from 3.0 to 6.0 will stabilize for 18 to 20 years. Numbers from 6.0 to 9.0 may be stable for 22 years, although numbers above nine may or may not be fully stable for 22 years or more.

- *No Cap Maximum Age* and at the age of 60, we did LASIK in individuals. It is a question of when one decides in life that enough is enough and that without these 'optical crutches' one would like to see the world. We have seen in our personal experience of 20 + years of LASIK that, by the age of 40, Indians typically consider glasses as part of their identity. Rarely have we seen people above this generation asking for LASIK. We have, however, witnessed a definite social shift in the last few years. Parents of children who have successfully done LASIK are now wondering if, at this point, they too can get rid of their glasses.
- *Ideal age: 20 to 40 years* When people experience like this is the perfect mature for LASIK, there is always an age band. We feel like this band is between 20 and 40 years old. The urge to look good without glasses is intense. during this time. Matrimony is a big cause, too. Though other factors such as lifestyle independence, sports, enhancement of personality and boost of self-confidence also play an important role in India.

10.2. Limitations on Pregnancy or Breastfeeding

During pregnancy or breastfeeding, LASIK is not advisable. Throughout this time, the hormonal levels in the womanly body are lofty, and relaxation of tissues is related to an increase in spectacular intensity. As this enlarge in spectacle power can occur in merely 10 percent of cases, this numeral is still very high to alert about LASIK all through this era. It is pragmatic that the spectacle power shift is habitually flanked by 0.5 and 1.0 D in those women, where the number increases throughout pregnancy. It is also pragmatic that in the first pregnancy, if the strength of the display increases, the subsequent pregnancy will increase similarly.

10.3. Corneal Thickness Limitations

To conduct LASIK, the cornea should be sufficiently dense. A cornea that is too thin becomes a limiting factor. The central thickness of a typical Indian cornea is 530 microns, or 0.53 mm. SBK (thin flap LASIK) or the Bladeless Femto LASIK will safely change the power of -8.0 to this thickness.

A cornea that is less than 495 microns is known to be thin, while a 'no go' is less than 450 microns thick. The obvious inference from these statistics is that if the cornea is thicker than 530 microns, it is possible to correct the number of spectacles. It is not right because power treatment greater than -8.0 results in unnecessary flattening of the cornea and associated vision disturbances called spherical aberration.

The optimal upper limit is therefore suggested to be -8.0, while the appropriate upper limit is -10.0.0 LASIK should be avoided beyond this amount, and it would be safer to go in for an ICL implant.

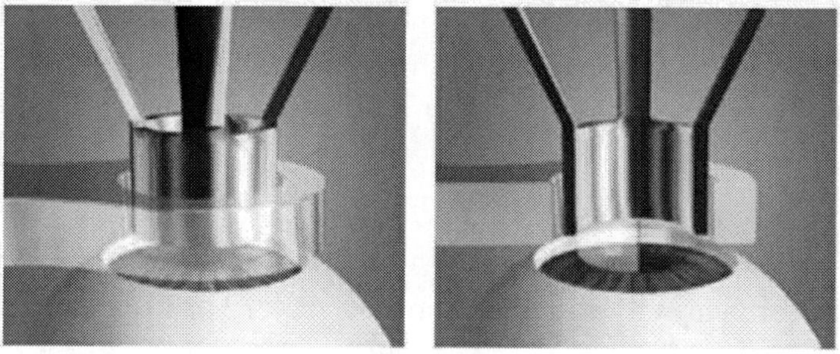

Figure 5. Laser LASIK for corneal flap making.

10.4. Corneal Curvature Limitations

A limiting factor may also be too flat a cornea or too steep a cornea.

- *Flat Cornea:* The curvature of a normal human cornea is 44,0 D. A flat cornea is assumed to be a cornea with a curve of 41.0 D or less. LASIK requires raising the corneal flap, and the size of the raised flap can be too small in very flat corneal situations. This means that the area of the cornea available for laser treatment can need to be limited, leading to visual issues such as halos and nighttime glare around lights. Also in the flat cornea, Femto Second Laser engineered flaps do better.
- *Steep Cornea:* A cornea is known to be a steep cornea that is more than 48.5 D. In such situations, the buttonholes of the flap or the irregular thickness of the flap may result from raising the flap. In just a very small percentage of steep corneas, it occurs. The flap is re-positioned bask without doing the laser treatment in case of buttonholing the flap and allowed to recover. After three months, the flap can be re-lifted, ideally with a Femto Second Laser, as the latter gives more effective flaps at corneal curvature extremes.
- *Corneal Pathology Weaknesses:* Keratoconus is a corneal disease in which naturally poor corneal tissue is present. The cornea begins bulging out because of the usual eye pressure inside the eyeball. This makes it steep and uneven for the cornea. Rays of light entering the eye through such corneas are spread irregularly, leading to a loss of focus quality and a reduction in vision. To adjust its curvature, LASIK involves ablating the cornea. Ablating the cornea thinens the cornea. The appropriate amount of thinning of a healthy cornea does not damage it. In an inherently weak cornea, however, the thinning caused by LASIK can weaken the cornea to the degree that it begins to bulge, causing optical distortions and vision reduction. 'C3R' or what is called Collagen Cross-Linking can then avoid this irregular bulging of the cornea. Cornea screening is critical in detecting subclinical or concealed

keratoconus and rejecting these cases so that the rest of the eyes receiving treatment with LASIK are healthy. With modern corneal scanning methods such as Pentacam, most of these secret cases of Keratoconus can be detected, thus making LASIK very clean. Quite rarely, however, one will still have to face a challenging situation, and it would then be appropriate to do Collagen Cross-Linking to stop the disease's development.

CONCLUSION

It has been shown by study and experiences that breastfeeding and human milk may provide large quantities of for the baby, nutritional and no nutritional benefits and the mother and set the perfect practicalities health for babies, children and adults, and for youth evolution. The encouragement of breastfeeding, therefore, It ought to be taken acutely as a global communal health concern. A crisis. Breastfeeding-reinforcing measures are comparatively straightforward and cheap. The impassioned shore up and engagement by pediatricians and the scheme Wide-scale sustain can be offered by the Baby-Friendly Hospital, Be effective in supporting breastfeeding. Additionally, Good laws for inspection and inspection should be implemented. Limit the use of chemical substances present in breast infections Milk, to trust In any case, this low-tech life hoarder is not destabilized. The use of a breastfeeding pillow substantially reduces maternal distress encountered during the process of breastfeeding. It is anticipated that maternal comfort Improve the consistency of breastfeeding by enhancing the mother baby's role and connexion during the breastfeeding process, raising the sucking capacity of the baby and the breastfeeding time of the baby to ensure adequate nutrition or boost the suckling needs of the baby. The release of stress hormones can also be suppressed by a secure and relaxed environment and the hormones that play a role in producing breast milk can be increased. Therefore, the use of a breastfeeding pillow by postpartum mothers should be enforced.

References

[1] Woreta KB, Woreta F. Update on contraindications for laser-assisted in situ keratomileusis and pho- torefractive keratectomy. *Curr Opin Ophthalmol*. 2014;25(4):251–7. https://doi.org/10.1097/icu.000000 0000000055.

[2] Tal R, Taylor HS, Burney RO, Mooney SB, GiudiceLC. *Endocrinology of pregnancy*. MDText.com, Inc.; 2000. http://www.ncbi.nlm.nih.gov/pubmed/ 25905197. Accessed 18 May 2019.

[3] Hafezi F, Iseli HP. Pregnancy-related exacerbation of iatrogenic keratectasia despite corneal collagen cross linking. *J Cataract Refract Surg*. 2008; 34(7):1219–21. https://doi.org/10.1016/j.jcrs. 2008.02.036

[4] Hendrick V, Altshuler LL, Suri R. Hormonal changes in the postpartum and implications for postpartum depression. *Psychosomatics*. 1998; 39(2):93–101. https://doi.org/10.1016/S0033-3182(98)71355-6.

[5] *The physiological basis of breastfeeding*. 2009. https://www.ncbi.nlm.nih.gov/books/NBK148970/. Accessed 19 May 2019.

[6] Pillay J, Davis TJ. *Physiology, lactation*. StatPearls Publishing; 2019. http://www.ncbi.nlm.nih.gov/pubmed/29763156. Accessed 19 May 2019

[7] Suzuki T, Sullivan DA. Estrogen stimulation of proinflammatory cytokine and matrix metalloproteinase gene expression in human corneal epithelial cells. *Cornea*. 2005; 24(8):1004–1009. http://www.ncbi.nlm.nih.gov/pubmed/16227852. Accessed 20 May 2019.

[8] López-Prats MJ, Hidalgo-Mora JJ, Sanz-Marco E, Pellicer A, Perales A, Díaz-Llopis M. Influencia del embarazo sobre los parámetros refractivos tras cirugía laser in situ keratomileusis. *Arch Soc Esp Oftalmol*. 2012; 87(6):173–8. https://doi.org/10.1016/j.oftal.2011.09.021.

[9] Dinn RB, Harris A, Marcus PS. Ocular changes in pregnancy. *Obstet Gynecol Surv*. 2003;58(2):137–44. https://doi.org/10.1097/01.OGX.0000047741.79433.52.

[10] Bahadir Kilavuzoglu AE, Cosar CB, Bildirici I, Cetin O, Ozbasli E. Estrogen- and progesterone-induced variation in corneal parameters according to hormonal status. *Eye Contact Lens Sci Clin Pract.* 2017;44(Suppl 1):1. https://doi.org/10.1097/ICL.0000000000000376.

[11] Kiely PM, Carney LG, Smith G. Menstrual cycle variations of corneal topography and thickness. *Am J Optom Physiol Opt*. 1983; 60(10): 822–829. http://www.ncbi.nlm.nih.gov/pubmed/6650653. Accessed 19 May 2019.

[12] Park SB, Lindahl KJ, Temnycky GO, Aquavella JV. The effect of pregnancy on corneal curvature. *CLAO J.* 1992; 18(4):256–259. http://www.ncbi.nlm.nih.gov/pubmed/1424062. Accessed 14 May 2019.

[13] Manges TD, Banaitis DA, Roth N, Yolton RL. Changes in optometric findings during pregnancy. *Am J Optom Physiol Opt*. 1987;64(3):159–166. http://www.ncbi.nlm.nih.gov/pubmed/3578480. Accessed 14 May 2019.

[14] Stahl B, Thurl S, Zeng J, Karas M, Hillenkamp F, Steup M, Sawatzki G. Oligosaccharides from human milk as revealed by matrix-assisted laser desorption/ionization mass spectrometry *Anal Biochem*. 1994; 223(2):218-26.

[15] American Academy of Pediatrics, Section on Breastfeeding. Breastfeeding and the use of human milk. *Pediatrics.* 2012; 129(3):e827-41.

[16] Ip S, Chung M, Raman G, Trikalinos TA, Lau J. A summary of the Agency for Healthcare Research and Quality's evidence report on breastfeeding in developed countries. *Breastfeed Med*. 2009; 4(Suppl 1):S17-30.

[17] Hambraeus, Forsum E, Lönnerdal B. Nutritional aspects of breast milk and cow's milk formulas. In: Hambraeus L, Hanson L, MacFarlane H. *Symposium on Food and Immunology*. Stockholm: Almqvist and Wiksell,1975.

[18] Moro G, Minoli I, Boehm G, Georgi G, Jelinek J, Sawatzki G. Postprandial plasma amino acids in preterm infants: influence of the protein source. *Acta Paediatr*. 1999; 88(8):885-9.

[19] Kramer MS, Chalmers B, Hodnett ED, Sevkovskaya Z, Dzikovich I, Shapiro S, Collet JP, Vanilovich I, Mezen I, Ducruet T, Shishko G, Zubovich V, Mknuik D, Gluchanina E, Dombrovskiy V, Ustinovitch A, Kot T, Bogdanovich N, Ovchinikova L, Helsing E; PROBIT Study Group (Promotion of Breastfeedin Intervention Trial). Promotion of Breastfeeding Intervention Trial (PROBIT): a randomized trial in the Republic of Belarus. *JAMA.* 2001; 285(4): 413-20.

[20] Labbok MH. Effects of breastfeeding on the mother. *Pediatr Clin North Am.* 2001; 48(1):143-58.

[21] Kurath S, Halwachs-Baumann G, Müller W, Resch B. Transmission of cytomegalovirus via breast milk to the prematurely born infant: a systematic review. *Clin Microbiol Infect.* 2010; 16(8):1172-8.

[22] American Academy of Pediatrics, Subcommittee on Hyperbilirubinemia. Management of hyperbilirubinemia in the newborn infant 35 or more weeks of gestation. *Pediatrics.* 2004; 114(1):297-316.

[23] Kearvel H, Grant J. Getting connected How nurses can support mother/infant attachment in the neonatal intensive care unit. *Aust J Adv Nurs* 2010; 27:75-82.

[24] Holdcroft A, Snidvongs S, Cason A, et al. Pain and uterine contractions during breastfeeding in the immediate post partum period increase with parity. *Pai* 2003; 104:58996.

[25] Aksu H, Küçük M, Gülergün DüzgünM. The effect of postnatal breastfeeding education/support offered at home 3 days after delivery on breast- feeding duration and knowledge: A ran- domized trial. *J Matern Fetal Neonatal Med* 2011; 24:354-61.

[26] Corlett EN, Bishop RP. A technique for assessing postural discomfort. *Ergonomics.* 1976; 19:175-82.

[27] Cameron JA. Assessing work-relate body-part discomfort: Current strategies and a behaviorally oriented assess- ment tool. *Int J Ind Ergonom* 1996; 18:389-98.

[28] Butchan P, Chamusri S, Singhala K. Effects of breastfeeding promoting program on family members self-efficacy and

ecific disease easy in clinical situations. Moreover, these algorithms are nplemented in the area of the healthcare system to allow health ecialists and professionals to diagnose, monitor, and focus on the nportant features or regions of the problem and provide an accurate rediction. In fact, the AI-based techniques are proactive and predictive fesaving in which is an essential ability of every healthcare system. In his chapter, we explored potential applications of AI-based approaches in ne smart healthcare system and how these approaches could improve ealthcare industries by improving health care services. We have lescribed how these computational models can impact medical diagnosis n healthcare. In the literature review, a comprehensive study of sixteen papers is carried out which includes a few key diseases such as Alzheimer's, Glaucoma, Coronavirus, Arrhythmia, and Diabetes disease. Many questions have been raised in this study regarding the best ML and DL approaches on various disease datasets and the solutions to overcome those issues for better performance.

words: artificial intelligence, machine learning, deep learning, smart healthcare, disease diagnosis

Introduction

Healthcare is described as the amelioration of health all through the oidance, cure, and investigation of mental damage, physical damage, ury, sickness, virus, and disease [1]. The industry of Healthcare is huge hich is dealing with drugs, patients, different kinds of diseases, omedical experts, the academic world, pharma, research laboratories, etc. ealth is wealth, as there is nothing more precious than being healthy. here are different definitions and interpretations of a "smart city." In this hapter, smart healthcare is seen as having some characteristics such as nticipatory, context-aware, responsive, adaptive, intelligent, personalized, nd transparent [2]. Researchers and Scientists have dedicated huge efforts o smart healthcare by proposing and recommending new algorithms, olicies, system architectures for smart healthcare. One major purpose of Healthcare is the disease-free nation-state. To accomplish this, aim all elements are working extremely tough day and night. Even so, many

breastfeeding promotion behavior in community. *J Nursing Health Care* 2016; 34(4):97-105.

[29] Mehdizadehkashi K, Chaichian S, Mehdizadehkashi A, et al. Visual acuity changes during pregnancy and postpartum: a cross-sectional study in Iran. *J Pregnancy*. 2014; 2014: 675792. https://doi.org/10.1155/2014/675792

[30] Suzuki T, Sullivan DA. Estrogen stimulation of proinflammatory cytokine and matrix metalloproteinase gene expression in human corneal epithelial cells. *Cornea*. 2005; 24(8):1004–1009. http://www.ncbi.nlm.nih.gov/pubmed/16227852. Accessed 20 May 2019.

[31] Sharif K. Regression of myopia induced by pregnancy after photorefractive keratectomy. *J Refract Surg*. 1997; 13(5):S445–6. https://doi.org/10.3928/1081-597X-19970801-13.

[32] Khakhong S, Nirattharadorn M. The effects of promoting self-efficacy program on breast feeding behavior among adolescent mothers in community. *J Public Health* 2017; 47(1):31 43.

[33] Atas¸ M, Duru N, Ulusoy DM, et al. Evaluation of anterior segment parameters during and after pregnancy. *Cont Lens Anterior Eye*. 2014; 37(6):447–50. https://doi.org/10.1016/j.clae.2014.07.013.

[34] Mehdizadehkashi K, Chaichian S, Mehdizadehkash A, et al. Visual acuity changes during pregnancy and postpartum: a cross-sectional study in Iran. *J Pregnancy*. 2014; 2014:675792. https://doi.org/10.1155/2014/675792.

[35] Anderson PO. Alcohol and breastfeeding. *J Human Lact.* 1995; 11:321-3.

[36] American Academy of Pediatrics, Subcommittee on Hyperbilirubinemia. Management of hyperbilirubinemia in the newborn infant 35 or more weeks of gestation. *Pediatrics.* 2004; 114(1):297-316.

[37] American Academy of Pediatrics, Section on Breastfeeding Breastfeeding and the use of human milk. *Pediatrics.* 2012; 129(3):e827-41.

[38] Corlett EN, Bishop RP. A technique for assessing postural discomfort. *Ergonomics*. 1976; 19:175-82.

[39] Wallenborn JT, Ihongbe T, Rozario S, et al. Knowledge of breastfeeding recommendations and breastfeeding duration: A survival analysis on infant feeding practices II. *BREASTFEED MED* 2017; 12(3):156-62.

[40] Starr MB. Pregnancy-associated overcorrection following myopic excimer laser photorefractive keratectomy. *Arch Ophthalmol* (Chicago, Ill 1960). 1998; 116(11):1551. http://www.ncbi.nlm.nih.gov/pubmed/9823373. Accessed 19 May 2019.

ISBN: 97
In: Mobile Health
Editors: G. Gupta, N. Kumar et al. © 2021 Nova Science

Chapter 6

A PROSPECTIVE AND COMPARAT STUDY OF MACHINE AND DEE LEARNING TECHNIQUES FOR SM HEALTHCARE APPLICATIONS

Ahmad Waleed Salehi*, Gaurav Gupta and S
Yogananda School of AI Computers and Data Scienc
Shoolini University, Solan, Himachal Pradesh, India

ABSTRACT

Artificial Intelligence (AI)-based technologies have attr considerable attention in the past recent years in the healthcare systen their potential to ease the strain on healthcare systems. Advar healthcare systems protect the lives of a human being as it improves life quality of humans. Machine Learning (ML) and Deep Learning (I is an emerging era for smart healthcare. These AI-based methods enab us to uncover patterns of different types of disease scan images such MRI, PET, X-Ray, and make healthcare prediction and diagnosis of

* Corresponding Author's Email: ahmadwaleed.sediqi18@gmail.com.

diseases are on the scene and many others are treating in the right way to cure.

By the year 2025, it has been observed that artificial intelligence in the sector of healthcare is going to be increased from 2.1 billion dollars (as of 2018) to 36.1 billion dollars at 50.2 of a CAGR [3]. AI-based techniques including machine and deep learning are used in making more successful clinical trials. These techniques are very useful and robust but taking more time and assist in the roadmap of each conduct experiment a success. When we say machine learning it is referring to learning the tasks from its past experiences, it is the algorithms that are used to do this task and give the ability to the machine to learn and to make the prediction. A common definition of a machine and deep learning is given in Wikipedia [4]; "Machine learning is sub-field of AI that deals with the study of computer algorithms which then automatically improve through experience. Machine learning algorithms work based on a sample of data which is called training data to build a mathematical model in order to make decisions or predictions without the intervention of humans. And deep learning is a broader field of machine learning techniques based on the artificial neural network" [5]. The learning methods of these techniques can be unsupervised, semi-supervised, or supervised [6]. These methods are the reason for smart healthcare systems to become intelligent, robust, and effective enough to operate. This is all become possible where ML and DL come into existence that is now playing a wonderful role in healthcare systems. An important benefit of these methods is to shift the tasks from hectic, time consuming manual methodology to a better, time-efficient, and automated one. The development of IoT (Internet of Thing) devices and machine-based AI techniques, takes smart healthcare to another level from alerting the doctors, caretakers using an alert system, to monitoring continuously to aid in the detection of disease. By using some kind of Decision Support system these devices and tools can also help in decision making very well [7]. Machine and deep learning used in healthcare deals with developing and designing algorithms that can enable the machine or the system to predict or detect a specific disease based on given and empirical data [8]. Recently ML and DL play a very useful role in smart healthcare, which can bring more quality to the services of healthcare by providing disease prediction and disease analysis in the early stages and delivering an accurate diagnosis.

The focus of this chapter is on different disease prediction using ML, and DL algorithms. The main reason more stresses on the machine and deep learning techniques in the area of healthcare is due to the high-speed generation of data [9]. There are three major challenges the world is experiencing today in the area of healthcare: the shortage of medical staff, the elderly, and high overall expenses on healthcare. But the good news is with the rapid rise in computation capacity and health data availability, applications of healthcare can contain AI and therefore become smart healthcare [1]. This can surely help out in solving some of the challenges in healthcare that are mentioned earlier. In addition to that, this will facilitate and accelerate sustainable development [10]. Machine and deep learning techniques are essential tools that can be very beneficial in healthcare industry applications.

The chapter is organized as follows-

- Section two represent the use of deep learning and machine learning in the medical diagnosis field and their applications in various diseases and virus.
- Section two gives an overview of machine learning and different types and their applications.
- Section three consists of a comparative study between various models/algorithms that are implemented in healthcare for medical diagnosis.
- Section four summarize, conclude the chapter with future work.

Machine and Deep Learning in Medical Diagnosis

The ever-growing population in the globe has been put huge pressure and burden on the healthcare industry to provide healthcare services with quality treatment. The century we live in today is the century of technology more than ever, so the demand is increasing by the people for smart healthcare services, wearable devices, and applications that will lead them into a better living and extend their lifetime [11]. So, the application of AI-based techniques such as machine learning, deep learning brings a transformation in detection, prediction. These techniques integrated with different interdisciplinary areas such as games, healthcare, self-driving cars, and many other fields [12]. The main focal point on the need for machine and deep learning techniques in healthcare is the ability to process or work with a huge and complex dataset, features selection, and to get out of that data analysis into useful clinical insights which then can be used aid clinicians in providing and plaining proper care.

Table 1. Major applications of ML and DL in healthcare

No	Applications	
1	Disease Diagnosis	In the current situation, human doctors cannot remember all the necessary information about a patient to make a quick but accurate analysis and diagnosis. In the modern and advanced plenty of research papers, case studies, and textbooks, it is very difficult for a doctor to recall and remember each detail of the cases which are similar [13, 14]. But yes, with AI it is possible to feed or train an AI-based model with relevant data and let the AI-based system do prediction and diagnosing [15].
2	Personalized Treatment	Personalized or precision medicine, is a more effective way of treatment that uses information about individual health to diagnose and prevent disease [13]. The most dominant machine learning technique is used is supervised learning, this enables a physician to estimate the risk of a patient based on some genetic information and likeness of signs or symptoms.
3	Drug Manufacturing	In the drug discovery area, machine and deep learning are the most powerful tools in preliminary stage drug discovery that can be useful in a variety of activities like, drug compounds initial screening [16].
4	Clinical Trial Research	Machine and deep learning have the number of potential applications and objectives in clinical trial research. ML and DL can help in the outcome prediction of clinical trials, which help in faster approval times and lower costs of the drug [17].
5	Prediction of Epidemic Outbreak	One of the most effective and important applications of AI-based technologies such as machine and deep learning is to monitor and predict the epidemic outbreaks. The data used for this purpose can be historical information, which is available on the web, satellites, social media real-time updates [13]. Like coronavirus outbreak which is a deadly disease around the world, these AI-based techniques can help in predicting the next outbreak [8].

The advances of AI-based methods in healthcare have been significantly improved over the past years and almost a possibility that AI can replace human physicians in the coming future. The major applications of AI for healthcare are given abow.

OVERVIEW OF ML AND DL TECHNIQUES

Machine learning is a field and application of AI, while deep learning is a subfield of ML. These approaches deal with the developing and designing algorithms that allows system to grow their behaviors based on past or empirical data [14]. Machine and deep learning approaches are progressing rapidly as a result of the advancement of the ML and DL algorithms, improved in computer networks, methods of data capturing enhanced, new units of sensors/IO [18].

In general, machine learning is categorized into three categories namely, supervised learning, unsupervised learning, and reinforcement learning. While machine learning is using simpler concepts, on the other hand, deep learning works with ANN (Artificial Neural Networks) that are designed to mimic the way humans learn and think. Deep learning can be used in solving any kind of pattern recognition problem without any intervention of humans.

Supervised Learning

In supervised learning, the model is going to be train based on a labeled dataset. In this, the data is split into two sets the training set and test set in which the network or the model is trained using the train set and for prediction or to see the result accuracy of the model the test dataset is used. There are two further groups in supervised learning, that are Regression and Classification.

Unsupervised Learning

The second category of machine learning is unsupervised learning which deals with the information that is neither labeled nor classified in the dataset. Unsupervised learning uses unlabeled data and tries to discover the hidden structure out of it. When the model learns to develop the patterns, then the model can predict the patterns in the form of clusters for any new dataset. There are two groups in unsupervised learning, which are Association and Clustering.

Reinforcement Learning

Reinforcement learning is another paradigm in machine learning which enables the machines and software agents to automatically take actions in an environment so that to maximize the notion of cumulative reward.

Table 2. Types of machine learning algorithms and their applications

SN	Major types of ML Learning	ML & DL Algorithms	Usage and Application
1	Supervised Learning	Support Vector Machine	This technique is used for both regression and classification problems. But in general, it is usually used for classification. The main goal of this technique is to divide all the data into different classes to find a maximum marginal hyperplane [19]. Applications of SVM are cancer prognosis and diagnosis, facial expression and text classification, speech recognition, etc.
2		Decision Tree	It is also used for both regression and classification problems but mostly used for classification. This classifier is tree-structured, where internal nodes in the tree represent all the features of a dataset, the decision rules are represented by branches and the outcome is represented by each leaf node [20]. Some applications are resources management, mineral identification [21].
3		Naïve Bayes	It is a classification method that is based on the theorem of Bayes.' It is working by assuming a particular feature present in a class is unrelated to any other feature presence. Applications are spam filtering, sentiment analysis, text classification [22].

Table 2. (Continued)

SN	Major types of ML Learning	ML & DL Algorithms	Usage and Application
4		Random Forest	Random forest is also a supervised learning technique, it builds an ensemble of decision trees based on samples of data and then provides prediction from each decision tree, and finally provides the optimal solution [23]. Application for example in the bank to find out the loyal customers, for the purpose of giving loans.
5		Linear Regression	It is a statistical technique that is used to produce insights on the basis of understanding business, consumer behavior [24]. The main business usage of this technique in the evaluation of trends and to make estimation or forecasting.
6	Unsupervised Learning	k-means	It is unsupervised learning which uses clusters in order to classify dataset using a number of groups or clusters. Market segmentation, image [25] compression, and segmentation are some of the application of k-means.
7		PCA	Used for dimensionality reduction which is known as Principal Component Analysis (PCA). A major application of this technique is to filter and remove noisy datasets.
9	Deep Learning	CNN	It is a type of artificial neural network which is used for different classification task like image, audio, etc. this algorithm is useful for two-dimensional data [15].
10		RNN	It is also a type of artificial neural network which is commonly used for natural language processing and speech recognition.
11		DBN	It is a generative graphical paradigm; in this algorithm, the hidden layers are linked unidirectional and used for both unsupervised and supervised learning.

Literature on This Area

There is an increasing number of papers related to machine and deep learning in healthcare. In this section, we presented a comprehensive study of various recent research work, in which they have used ML and DL approaches for disease prediction. We then categorize some of the algorithms that can lead to a substantial increase in prediction accuracy and various disease detection and diagnosis improvements through machine learning and deep learning. For the review of different disease predictions, the total number of articles that are considered in this chapter for the review process is shown in Figure 1. We have searched and found a huge number of paper related to disease prediction, the keywords used in the search engine were machine learning, deep learning, disease prediction and prognosis or diagnosis, Healthcare, Alzheimer disease, Coronavirus, Arrhythmia, Glaucoma, and diabetes disease. We have searched from different search platforms like Google scholar, IEEE, and Science Direct.

The main purpose and focus were on the articles that are related to the prediction of various disease prediction using the machine and deep learning approaches.

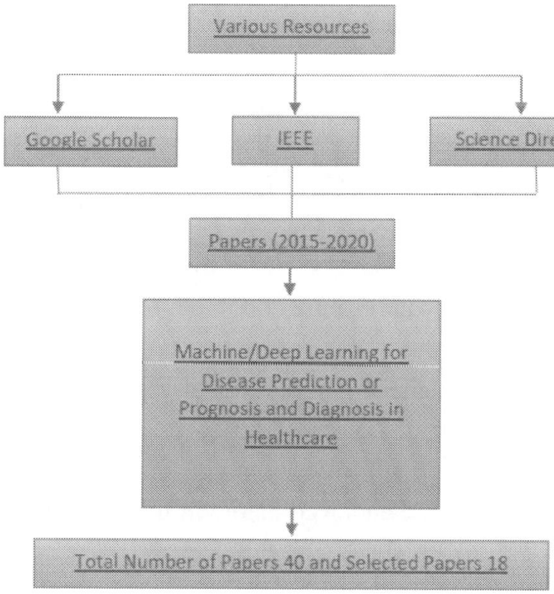

Figure 1. Process of searching and selection of the relevant papers.

Alzheimer's Disease

Alzheimer's disease is a type of dementia that leads to neurological or brain disorder in which the death of brain cells causes cognitive impairment and gradual memory loss. It is likely that early diagnosis and treatment of AD is a successful treatment [26]. Particularly at an early stage of AD diagnosis, it is a difficult task. With the rapid growth in the development of machine and deep learning techniques, researchers proposed different techniques with the help of medical images to detect and predict the diseases.

[27] In this paper, they used a new technique of deep learning approach to primary identify the mild cognitive impairment (MCI) patients with more risk to convert into AD within 3 years. Using the ADNI database they combine the base-line structural MRI, neuropsychological, demographic, and APOe4 genetic data. And it is the primary aim to discriminate an AD patient from a healthy control. They achieved predictions with very high performance with an average of 0.924 AUC, 86% prediction accuracy, 87.5% of sensitivity, and 85% specificity.

[28] This paper proposed CNN based technique using structural MRI to extract its discriminative features. With the aim of the diagnosis of Early Mild Cognitive Impairment (EMCI), Late Mild Cognitive Impairment (LMCI), and classification method among healthy subjects and the two groups. They implemented on 600 subjects from the ADNI database and the model for classification and feature extraction provided a high accuracy result for these three groups (EMCI, LMCI, CN (Cognitively Normal)). The best result has been achieved in the sagittal view for the classification between CN and LMCI groups and a slightly better accuracy was achieved for the EMCI/LMCI than CN/EMCI pairs concerning all views of MRI. All the mentioned results are achieved below in the table from the sagittal view.

[29] This paper proposed an efficient deep convolutional neural network technique using brain MRI data analysis for diagnosis of AD and the main focus of this research work is on structured magnetic resonance image (sMRI). The model offers a significant improvement for multi-class classification, while most of the existing proposed research works accomplish binary classification. It can identify different stages of AD and achieves higher performance in the diagnosis of early stage. The training model is done on a smaller dataset which is taken from the OASIS dataset that contains 416 data samples.

A multiple state-of-the-art ML technique used in [30] the algorithms are such as k-nearest neighbor (kNN), SVM, backpropagation neural network (BP-NN) for the purpose of discriminating AD and mild from normal controls. The performance of prediction was compared using sensitivity, specificity, and accuracy. So, the result has sown that AD patients can be distinguished from normal controls magnificently using ML tools and multivariate morphological features. According to the experiment, the most successful classifier for AD detection was SVM with up to 82% accuracies. In this work common structural brain measures for example thickness of anatomical structure and volumes which are acquired from OASIS data source.

Another method is used in [31] 8 layer of convolutional neural network with three activation function of Rectified Linear Unit (ReLU), sigmoid and Leaky Rectified Linear Unit and three pooling functions such as max, average, and stochastic pooling. The mathematical experiments have shown that in terms of performance the max pooling and leaky ReLU delivered the higher results. 97.96% sensitivity, 97.35% specificity, and accuracy of 97.65% have been obtained, respectively. And they have compared the proposed method with 8 state-of-the-art methods in which the proposed approach accuracy increased by around 5%. There are two different sources used for data collection. OASIS is one of them.

[32] a CNN architecture is also known as (DemNet) proposed in this paper with alteration of 16-layered of VGGNet for AD, MCI, and HC 3-way classification of MRI images. The images were obtained from the ADNI data source. And the result outperforms other classification techniques from previous related experiments. Total 91.85% accuracy has been achieved. It is also expressed in this research work that 17 slices of coronal from the middle portion of the brain are sufficient enough for classification.

Coronavirus

Coronavirus is also known as Covid-19 which has quickly spread to all countries around the world to this date. Coronavirus is a wide family of viruses that, beginning from the very common cold to very more acute or serious illness, cause disease or sickness. And yet there is not any therapeutic vaccine or drug for this. The Coronavirus can be the start of an exciting time or decade in science and medicine since it can be used and used to tackle various diseases and major clinical problems through the advancement and enhancement of various digital technologies [8].

[33] Has proposed a deep learning-based technique called deep transfer learning, which can predict patients with Coronavirus disease automatically. It uses images of chest X-ray obtained from patients with Coronavirus and a healthy person. Dataset of 50 patients, with Coronavirus, images of X-Ray were taken from a shared GitHub repository and 50 X-ray images of healthy human shave taken from a repository in Kaggle. In this study, results showed that the pre-trained model, ResNet50, yielded 98% accuracy among the other three models. They have also stated that we believe in our findings and this can help the public health care workers to decide clinical practice because of its high performance and accuracy. Also, for patients with Coronavirus, early prediction of the infection can avoid the rapid spreading of the disease.

This paper [34] established a deep learning paradigm for the screening of Coronavirus patients at an early stage. The main aim of this paper is to distinguish Coronavirus from Influenza-A viral pneumonia and normal cases with the use of CT images. CT samples have been taken from three hospitals designated to Coronavirus from China, Zhejiang Province. A total number of 618 samples was collected, which includes 219 from 110 Coronavirus patients, 224 samples of CT from patients with the viral pneumonia Influenza-A and CT samples of 175 healthy people. The experiments result of this study shown an overall 86.7% accuracy from the viewpoint of CT cases as a whole. They demonstrated that it can be a promising accompanying diagnostic tool for the clinical frontline doctors.

Glaucoma

Glaucoma is an eye disease that, due to risen Intraocular pressure leads to damage to the eye's optic nerve, and it is the leading cause of permanent blindness [35]. The very common method for glaucoma progression diagnosis is by examining the dilated pupil whish in the eye by the eye or ophthalmologist experts. But this way of diagnosing is very time consuming and laborious. Therefore, there are different AI-based techniques nowadays like ML, DL which very helpful automation models to solve these kinds of problems.

Mamta Juneja [35] developed an architecture of deep learning which is CNN, also named as an Artificially Intelligent expert system based for the purpose of the optic disc and optic cup segmentation for glaucoma disease from fundus images. In this model, they have used two neural networks in which this network in combination with the optic cup and disc section. They have used a dataset from an eye hospital which is the DRISHTI-GS dataset which is consisting of a total of 101 images and is divided into the subset of two training 50 and the testing part is 51 Fundus images. The age of subjects ranges from 40-80 years. And they have achieved 93% accuracy for the segmentation of cups and 95.8$ accuracy for disc segmentation.

In [36] authors used RIM-ONE which openly available database consisting of 455 non-glaucoma and glaucoma images, normal with 255 and 200 glaucoma's are classified in this dataset. In order to differentiate between normal and glaucomatous patterns for diagnostic decisions, a completely CNN-based automated system has been developed. They have also utilized CNN to automatically extract optic disc features from the unprocessed images without the need for human intervention. Then they have a machine learning classifier called Support Vector Machine (SVM) to feed those features to it in order to classify those images into abnormal or normal. The accuracy achieved in this paper 88.2%.

A CNN model is developed in this paper [37] to discriminate non-glaucoma and glaucoma patterns decisions of diagnostic. The architecture of the proposed model includes 6 layers of learning, 4 Conv-layers, and 2 fully connected layers. For further boosting the performance they have adopted two more strategies data augmentation and Dropout. The area under the curve (AUC) of the receiver operating characteristic curve for detection of glaucoma at 0.887 and 0.831 in the two databases.

Arrhythmia

Many cardiovascular conditions or illnesses may be avoided, but due to misdiagnosis, mortality tends to increase due to insufficient treatment. Arrhythmia is one of these cardiovascular diseases [38]. An arrhythmia is a heart condition affecting the rate or rhythm at which the heartbeats. This occurs when there are not properly working electrical impulses that direct and regulate heartbeats [39]. This triggers the pounding of the heart. Electrocardiogram (ECG) monitoring for Arrhythmia Diagnosis is often difficult to observe. Electrocardiogram (ECG) monitoring for Arrhythmia Diagnosis is often difficult to observe. Therefore, for this disease also there are many papers published in which they have proposed different AI-based algorithms for detection of this disease [40].

In this paper [41] a deep learning 1D-CNN was developed that can effectively identify cardiac arrhythmias (17 diagnostic groups comprising "normal sinus rhythm," "pacemaker rhythm" and 15 other rhythm disorders) from long-term (10-s) ECG signal fragment analysis. For 17 cardiac arrhythmias (classes), the D-CNN model achieved an overall classification accuracy of 91.33 percent with a classification time of 0.015 s for analysis of each 10-s ECG sample. The findings are one of the best to date relative to published research and our approach can be applied feasibly in cloud computing [42] and mobile devices. The PhysioNet ECG signals were collected from the MIT-BIH Arrhythmia database hosted by PhysioNet.

Hilmy Assodiky [40] ECG data from the machine learning UCI Repository has been used in this work. This paper used the deep learning technique and compare it to some well-known classification techniques in which the proposed model performed better, such as K-Nearest Neighbor, SVM. The accuracy was achieved is 76.51%.

The HRV (Heart Rate Variability) signal is often noted for the identification and classification of cardiac arrhythmias. To predict cardiac arrhythmias, the Neural Network has been used in this paper. The ECG data from the repository of the UCI ML arrhythmia dataset is used to obtain the HRV data and RR interval time series. Naïve Bayes and SVM classifier also used for classification but the Extreme Learning Machine (ELM) provided an effective result in contrast to other techniques used in this paper [43].

[44] This paper used different machine learning algorithms such as Naïve Bayes, OneR, and J48 for the task of arrhythmia classification. They have used the dataset of ECG from ML Datasets archives at the California University, Irvine. They have evaluated these three algorithms and out of these, the experiment results show that Naïve Bayes and OneR perform better and have a stable accuracy rate. This is not true about the J48 algorithm. The accuracies are 56.04 OneR, 67.03 J48, and 74.73 Naïve Bayes in which it is implemented in testing criterion the percentage of training was 80% and 20% was the testing set.

Diabetes

Diabetes is a chronic condition that progresses with time and causes other problems if this disease is not treated at an early stage. The early death of diabetes patients is the reason due to other complications. All over the world many people are also undiagnosed and suffering from this disease [45]. There are many papers in which they have implemented machine learning techniques for the early detection and prediction of this disease. Below, we have mentioned two papers which are implemented computational methods for the detection and prediction of diabetes disease.

The first paper [46] has used two machine learning techniques such as Naïve Bayes and Decision Tree algorithm with the use of a dataset from Pima Indians Diabetes Database (from UCI ML Repository). And they have used the achieved result of both techniques for the comparison of each other and to find a better and suitable technique for the detection of diabetes. 80.0% accuracy achieved with Naïve Bayes which is higher than the Decision tree with 78.3%. And it is also stated that the Decision tree can perform better when it comes to the classification of negative instances, but the Naïve Bayes performed better when it comes to negative instances.

In another paper [47] they have stated that many researchers developed different techniques for diagnosing diabetes but they have trained and tested their models only on a single dataset. But there is a need for such a model to work with all types of datasets. This paper developed a machine learning algorithm with the usage of a combination of datasets. The dataset they have used was gathered from the UCI ML repository. A dataset of 13-US hospitals for the years 1999 up to 2008 contains more than ten thousand instances. The other dataset consists of 768 instances. Based on some common features in these datasets, the datasets combined with each other. The SVM algorithm is used as a classifier in this paper and a 72% accuracy is achieved.

Result and Discussions

In the last few years, the Creation of automated computer-based methods for the precise and accurate classification of different diseases from clinical data has drawn strong attention from the clinical community. As we have seen and reviewed various papers on disease diagnosis and prediction using the machine and deep learning, many of these techniques for classification are based on CNN deep learning-based technique in which can be used to take an image as an input, assigning importance like biases, and learnable weights to the various objects of the image and in order to distinguish one from the other. And SVM is also mostly used algorithm in which it is supervised learning used to build such classifier which then can predict the class to which a new example belongs. Table 3 shows that how these ML and DL techniques are utilized data from various sources and perform very well in the prediction of various diseases such as Glaucoma diagnosis, Alzheimer's disease, Coronavirus, Arrhythmia, Diabetes.

Table 3. Various techniques are used for different disease detection and the accuracy they have achieved

Ref	Disease Type	Technique	Data Source	Accuracy
[27]	Alzheimer's Disease	Deep Learning-based Approach	ADNI Base-line Structural MRI	Accuracy = 86%
[28]		Convolutional Neural Network	ADNI Structural MRI	Accuracy = 94.5%
[29]		Convolutional Neural Network	OASIS Structural MRI	Accuracy = 93.18
[30]		KNN, SVM, and Backpropagation neural network	OASIS	SVM Accuracy = 82%
[31]		8-layer CNN with three different activation function and three different pooling function	OASIS MRI	Accuracy= 97.65%
[32]		CNN (DemNet)	ADNI MRI	Classification of 3-way overall Acc= 91.85%
[33]	Coronavirus	Deep Transfer Learning	GitHub Repository X-ray Images	Accuracy = 98%
[34]		Deep Learning Paradigm	3 Hospital, Zhejiang, China Computed Tomography (CT) Samples	Accuracy = 86.7%
[35]	Glaucoma Disease	Convolutional Neural Network	Eye Hospital DRISHTI-GS dataset	Accuracy = 93%
[36]		Support Vector Machine And Convolutional Neural Network	RIM-ONE openly available database Glaucoma and non-Glaucoma Images	Accuracy = 88.2%
[37]		CNN	Fundas Images from SCES and ORIGA datasets	AUC SCES = 0.887% AUC ORIGA = 8.831%
[41]	Arrhythmia Disease	1D-CNN (One Dimensional Convolutional Neural Network)	MIT-BIH database hosted by PhysioNet. PhysioNet ECG	Accuracy = 91.33%
[40]		Deep Learning Technique	ECG data from Machine Learning UCI Repository	Accuracy = 76.51%
[43]		Extreme Learning Machine	UCI ML Repository HRV data & RR interval time series.	Null

Table 3. (Continued)

Ref	Disease Type	Technique	Data Source	Accuracy
[44]		Naïve Bayes, OneR, and J48 Machine learning algorithms	ECG ML dataset archives at California University.	Naïve Bayes = 74.73% OneR = 56.04% J48 = 67.03%
[46]	Diabetes Disease	Decision Tree and Naïve Bayes for detection of diabetes	Machine Learning UCI Repository (diabetes dataset)	Naïve Bayes = 80.0% Decision Tree = 78.3%
[47]		SVM Machine Learning	UCI ML Repository (diabetes dataset)	SVM = 72%

In several s-Health applications, such as Various Disease Detection and Prediction, we can find from the above Table that the ML and DL are used methods. The SVM, Artificial Neural Network (ANN) algorithms, and in particular CNN Deep learning-based technique, are the most widely used approaches in machine learning where in most cases, they have proved and to get higher performance evaluation.

Deep learning has appealed intuitively to healthcare applications, Deep learning-based techniques scale to larger datasets, partly because of their capability to operate on specialized computer hardware resources and continue to enhance with more data, allowing them to surpass many classical ML approaches. And these techniques could be very useful in smart healthcare, particularly in medical imaging which can considerably benefit from the current advances and development in object detection and classification of images [48]. As we have reviewed many studies and papers have been adopted deep learning-based models and demonstrated promising outcomes in complex medical diagnostics such as Alzheimer's [26], Arrhythmia [40], Glaucoma [35], Coronavirus [8], diabetes [45]. These techniques could be very useful and helping clinicians by having second thoughts and flagging different parts of the image.

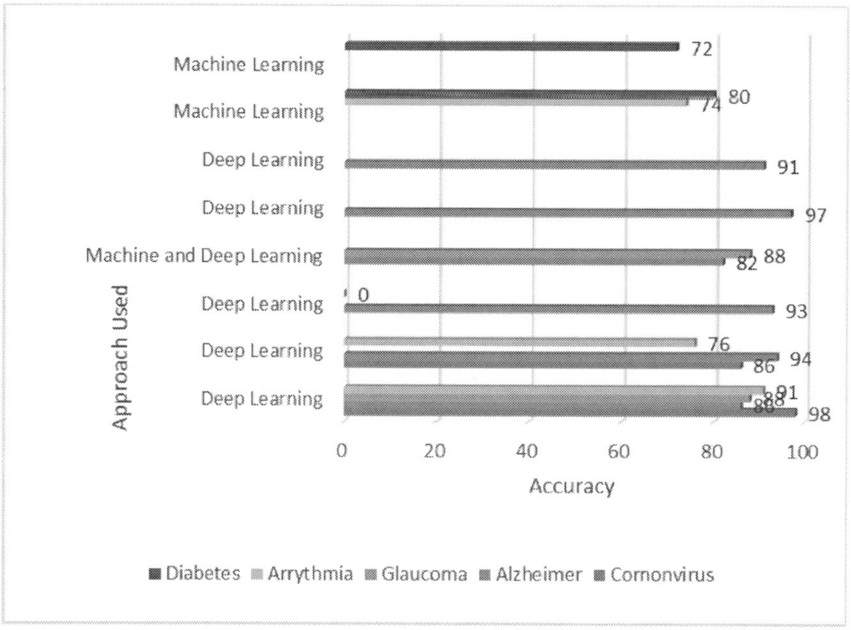

Figure 2. Utilization of deep and machine learning approaches for various diseases with their accuracies.

Deep Learning over Machine Learning

There are two big reasons why deep learning over machine learning the first reason is the huge amount of data, the data is surprisingly increasing and there is a lot of data which is generated nowadays. As the data increased the traditional machine learning algorithms will not work efficiently that is why another concept came into existence which is known as the artificial neural network in which the idea is taken from the human brain. How the neurons work, how the neurons are communicating with each other, and generating results. This is how artificial neural networks are made up of multiple neural networks. The more data there will be more layers of neural networks and complected artificial neural networks to solve complex problems. Extracting features automatically and feeding the network automatically.

For this huge data, complex neural networks there is also a need for high-end systems that can deal and analyze this large amount of data. Due to the advancement of technology for that also we can say for sure that we have very much powerful systems nowadays.

A large neural network can have a lot more hidden layers, and, in each layer, there is a lot of nodes as well. We cannot learn the model efficiently without enough medical data. and also learning would be too slow and inadequate without strong computers. That is why we are moving towards new technologies and new algorithms [48].

"Nuts and Bolts" [48] have presented the relationship between the performance of the model and the scale of the data in the following graph. They have used different traditional machine learning techniques like, Random Forests, Regression, SVM, etc. on a small dataset which does an excellent job by these statistical methods. But once data is increasing or scale-up, the neural network is which outperforms the other techniques.

In part, a deep neural network approaches have the potential to learn more complex types of patterns like non-linear patterns as compared to conventional ML models. Therefore, deep neural networks are the best and helpful in extracting the features and picking up the most useful features on their own without even much manual extraction of features by an expert in the particular field.

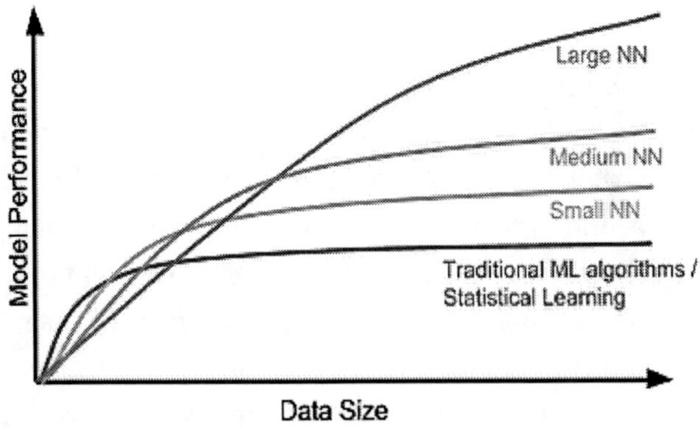

Figure 3. The scale of data vs the model performance [48].

CONCLUSION

Healthcare is one of today's economy's quickest growing areas in a country, more citizens need care and treatment, and it is turn out to be more and more costly. In terms of improved care and reduced costs, innovations such as big data, deep and machine learning have the ability to assist in the area of smart healthcare. Smart healthcare systems now having huge data, needs such kind technologies as machine and deep learning in order to interpret, analyze huge data which is generated in the healthcare sector.

In this chapter, we have discussed the importance and application of AI-based deep and machine learning approaches in medical diagnosis and the smart healthcare domain. The three types of learning including, supervised, unsupervised and reinforcement learning and the algorithms that are present such as, SVM, Regression, K. Means, Random Forest, Decision Tree, Naïve Bayes, CNN, RNN, and so on, and we have addressed how these algorithms are used in various real-world problems, particularly in healthcare. The impact of deep learning and machine learning in a smart healthcare system and how these enabling algorithms are efficient in the prediction and detection of various diseases and viruses. There is no other technique that has such potential as these AI-based methods transform health care services.

While machine learning techniques in the healthcare domain have already shown good results and performance, but based on recent rising trends, due to the predominant nature of data, and based on this study after the review pervious works that deep learning techniques surely hold considerable promise in the creation of an intelligent application for smart healthcare domain. From the literature, the highest accuracies are mentioned that deep transfer learning provides 98% of accuracy for the prediction of Covid-19 patient, similarly, another model called convolutional neural network obtained an accuracy of 97.65% for Alzheimer's Disease diagnosis. SVM with CNN gives 88.2% accuracy for the classification of Glaucoma disease. By this literature, in this chapter, it is revealed that deep learning-based technique particularly CNN is the most widely used and successful technique for various disease detection and prediction.

References

[1] Chui, K. T., and W. Alhalabi, "*Disease Diagnosis in Smart Healthcare : Innovation, Technologies and Applications*," pp. 1–23, doi: 10.3390/su9122309.

[2] Sundaravadivel, B. P., E. Kougianos, S. P. Mohanty, and M. Ganapathiraju, "*Everything You Wanted to Know about Smart Healthcare*," pp. 1–10.

[3] "*Artificial Intelligence in Healthcare Spending to Hit $36B*." 2018.

[4] "*Machine learning - Wikipedia*."

[5] Baglat G. G., P., Salehi A. W., Gupta A., "Multiple Machine Learning Models for Detection of Alzheimer's Disease Using OASIS Dataset," *IFIP Adv. Inf. Commun. Technol. Springer, Cham*, vol. 617, pp. 614–622, 2020, doi: https://doi.org/10.1007/978-3-030-64849-7_54.

[6] Savio, A. "Supervised classification using deformation-based features for Alzheimer's disease detection on the OASIS cross-sectional database," *Front. Artif. Intell. Appl.*, vol. 243, pp. 2191–2200, 2012, doi: 10.3233/978-1-61499-105-2-2191.

[7] Durga, S. and E. Daniel, "Survey on Machine Learning and Deep Learning Algorithms used in Internet of Things (IoT) Healthcare," *2019 3rd Int. Conf. Comput. Methodol. Commun.*, no. Iccmc, pp. 1018–1022, 2019.

[8] Salehi, A. W., P. Baglat, and G. Gupta, "Materials Today : Proceedings Review on machine and deep learning models for the detection and prediction of Coronavirus," *Mater. Today Proc.*, no. xxxx, 2020, doi: 10.1016/j.matpr.2020.06.245.

[9] Salehi, A. W., P. Baglat, B. B. Sharma, G. Gupta, and A. Upadhya, "*A CNN Model: Earlier Diagnosis and Classification of Alzheimer*

Disease using MRI," no. Icosec, pp. 156–161, 2020, doi: 10.1109/icosec49089.2020.9215402.

[10] Du, G. and C. Sun, "*Location Planning Problem of Service Centers for Sustainable Home Healthcare: Evidence from the Empirical Analysis of Shanghai,*" pp. 15812–15832, 2015, doi: 10.3390/su71215787.

[11] "*12+ Machine Learning Applications Enhancing Healthcare Sector 2020 upGrad blog.*"

[12] Care, S. H., "*Everything You,*" no. january, pp. 18–28, 2018.

[13] Sciforce, "*Machine Learning and AI Technologies in the Healthcare Industry by Sciforce Sciforce Medium.*" 2018, [Online]. Available: https://medium.com/sciforce/machine-learning-and-ai-technologies-in-the-healthcare-industry-ad824211be19.

[14] Gupta, G., A. Gupta, P. Barura, V. Jaiswal, C. S. Engineering, and N. Delhi, "*Mobile Health Applications and Android Toolkit for Alzheimer Patients, Caregivers and Doctors,*" vol. 11, no. 1, pp. 199–205, 2019.

[15] Salehi, A. W., P. Baglat, and G. Gupta, "Alzheimer's Disease Diagnosis using Deep Learning Techniques," *Int. J. Eng. Adv. Technol.*, vol. 9, no. 3, pp. 874–880, 2020, doi: 10.35940/ijeat.c5345.029320.

[16] Shah, P., et al., "Artificial intelligence and machine learning in clinical development: a translational perspective," *npj Digit. Med.*, no. February, 2019, doi: 10.1038/s41746-019-0148-3.

[17] Spinner, Jenni, "*Artificial intelligence technology improves clinical trials.*" 2020, [Online]. Available: https://www.outsourcing-pharma.com/Article/2020/05/12/Artificial-intelligence-technology-improves-clinical-trials.

[18] Rayan, Z., M. Alfonse, and A. M. Salem, "ScienceDirect ScienceDirect ScienceDirect Machine Learning Approaches in Smart Health Machine Approaches in Smart Health on the Learning Innovation of Protecting Intangible Cultural Heritage in the " Internet Plus " Era," *Procedia Comput. Sci.*, vol. 154, no. 1985, pp. 361–368, 2019, doi: 10.1016/j.procs.2019.06.052.

[19] "*ML - Support Vector Machine(SVM) - Tutorialspoint.*"

[20] "*Machine Learning Decision Tree Classification Algorithm - Javatpoint.*"

[21] Akkaş, E., L. Akin, and H. E. Çubukçu, "Author's Accepted Manuscript," *Comput. Geosci.*, 2015, doi: 10.1016/j.cageo.2015.03.015.

[22] Wei, W., S. Visweswaran, and G. F. Cooper, "*The application of naive Bayes model averaging to predict Alzheimer's disease from genome-wide data,*" pp. 370–375, 2011, doi: 10.1136/amiajnl-2011-000101.

[23] Zou, R., M. Schonlau, and D. Ph, "*Applications of Random Forest Algorithm Stata Syntax Classification Example : Credit Card Default Regression Example : Consumer Finance Survey,*" pp. 1–33.

[24] Naseem, I., R. Togneri, S. Member, and M. Bennamoun, "*Linear Regression for Face Recognition,*" vol. 32, no. 11, pp. 2106–2112, 2010.

[25] Sharma, A., D. Kaur, A. Gupta, and V. Jaiswal, "Application and Analysis of Hyperspectal Imaging," *Proc. IEEE Int. Conf. Signal Process. Control*, vol. 2019-Octob, pp. 30–35, 2019, doi: 10.1109/ISPCC48220.2019.8988436.

[26] Khachaturian, Z. S., "Diagnosis of Alzheimer's Disease - Neuropsychological Testing," *Arch Neurol*, vol. 4, pp. 1097–1105, 1985.

[27] Spasov, S., L. Passamonti, A. Duggento, P. Liò, and N. Toschi, "A parameter-efficient deep learning approach to predict conversion from mild cognitive impairment to Alzheimer's disease," *Neuroimage*, vol. 189, no. August 2018, pp. 276–287, 2019, doi: 10.1016/j.neuroimage.2019.01.031.

[28] Gorji, H. T. and N. Kaabouch, "*brain sciences A Deep Learning approach for Diagnosis of Mild Cognitive Impairment Based on MRI Images,*" 2019.

[29] Islam, J. and Y. Zhang, "Brain MRI analysis for Alzheimer's disease diagnosis using an ensemble system of deep convolutional neural

networks," *Brain Informatics*, vol. 5, no. 2, 2018, doi: 10.1186/ s40708-018-0080-3.

[30] Demirhan, A. "Classification of Structural MRI for Detecting Alzheimer s Disease," *Int. J. Intell. Syst. Appl. Eng.*, vol. 4, no. Special Issue-1, pp. 195–198, 2016, doi: 10.18201/ijisae.2016 specialissue-146973.

[31] Wang, S. H., P. Phillips, Y. Sui, B. Liu, M. Yang, and H. Cheng, "Classification of Alzheimer's Disease Based on Eight-Layer Convolutional Neural Network with Leaky Rectified Linear Unit and Max Pooling," *J. Med. Syst.*, vol. 42, no. 5, p. 85, 2018, doi: 10. 1007/s10916-018-0932-7.

[32] Billones, C. D., O. Jan, L. D. Demetria, D. E. D. Hostallero, and P. C. Naval, "*DemNet : A Convolutional Neural Network for the Detection of Alzheimer's Disease and Mild Cognitive Impairment*," pp. 3724–3727, 2016.

[33] Apostolopoulos, I. D. and T. A. Mpesiana, "Covid-19: automatic detection from X-ray images utilizing transfer learning with convolutional neural networks," *Phys. Eng. Sci. Med.*, vol. 43, no. 2, pp. 635–640, 2020, doi: 10.1007/s13246-020-00865-4.

[34] Xu, X. et al., "A Deep Learning System to Screen Novel Coronavirus Disease 2019 Pneumonia," *Engineering*, p. 10489, 2020, doi: 10. 1016/j.eng.2020.04.010.

[35] Juneja, M. et al., "Automated detection of Glaucoma using deep learning convolution network (G-net)," *Multimed. Tools Appl.*, vol. 79, no. 21–22, pp. 15531–15553, 2020, doi: 10.1007/s11042-019-7460-4.

[36] Al-Bander, B., W. Al-Nuaimy, M. A. Al-Taee, and Y. Zheng, "Automated glaucoma diagnosis using deep learning approach," *2017 14th Int. Multi-Conference Syst. Signals Devices, SSD 2017*, vol. 2017-Janua, pp. 207–210, 2017, doi: 10.1109/SSD.2017. 8166974.

[37] Lu, Y., J. Sun, and S. Ma, "Moving ObjectDetection Based on Deep Convolutional Neural Network," *Xitong Fangzhen Xuebao / J. Syst.*

Simul., vol. 31, no. 11, pp. 2275–2280, 2019, doi: 10.16182/j.issn 1004731x.joss.19-FZ0368.

[38] Takac, P., Skorodenský, M., Pilipcincova, A., & Pella, J. (2007). Evaluation of risk factors in cardiovascular diseases with examination of heart rate variability in behavioral medicine and health psychology. *Studia Psychologica*, 49(2), 117.

[39] Saboori, R., B. B. Sharma, N. Kumar, and G. Gupta, "*IoT-Based Healthcare Support Services for Arrhythmia : A Review Page No : 1035,*" vol. XII, no. Iv, pp. 1035–1039, 2020.

[40] Assodiky, H., I. Syarif, and T. Badriyah, "Deep learning algorithm for arrhythmia detection," *Proc. - Int. Electron. Symp. Knowl. Creat. Intell. Comput. IES-KCIC 2017*, vol. 2017-Janua, pp. 26–32, 2017, doi: 10.1109/KCIC.2017.8228452.

[41] Yıldırım, Ö., P. Pławiak, R. S. Tan, and U. R. Acharya, "Arrhythmia detection using deep convolutional neural network with long duration ECG signals," *Comput. Biol. Med.*, vol. 102, pp. 411–420, 2018, doi: 10.1016/j.compbiomed.2018.09.009.

[42] Salehi, A. W., F. Noori, and R. Saboori, "*Cloud Computing Security Challenges and its Potential Solution American Journal of Engineering Research (AJER) Cloud Computing Security Challenges and its Potential Solution,*" no. June, pp. 165–175, 2020.

[43] Gupta, V., S. Srinivasan, and S. S. Kudli, "*Prediction and Classification of Cardiac Arrhythmia,*" vol. 1, no. January, pp. 1–5, 2015, [Online]. Available: https://archive.

[44] Soman, T. and P. O. Bobbie, "Classification of arrhythmia using machine learning techniques," *WSEAS Trans. Comput.*, vol. 4, no. 6, pp. 548–552, 2005.

[45] Kavakiotis, I., O. Tsave, A. Salifoglou, N. Maglaveras, I. Vlahavas, and I. Chouvarda, "Machine Learning and Data Mining Methods in Diabetes Research," *Comput. Struct. Biotechnol. J.*, vol. 15, pp. 104–116, 2017, doi: 10.1016/j.csbj.2016.12.005.

[46] Stigeborn, O. "*Detecting diabetes with Machine learning Detecting diabetes with Machine Learning,*" 2020.

[47] Negi, A. and V. Jaiswal, "A first attempt to develop a diabetes prediction method based on different global datasets," *2016 4th Int. Conf. Parallel, Distrib. Grid Comput. PDGC 2016*, pp. 237–241, 2016, doi: 10.1109/PDGC.2016.7913152.

[48] Esteva, A. et al., "A guide to deep learning in healthcare," *Nat. Med.*, vol. 25, no. 1, pp. 24–29, 2019, doi: 10.1038/s41591-018-0316-z.

In: Mobile Health
Editors: G. Gupta, N. Kumar et al.
ISBN: 978-1-53619-420-3

Chapter 7

CONTEXT-AWARE MOBILE HEALTHCARE FOR SMART HEALTH SERVICES IN NURSING HOMES

Kalpana Verma*
Kasturba Medical College, Mangalore, India

ABSTRACT

Context-Aware mobile healthcare applications exist to help human health services like those applications developed for the National Health Mission of India based on center frameworks of patient and supplier vaults. It involved the clinical and analytic imaging frameworks based on clinical reports and past disease data. Mobile healthcare for smart health services has a key focus area for the development and effective treatment system. Mobile devices such as smart mobile devices have been transforming healthcare with consulting and medical treatment at home. It has been a trend that medical facilities have been integrating mobile devices in their infrastructure. Mobile health is a term synonymous with the utilization of cell phones and remote advances to guarantee a solid way of life, including genuine clinical consideration. The most

* Corresponding Author's Email: kalpana.verma.lko@gmail.com.

recognizable to numerous instances of mobile health innovations are various kinds of medical services applications planned to help control an individual's state of being. For medical patients, a significant advantage of mobile health is its accommodation at their place of choice. Wearable gadgets and other portable innovations permit clients to ceaselessly follow and deal with certain health information without seeing their medical care supplier. There are additionally plenty of applications to browse that were thousands of mobile health applications accessible for download from application stores, as per computerized health counseling firm. This chapter shall describe the mobile healthcare services in the context of nursing home and discuss a case study on nursing home in digital healthcare.

Keywords: digital health, mHealth, health care system, smart nursing home, mobile health

1. Introduction

Medical services frameworks will incorporate new registering ideal models in the coming years. Setting mindfulness registering is an exploration field that regularly alludes to medical care as a fascinating and rich territory of use. Through a review of the examination writing, we planned to infer a target perspective on the genuine dynamism of setting mindfulness in medical services and to recognize qualities and shortcomings in this field. In the wake of talking about the meanings of setting, we discuss a straightforward system to examine and describe the utilization of setting through three fundamental points. We at that point zeroed in on setting mindfulness figuring and technology that the principle groups working in healthcare. We depicted a portion of the setting of mindfulness ventures in medical services. A more profound investigation of the clinic-based undertakings exhibited the hole between mobile communication for understanding setting mindfulness and the genuine use in a model. At last, we recognized that traps experienced a world of exploration in mobile healthcare. Various open doors stay for this developing field of examination. We discovered generally hardly any gatherings with such a particular core interest. So far there is no agreement for the most fitting, models, or ascribes to remember for setting mobile health. We infer that a more prominent comprehension of which parts of setting are significant in a medical services setting is required; the innate socio-technical nature of setting mindful applications in medical services; and the need to draw on various controls to lead real-world examination using mobile devices.

1.1. Mobile Healthcare

Mobile health is a term utilized for the act of medication and general health upheld by cell phones. Mobile health is often termed mHealth. The term is most normally utilized concerning utilizing versatile specialized gadgets, for example, cell phones, tablet PCs and individual computerized colleagues like PDA, and wearable gadgets. Some wearable gadgets that are widely adopted are smart watches and bands for health administrations, data, and information storage. The mHealth field has ascended as a sub-segment of eHealth, the usage of information and correspondence development that incorporates ICT, for instance, PCs, phones, trades satellite, getting screens, etc., for medical organizations and information. Mobile health applications remember the utilization of cell phones for gathering network and clinical health information, conveyance of medical services data to professionals, scientists and patients, constant observation of patient imperative signs, the immediate arrangement of care through mobile telemedicine just as preparing and cooperation of medical staff.

Admittance to medical care may change across nations, networks, and people, impacted by social and financial conditions just as health strategies. Giving medical care administrations signifies "the convenient utilization of individual health administrations to accomplish the most ideal health results." Components to consider as far as medical care access incorporate monetary impediments, (for example, protection inclusion), geographic hindrances, (for example, extra transportation costs, plausibility to take took care of season of work to utilize such administrations), and individual restrictions (absence of capacity to speak with medical care suppliers, unexpected frailty education, low salary). A restriction to medical services administrations influences the utilization of clinical administrations, the viability of therapies, and the result (prosperity, death rates).

Medical services frameworks are associations set up to meet the health needs of focused populaces. As indicated by the WHO, a well-working medical care framework requires a financing system, a very much prepared and enough paid workforce, solid data on which to base choices and strategies, and all around kept up health offices to convey quality medications and advancements.

An effective medical services framework can add to a critical aspect of a nation's economy, improvement, and industrialization. Medical care is ordinarily viewed as a significant determinant in advancing the overall physical and psychological well-being and prosperity of individuals around the globe. A case of this was the overall annihilation of smallpox in 1980, pronounced by the WHO as the main malady in humankind's history to be wiped out by intentional medical services intercessions.

Mobile medical services are a significant expansion of electronic medical care. It empowers the guardians to have a universal and continuous admittance to patients' clinical information and the most recent clinical information; simultaneously, it permits patients with ceaseless conditions to stay under steady perception without waiting to be genuinely present at the center. The basic difficulties to a full-scale usage incorporate setting up interoperability among electronic health records, growing better presentation advancements and security controls for cell phones and creating brilliant calculations to distinguish clinically noteworthy occasions before informing parental figures.

1.2. Introduction to Mobile Healthcare

Mobile health comprehensively envelops the utilization of portable media transmission and sight and sound advancements, as they are coordinated inside progressively versatile and remote medical care conveyance frameworks. The field extensively envelops the utilization of versatile media transmission and sight and sound innovations in medical services conveyance. The term Mobile health was instituted by Robert Istepanian as utilization of mobile devices that are networked with system innovations for medical care. It is characterized as the conveyance of medical care administrations through portable specialized gadgets.

While there are a few ventures that are considered exclusively inside the field of Mobile health, the linkage between health and cares delivery systems. For instance, a Mobile health venture that utilizes cell phones to get information on COVID-19 spread rates would require an eHealth framework to oversee, store, and evaluate the information. Consequently, eHealth ventures commonly work as the foundation of mobile health ventures.

Mobile healthcare is the conveyance of health-related administrations and data through electronic data and media transmission advancements. It permits significant distance patient and clinician contact, care, guidance, updates, instruction, intercession, observing, and far off confirmations. Mobile healthcare has been utilized as an equivalent or greater in a more medical treatment to depict far off clinical administrations, for example, analysis and checking. At the point when rustic settings, absence of transport, an absence of portability, diminished subsidizing, or an absence of staff limit admittance to mind, Mobile healthcare may overcome any barrier. It has supplier separation learning; gatherings, oversight, and introductions between online data and health information. It is the executives and medical care framework incorporation. Mobile healthcare could incorporate two clinicians talking about a case over video meetings. An automated medical procedure happening through far off access; exercise based recuperation done using advanced checking instruments live feed and application blends; tests being sent between offices for understanding by a higher expert; home observing through constant sending of patient health information; customer to specialist online gathering; or even videophone translation during a counsel.

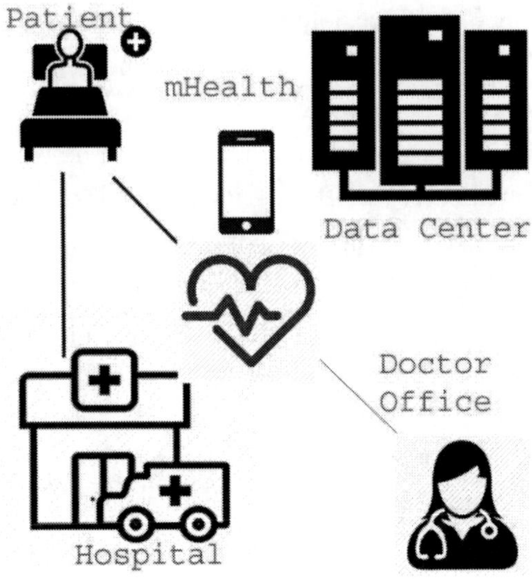

Figure 1. Mobile healthcare in smart health services.

Mobile healthcare has been considered a key pillar of smart health services as illustrated in Figure 1. In a comparable vein, while mistakably bifurcated by such a definition, eHealth can largely be seen as an innovation that underpins the capacities and conveyance of medical services, while mobile health lies generally on giving medical services access. Since mobile health is by definition dependent on portable innovation, for example, cell phones, medical services, through data and conveyance, can more readily arrive at zones, individuals, or potentially medical care professionals with a recently restricted presentation to specific parts of medical care.

1.3. Significance of Mobile Healthcare

The intensity of getting to anything anywhere whenever is the thing that portable innovation offers to shape our future and health objectives. Regardless of whether it is going to keep a tab on dozing examples or determination of any physical afflictions, the health-based applications have now become a standard to give better minds and health offices directly at the fingertips of the clients.

A ton of medical services portable applications are accessible in the market that encourages clients to book arrangements and pose inquiries identified with medical problems nonstop.

Mobile health has diminished the risks of diagnostic errors. A blunder in the clinical conclusion of an individual can make extreme harm to a patient's health condition. Medical services versatile applications had with smart demonstrative capacities can lessen the mistake rate and give drug expectations. The component is not restricted to exact analysis, the medical care versatile application advancement organizations coordinate extra highlights that likewise help doctors to utilize portable applications with cloud offices to store persistent records. Hence, blunders originating from helpless allowance from persistent history or blended/missing records can be limited largely.

It helps Patients to take ownership of their health. The rising waves of health wearable and medical status trackers have guaranteed self-observing capacities that patients can use to screen their health conditions on a predictable premise. It is not just giving them possession to screen their health to remain dynamic yet additionally helping them to accomplish better outcomes. With these incredible things, clients are getting more dedicated to whatever activity/action they are on by settling on their choices, which thus, help them to dodge any maladies or medical problems. Measurements that clients can follow through such wearable are practice schedules, diet system, calorie utilization, heartbeat, diabetes, etc.

It is smoothing out the clinical processes. As a figure says, the IoT medical care market is going to reach multi-billion in the future, it is very evident that clinical specialists/clinicians are intensely putting resources into the inventive medical care application thoughts to bring an ocean change in the business. There is no hesitation that IoT innovation has improved the assignment of medical care experts by empowering them to gain admittance to all the data and information on their updated gadgets. These gadgets are associated with the patient's body to screen essential boundaries. Moreover, the IoT combination with medical services has given an approach to more readily deal with the assets. The clinical staff can keep a tab on their huge stocks effectively and keep it up methodically.

Take into account Patient Customization: Every patient involves an extraordinary rundown of past health records and that is the reason he requires explicit consideration and alternate treatment. To redo the treatment for every patient would be tedious, particularly in situations when there is a crowd of patients to manage. With redid versatile applications, doctors can rapidly stroll through a patient's clinical records, give custom-made treatment, pinpoint answers for every patient.

2. Digital Healthcare Services

Mobile health has changed the medical services in the positive effect of innovation in medical services. Telemedicine, synthetic consciousness (AI) - empowered clinical gadgets, and Blockchain electronic health records are only a couple of solid instances of advanced change in medical care.

Advancement is the situation here, with the primary objective of smoothing out doctors' work, streamlining frameworks, improving patient results, decreasing human error, and bringing down expenses through stunning web and versatile encounters.

Tragically, the medical services and drug businesses have failed behind concerning executing computerized systems. Indeed, in an ongoing review, just seven percent of medical care and drug organizations said they had gone advanced, contrasted with 15 percent of organizations in different businesses.

Notwithstanding that, the developed countries medical services market is huge; with the public health, spending extended to reach trillion by mid-2020. There is still an ideal opportunity for medical services to get knowledgeable in advanced innovation and use it to get an improvement in availability. Yet, to change medical services standard practice into a flourishing, computerized machine in 2020, medical services first need an exhaustive image of the advanced medical care outlook.

2.1. Various Digital Healthcare Services

Mobile health applications have been raised as critical instruments in the everyday patient consideration and medical services of executives over various offices everywhere on over the globe. The guarantee of versatile applications in the medical services biological system is not just restricted to better therapy, yet these applications likewise contributed enormously to make medical services more reasonable and open.

A large number of cell industries displaying advantageous features in any event are their use in health application. Rapid development of health applications in numbers is very admirable in their usage in medical care. A medical services environment is not conceivable now without the part of versatile health applications. For application engineers around the world, health applications bring a sizable development opportunity. The effect of health applications has gotten so boundless and time characterizing that any medical care office that does not grasp mHealth applications are showing the danger of being abandoned to the patients.

Advancement innovations and digitization have affected every industry in the previous hardly any years. We have additionally begun to observe a broad advanced change that has been acquired in the medical services industry. With the selection of new advancements like AI, Big Data, Cloud Computing, CRM and IoT that involves medical care is receiving huge rewards.

Rapid Value gives unrivaled arrangements and administrations that are fundamental for the advancement of computerized change activities while guaranteeing basic assistance execution to the medical services industry. It endeavors to engage medical care associations to defend basic medical care benefits and convey top-notch persistent consideration while at the same time enhancing its advanced worth chain. This causes patients to have better admittance to qualified specialists and speedier health.

Mobile health helps to modernize inheritance frameworks to help bound together with the information stage and online patient assets. From creating installment and protecting the executives' entry to review and consistency of the board apparatus, mobile health assists patients with building versatile electronic arrangements.

Creating tolerant experience applications for arrangement, the executives, online meetings, are overseeing lab test results. Self-improvement and mindfulness are these applications incorporate a few highlights of constant cooperation, specialized apparatuses, resource the board and following basic undertaking agenda.

Mobile health influence progressed examination and AI answers to gain bits of knowledge for measure streamlining. Mobile health has executed new-age medical services arrangements that incorporate highlights like geo-fenced following of high qualities things, following staff within emergency clinic premises, empowering simple routes for contrastingly able patients. The health institutes coordinate investigation answers for lessening inconstancy in clinical practices.

2.2. Telehealth and Telemedicine

The term telehealth incorporates an expansive scope of advances and administrations to give a tolerant mind and improve the medical care conveyance framework overall. Telehealth is not the same as telemedicine because it alludes to a more extensive extent of distant medical care administrations than telemedicine. While telemedicine eludes explicitly too far off clinical administrations, telehealth can allude to distant non-clinical administrations. Its examples are supplier preparation, managerial gatherings, and proceeding with clinical training, notwithstanding clinical administrations. UN health organizations have promoted the use of advanced technologies in health care like mobile health.

Telehealth is a subset of E-Health, which incorporates the conveyance of health data, for health experts and health purchasers, instruction and preparation of health laborers and health frameworks the executives through the web and broadcast communications.

Telemedicine is a subset of medicine that uses modern communication technology video conferencing to connect two places for medical treatment. Telemedicine includes the utilization of electronic interchanges and programming to offer clinical types of assistance to patients without an in-person visit. Telemedicine innovation is oftentimes utilized for follow-up visits, the executives of ceaseless conditions, prescription administration, pro discussion and a large group of other clinical administrations that can be given distantly through secure video and sound associations.

Just to toss another term in with the general mish-mash, we should take note that the WHO additionally utilizes the expression "telematics." According to them, telematics for health is a composite term for both telemedicine and telehealth, or any health-related exercises did over separation by methods for data correspondence innovations.

Therefore, all telemedicine is telehealth, however not all telehealth is telemedicine. Both are important for the bigger exertion to grow admittance to mind, make health the board simpler for patients and improve the effectiveness of the medical services conveyance organize. mHealth with mapping intended to help telemedicine for specialists would construct a smart health services.

2.3. Electronic Health Record

An electronic health record (EHR) is an advanced form of a patient's paper details. EHRs are progressing, understanding centered records that make information open in a brief instant and securely to endorsed customers. An EHR contains the clinical and treatment accounts of patients and an EHR structure is endeavored to go past standard clinical information collected in a supplier's office and can be intensive from a wider perspective on an idea of the patient. EHRs are an imperative piece of health IT and can:

- Contain a patient's clinical history, analyze, prescriptions, treatment plans, vaccination dates, sensitivities, radiology pictures, and research center and test outcomes

- Permit admittance to confirm based devices that suppliers can use to settle on choices about a patient's consideration
- Mechanize and smooth out the supplier work process

While there is yet a lot of discussion around the prevalence of electronic health records over paper records, exploration writing illustrates the advantages and drawbacks.

The expanded straightforwardness, convenience, and openness procured by the selection of electronic clinical records may build simplicity. They can be gotten to by medical services experts, yet additionally can build the measure of taken data by unapproved people or deceitful clients versus paper clinical records, as recognized by the expanded security prerequisites for electronic clinical records remembered for the Health Information and Accessibility Act and by huge scope breaks in secret records detailed by EMR clients. Worries about security add to the opposition that appeared to their adoption.

Transcribed paper clinical records might be ineffectively intelligible, which can add to clinical mistakes. Pre-printed structures, normalization of shortened forms and guidelines for handwriting were urged to improve the dependability of paper clinical records. Electronic records may help with the normalization of structures, phrasing and information input. Digitization of structures encourages the assortment of information for the study of disease transmission and clinical investigations. Nevertheless, normalization may make difficulties for a neighborhood practice. Those with EMRs that have robotized notes and records request passage, and clinical choice help had fewer inconveniences, lower death rates, and lower costs.

EMRs can be consistently refreshed inside certain legitimate impediments that examine in detail. If the capacity to trade records between various EMR frameworks culminated, it would encourage the coordination of medical services conveyance in non-partnered medical services offices. Besides, information from an electronic framework can be utilized secretly for factual revealing in issues, for example, quality improvement, asset the board, and general health transmittable illness reconnaissance. In any case, it is hard to eliminate information from its specific circumstance.

One of the key features of an EHR is that body information can be made and regulated by endorsed providers in a serious game plan fit for being granted to various providers across more than one clinical consideration affiliation. EHRs are attempted to bestow information to other clinical administration providers and relationships, for instance, labs, specialists, clinical imaging workplaces, drug stores, emergency workplaces, and school and workspace offices, so they contain information from all clinicians drawn in with a thought of the patient.

2.4. Pharmaceutical Record

The Pharmaceutical Record records all the restorative items gave to every patient in the course of the past treatment. This incorporates both therapeutic items endorsed by a specialist and those exhorted by a drug specialist. The Pharmaceutical Record has secured under protection law and its execution has been endowed to the experts in the data center of hospitals.

Each industry manages some documentation. The administration of that documentation, in shifting degrees, is fundamental to working an effective business. Notwithstanding, for certain divisions like the drug business, documentation and records the board can mean the contrast between drugs being affirmed and monstrous fines from controllers.

As an individual who works in the drug business will let you know, there is no deficiency of documentation associated with getting medication from innovative work to the solution counter of your neighborhood drug specialist. Given the idea of the business, a lot of it applies to administrative consistency. Notwithstanding, there are explicit kinds of documentation and records that are of specific significance.

Great assembling rehearsals are rules given by controllers that direct norms for producers in the food, medication, beauty care products, and clinical gadget fabricating enterprises. In developed countries, certain rules are set out in the Food and Drug Administration guideline. Most different nations either utilize the WHO standard or the EU-GMP of the European Union.

GMP rules expect to make a benchmark for quality affirmation and assembling consistency to guarantee those customer items are consistent with adequate quality. These rules expand well past basic sterilization or assembling principles, nonetheless, and are continually evolving. Indeed, they are all the more regularly alluded to as cGMP, or "current great assembling rehearses."

Because of the FDA, GMP rules set out the standard working methodology and least degrees of value control for every part of the assembling cycle.

Consistence for makers implies guaranteeing that each territory that is secured by GMP is at any rate inside the rules. Fortunately, the greater part of the rules is moderately open-finished, permitting space for producers to choose how best to satisfy the guideline in their office. In any case, that does not imply that they can be trifled with. The inability to fulfill guidelines in any territory can bring about noteworthy fines, huge loss of stock worth, and even prison time.

2.5. Significance of Digital Healthcare Services

Digital healthcare services have become an impacting factor in the present day. Patients utilizing computerized systems to speak with specialists are appreciating the advantages of inventive medical care understanding. It has changed medical services rehearsals by helping them conquer numerous conventional difficulties and cycles. It gives patients the ability to deal with their health by giving admittance to their health information from various sources, for example, specialist's centers, clinics, labs, drug specialists and even old clinical records. Yet, notwithstanding medical care is perhaps the biggest segment in India and a favored objective for clinical the travel industry around the world, the condition of medical services stays to depend on composing solutions, manual cycles, and paper documents.

Digitization is conceivably the most agreeable change that Indian specialists and patients are encountering. The multiplication of the web, infiltration of the worldwide market and rising utilization of mobiles is relied upon to fuel this pattern further. Training and data around the utilization of computerized health can bring the number of individuals under the umbrella of innovation benefits.

Imagine this to see more about advanced health: You have a place with a rustic region, where you cannot locate any clinical assistance after nightfall. One fine day you begin feeling sickly and you understand that the sun has just gone down. Hearing a touch of conventional guidance, you fly in a portion of "Paracetamol," trusting it would help. Following a couple of hours, your manifestations lose their cutoff points, and you are under uncommon torment at noon where you have no admittance to clinical offices.

Here comes the requirement for computerized health – In a similar situation, advanced health can assist you with bestowing the clinical guidance you need. You simply need to turn on your telephone and quest for specialists close to you and request that they associate over video visits. Where in the specialist can take a gander at your clinical history, get some information about your indications and give you exhortation you were hanging tight for better. He can likewise assist you with doorstep conveyance of endorsed medication from your closest drug store. Your telephone observes your clinical admission and passes the report of your recuperation to your primary care physician. In only a couple of days, you are back to your normal life where nightfall does not frequent you any longer.

This situation is not a scene from a fictional novel but a reality made possible by mobile health. This is advancement happening now, in the medical services space. This happens when advanced health comes to utility. Here is significant training to bestow to utilize advanced health in medical care.

2.6. Limitation of Digital Healthcare Services

One of the principal impediments is accessibility and cost. You might not approach digital healthcare services due to the high cost of gadgets. For the supplier, it tends to be costly to set up and keep up. Although an incredible and commendable help, digital healthcare services might be excessively exorbitant for littler medical services offices.

Digital healthcare services can open up numerous treatment entryways, yet it is not equivalent to a physical specialist office. On the off chance, that you favor a closer to home or vis-à-vis relationship, digital healthcare services probably will not be the alternative for you. You regularly do not get an opportunity to bond with your digital healthcare services specialist, and you may never get an opportunity of real-world contact with them.

3. Digital Healthcare Services Using Mobile Healthcare

Digital healthcare services using mobile healthcare is the same as different territories of ehealth in its need to receive worldwide-acknowledged principles and interoperable innovations, preferably utilizing open source engineering and cheap mobile devices. The utilization of normalized data and correspondence advancements would improve productivity and diminish cost. To achieve this, nations should work together in creating worldwide-prescribed procedures so information can move all the more adequately among frameworks and applications. Moving towards a more vital way to deal with arranging, improvement, and assessment of digital healthcare services using mobile healthcare exercises will enormously upgrade the effect of mobile healthcare. Expanded direction and data are expected to help adjust mobile healthcare with more extensive health needs in nations and coordinate digital healthcare services using mobile healthcare into endeavors to fortify health frameworks.

3.1. Mobile Healthcare Based Telemedicine

Mobile healthcare based telemedicine is a sort of versatile medical services that would incorporate utilizing an application to meet with your primary care physician by video, utilizing site based talk administrations to get clinical counsel, or getting to your clinical data using a protected online gateway gave by mobile devices in a mobile healthcare system.

Mobile health is likewise used to depict pulse screens, wearable blood glucose recordings, and different sorts of gadgets that empower a medical care supplier to follow a patient's health over a specific period without keeping the person in question in a clinical consideration office. This sort of versatile health is utilized to either help distinguish whether a specific medical problem may exist or to guarantee that appropriate therapy levels are being accomplished.

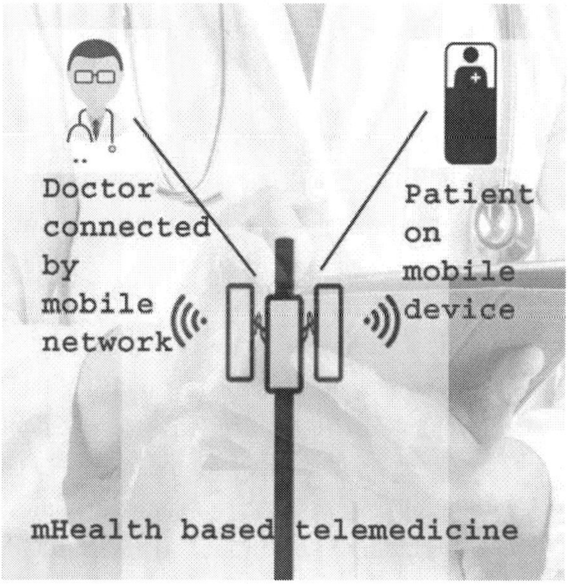

Figure 2. Doctor counseling a patient using a mobile device.

Doctors are counseling the patients using a mobile device as shown in Figure 2. A portion of these necessitates that people enter their health-related data and others gather the information themselves. In any case, applications like these furnish people with quick admittance to their medical services data whether they are home, grinding away, voyaging, or anywhere else on the planet. Another advantage of telehealth applications is that they permit people to all the more effectively track their health information. No additionally requesting that specialists forward test outcomes and not even more being uninformed of what changes your medical care supplier sees starting with one visit then onto the next. Presently, you can sign in to the frameworks and find that data for yourself.

3.2. Mobile Healthcare Based Electronic Health Record

The recent development of cell phones has opened additional opportunities for giving emphatically incorporated portable administrations in medical care. The goal of many types of research has been to depict the decision driver, improvement, and execution of an incorporated versatile Electronic Health Record (EHR) mobile healthcare application at many universities and hospitals. Some applications enable medical services suppliers to see patients' clinical records and data without a fixed PC workstation. Many engineers have built up multiple mobile application models that are intended to improve the versatility and ease of use of medical services suppliers during their everyday clinical exercises. The mobile application maker has been involved to make the mobile EHR application. The convenient EHR application offers lenient basic hints, determined data, text correspondence, and composed EHR. The application permits medical care suppliers to know the status of patients inside and outside the emergency clinic condition. These mobile healthcare applications give a reliable client condition on a few viable Android and iOS gadgets. Systems have been building up the coordinated versatile EHR application with the objectives of actualizing a situation that is easy to understand, executing a patient-focused framework, and expanding the clinic's intensity.

3.3. Mobile Healthcare Based Pharmaceutical Record

The introduction of portable wearable gadgets, followed by cell phones and tablet PCs has significantly affected numerous fields, including pharmaceutical records. Mobile healthcare based on the Electronic Pharmaceutical Record (ePR) has been created to enroll every medicine taken by mobile patients, to make allotment in-network drug stores safe. Medical care experts currently use cell phone or tablet PCs for capacities they used to require a pager, cell phone, and wearable devices to achieve. Cell phones and tablets consolidate both registering and correspondence highlights in a solitary gadget that can be held in a hand or put away in a pocket, permitting simple access and use at the purpose of care. Notwithstanding voice and text, new cell phone models offer further developed features including internet, navigation aid like GPS, great cameras, and sound recorders. With these advancements areas of groundbreaking processors, motherboard, large memory size and large screen size in cell phones, these phones have become handheld PCs.

Mobile device-based pharmacy is the conveyance of drug care using media communications to patients in areas where they might not have direct contact with a drug specialist. It is an occasion of the more extensive marvel of mobile health care, as executed in the field of drug store. Mobile device-based pharmacy administrations incorporate medication treatment checking persistent directing, earlier approval and reorder physician approval recommended medications and observing of model consistency with the guide of remotely coordinating or videoconferencing. Far off administering of prescriptions via mechanized bundling and naming frameworks can likewise be thought of as an example of mobile pharmacy. Mobile device-based pharmacy administrations can be conveyed at retail drug store destinations or through emergency clinics, nursing homes, or other clinical consideration offices.

4. Case Study of Mobile Healthcare in a Nursing Home

As of late, the fast development of versatile innovation that is of innovation that can be utilized "progressing" has been influencing nursing homes, and the medical services industry is not a special case. Indeed, the wide scale use of cell phones including tablets has the ascent in their selections has prompted the development in the number of versatile mobile health applications for nursing homes. In this sense, there is as of now a wide scope of versatile health applications that offer an assortment of highlights and, even more as of late, mobile health applications have been extending because of their capability to improve medical services conveyance in a nursing home.

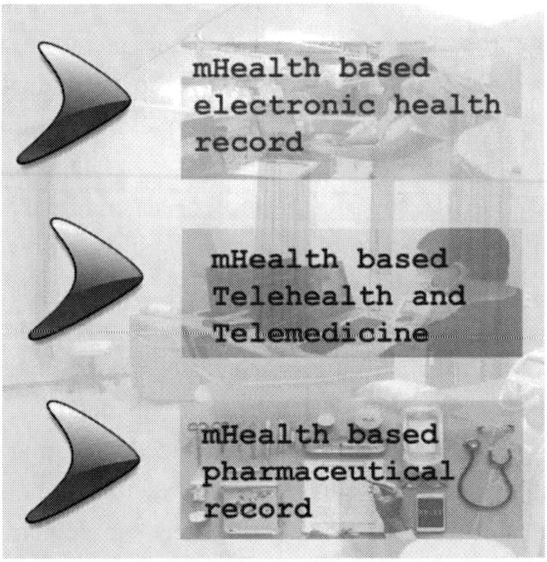

Figure 3. Utilization of mHealth in a medical care facility like nursing home.

In this specific situation, the utilization of mobile health as shown in Figure 3 that is cell phones and applications to help the clinical practice has been changing a few parts of the medical services industry and ending up being very encouraging and useful for nursing homes. It could be specific to assist them with executing their everyday undertakings, to oversee and screen patients, to get to and oversee clinical information, and to upgrade the dynamic cycle, among others. Nevertheless, mobile Health has not exclusively been invaluable for medical care suppliers yet additionally for the customers, permitting them to fortify their correspondence with medical care associations.

The primary advantages of mobile Health in a medical care facility like nursing home are as following:

- Helpful and quicker availability to data since all information is assembled in a solitary source, which can be utilized while away from patient that based on electronic health records
- Decrease of time-squander since Health experts can control data at the purpose of care, not interfering with their work process using mHealth along Telehealth and Telemedicine.
- Quicker and better dynamic cycle, since Health experts can approach state-of-the-art data at the purpose of care, prompting more educated and based choices stored on mHealth based pharmaceutical records.
- Quicker and improved correspondence since Health associates all the experts dispersed over the medical services association;
- Help medical care associations to fortify their correspondence with medical services customers by giving data to them at some random second through arrangement updates, test result notices, diagnostics, and illness control, among others;
- Abatement mistakes and unfriendly occasions; and
- Improve the nature of medical care conveyance and administrations.

Mention that the utilization of versatile applications in medical care settings is not proposed to supplant work area applications, which can be more remarkable and less prohibitive than mHealth applications, however, to supplement them and, particularly, to upgrade results at the purpose of-care. Truth be told, in circumstances where quick data trade is required, where data ought to be entered at the purpose of-care, and where Health experts are continually progressing and have, consequently, less an ideal opportunity to spend on PCs, mHealth innovation is profoundly helpful contrasted with work area applications as shown as Figure 4. In Figure 4, a mobile device displays all health data using a smart health band. For example, Health experts working in nursing homes could incredibly profit by portable innovation since they are continually moving and have a brief period to spend on PCs, which are frequently situated in nursing stations far away from the inhabitants.

Consequently, the unquestionable advantages of mobile healthcare in nursing homes show that a higher venture ought to be done in its reception as it can improve the nature of medical care conveyance. Nonetheless, mHealth applications should just be created after really understanding the requirements of the planned clients to grow high caliber and precise applications and maintain a strategic distance from their underutilization.

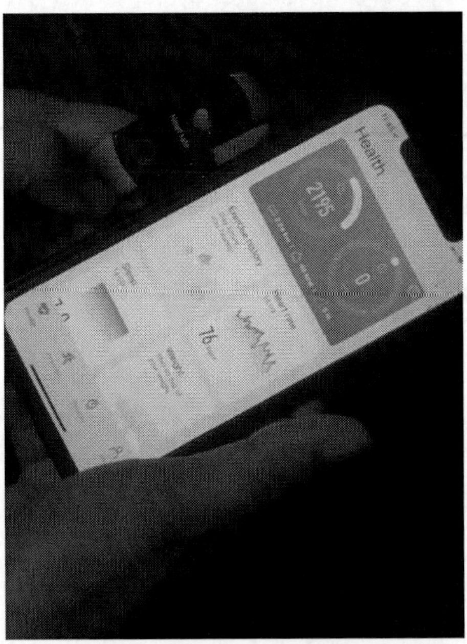

Figure 4. mHealth innovation is profoundly helpful contrasted with work area applications.

Conclusion

Mobile healthcare for smart health services in a nursing home has been vital features for the improvement of medical care services. This chapter has discussed all aspects of mobile healthcare for smart health services. A case study on the use of mobile healthcare in a nursing home has been studied to improve practical aspects.

Mobile health has shown a very promising aspect of improvement in the quality of health services. Mobile health has been improving health care services in both developed countries and developing countries. Overall, mobile health services had a great impact on the improvement of availability, timely delivery and quality for medical care.

Acknowledgments

We are appreciative of our families for their ethical help over the proper way of section composing. We are also grateful to the doctors of Kalpana Nursing Home for their cooperation in the case study. We likewise feel like we recognize the commitment of the considerable number of individuals engaged with their recommendation in improving this chapter distinction.

References

Verma, K. (2020). "Comprehend the COVID-19 Virus in the Human Body and Its Symptoms," *International Journal of Science and Research* (IJSR), Volume 9 Issue 7, July 2020, 1707 – 1709.

Verma, K. (2020). The mental health impact of the COVID-19 epidemic on college students in India. *Asian Journal of Psychiatry*.

Istepanian, R., Laxminarayan, S., & Pattichis, C. S. (Eds.). (2007). *M-health: Emerging mobile health systems.* Springer Science & Business Media.

Madden, M., Lenhart, A., Cortesi, S., & Gasser, U. (2010). *Pew Internet and American life project.* Washington, DC: Pew Research Center.

Steinhubl, S. R., Muse, E. D., & Topol, E. J. (2013). Can mobile health technologies transform health care?. *JAMA,* 310(22), 2395-2396.a.

Kumar, S., Nilsen, W. J., Abernethy, A., Atienza, A., Patrick, K., Pavel, M., & Hedeker, D. (2013). Mobile health technology evaluation: the mHealth evidence workshop. *American Journal of Preventive Medicine*, 45(2), 228-236.

Silva, B. M., Rodrigues, J. J., de la Torre Díez, I., López-Coronado, M., & Saleem, K. (2015). Mobile-health: A review of current state in 2015. *Journal of biomedical informatics*, 56, 265-272.

Steinhubl, S. R., Muse, E. D., & Topol, E. J. (2015). The emerging field of mobile health. *Science translational medicine*, 7(283), 283rv3-283rv3.

Eysenbach, G., & Consort-EHEALTH Group. (2011). CONSORT-EHEALTH: improving and standardizing evaluation reports of Web-based and mobile health interventions. *Journal of medical Internet research*, 13(4), e126.

Free, C., Phillips, G., Watson, L., Galli, L., Felix, L., Edwards, P., & Haines, A. (2013). The effectiveness of mobile-health technologies to improve health care service delivery processes: a systematic review and meta-analysis. *PLoS Med*, 10(1), e1001363.

Alexy, B. B., & Elnitsky, C. (1998). Rural mobile health unit: outcomes. *Public Health Nursing*, 15(1), 3-11.

Istepanian, R., Laxminarayan, S., & Pattichis, C. S. (Eds.). (2007). *M-health: Emerging mobile health systems*. Springer Science & Business Media.

Alexy, B. B., & Elnitsky, C. A. (1996). Community outreach: rural mobile health unit. *JONA: The Journal of Nursing Administration*, 26(12), 38-42.

Steinhubl, S. R., Muse, E. D., & Topol, E. J. (2013). Can mobile health technologies transform health care?. *JAMA*, 310(22), 2395-2396.

Shorey, S., Ng, Y. P. M., Danbjørg, D. B., Dennis, C. L., & Morelius, E. (2017). Effectiveness of the 'Home-but not Alone' mobile health application educational programme on parental outcomes: a randomized controlled trial, study protocol. *Journal of advanced nursing,* 73(1), 253-264.

Moon, R. Y., Hauck, F. R., Colson, E. R., Kellams, A. L., Geller, N. L., Heeren, T., & Corwin, M. J. (2017). The effect of nursing quality improvement and mobile health interventions on infant sleep practices: a randomized clinical trial. *JAMA,* 318(4), 351-359.

In: Mobile Health
Editors: G. Gupta, N. Kumar et al.
ISBN: 978-1-53619-420-3

Chapter 8

MACHINE LEARNING TECHNIQUES TO FIGHT AGAINST PANDEMIC: A REVIEW

Bharti Thakur* and Nagesh Kumar
Yogananda School of Artificial Intelligence,
Computers and Data Science, Bajhol, Himachal Pradesh, India
Shoolini University of Biotechnology and Management Sciences,
Solan, Himachal Pradesh, India

ABSTRACT

Pandemic has affected the world since 165 BC to till date. The Pandemic word comes from the Greek, which means about people. This pandemic has impaired all the countries which include the developed, developing and underdeveloped. Machine learning has played a significant role in predicting accuracy and finding solutions to various issues related to pandemics. We have divided this book chapter into three parts; first part describes all about the Pandemic; second part include the multiple papers related to Panademic based on machine learning techniques. In third part there is comparison of machine learning's algorithm. This review article analyses the accuracy, specification and sensitivity of different machine learning techniques over Pandemic. By

* Corresponding Auhtor's Email: hartithakur@shooliniuniversity.com.

reviewing all ML techniques, we find out that CNN gives the highest accurancy of 99% for monitoring Influenza A.

Keywords: pandemic, epidemic, COVID-19 and Machine Learning

INTRODUCTION

Pandemic has affected the world since 165 BC to till 2020. It did not leave any of the countries untouched, let it be developed, developing and underdeveloped. Almost all the countries have been affected so far and more than 350 Million lost their life even if the country has the best health care facility (Damir 2019).

Pandemic word crop up from a country or a region from southern Europe. This word broadly can be described as the total of two words joined together as Pan + Demons, Pan describe, all and demons describe people. (Qiu and Rutherford et al., 2016-2017). Although to make it simple we can say that Pandemic affect the more extensive area people opt, but Epidemic effects small portion of population. Example of epidemic is Malaria and T.B.

Pandemic Characteristics (Qiu and Rutherford et al., 2016-2017)

Infection Spread

This means the infection can be spread from one individual to another through respiratory infection like pandemic influenza and severe acute respiratory syndrome virus.

Vast Terrestrial Activity

Pandemic hold out to the broader area, for instance in fourteen century cholera, plague and influenza had affected the broader geographic region.

Lower Resistance Capacity

This virus reduce the capacity of individual immune system because that person cannot be able to fight against the virus. So it is simple for a vast community to get infected.

Unfamilarity

The name pandemic relates to the latest infection with an unfamiliar variant of live organisms.

Epidemic vs Pandemic

The main difference between the two terms is based on area and people they affect. Pandemic is like an Epidemic that spreads more than Epidemic. History is a great teacher, especially regarding diseases as it provides us information base for working further and invent new methods or medicines to prevent the outbreak of diseases (Quinn and Kumar 2014).

Machine Learning has always acted as great help for finding solutions to various diseases including Pandemics. This chapter has tried to acquire knowledge about the various use of machine learning algorithms to find answers to such diseases and Pandemic issues. It includes forecasting accuracy and methods to prevent the spread of Pandemics.

LITERATURE SURVEY

In our study we have divided the chapter into three parts. The first part throws light on the meaning of Pandemic and afterthat, D.N.A prints of Pandemics are traced from the pages of history. The second part consist of the various papers related to Pandemics, based on techniques, wherein ML methods are used for prediction or forecasting accuracy percentage about the Pandemics and analyzed papers based on different methods or machine learning techniques to find out answers to various other issues than accuracy prediction with regards to pandemics (Chamola and Hassija et al.,

2020). In the third part various, the different researchers performed various studies about their respective research on the past pandemics. Based on these discussions we have tried finding the best Algorithm used by various researchers or doctors to get highest accuracy in predicting any pandemic so that this metholdology or algorithm of machine learning can help us to find a cure against ongoing COVID-19 pandemic.

Part 1

The word Pandemic originated from a southern European country and indicated its span.

Below is the list of Pandemics and the death toll that has occurred to date which shows the overall history of Pandemic disease (Lepan 2020).

Table 1. Pandemic, time period and deaths reported

Type of Disease	Time Span	Appearance of Disease	Mortality Rate
Antonine Plague	165 to 180	It can be either smallpox or measle	5M
Japanese smallpox epidemic	735 to 737	Variola big virus	1M
Plague of Justinian	541 to 542	Yersinia pestis bacteria/Rats, fleas	30-50M
Black Death	1347 to 1351	Yersinia pestis bacteria/Rats, flea	200M
New World Smallpox Outbreak	1520 - onwards	Variola major virus	56M
Great Plague of London	1665	Yersinia pestis bacteria/Rats, fleas	100,000
Italian plague	1629 to 1631	Yersinia pestis bacteria/Rats, fleas	1M
Cholera Pandemics 1-6	1817 to 1923	V. cholerae bacteria	1M+
Third Plague	1885	Yersinia pestis bacteria/Rats, fleas	12M (China and India)
Yellow Fever	Late 1800s	Virus/Mosquitoes	100,000-150,000 (U.S.)
Russian Flu	1889 to 1890	Believed to be H2N2 (avian origin)	1M
Spanish Flu	1918 to 1919	H1N1 virus/Pigs	40-50M
Asian Flu	1957 to 1958	H2N2 virus	1.1M

Type of Disease	Time Span	Appearance of Disease	Mortality Rate
Hong Kong Flu	1968 to 1970	H3N2 virus	1M
HIV/AIDS	1981 to til date	Virus/Chimpanzees	25-35M
Swine Flu	2009 to 2010	H1N1 virus/Pigs	200,000
SARS	2002 to 2003	Coronavirus/Bats, Civets	770
Ebola	2014 to 2016	Ebolavirus/Wild animals	11,000
MERS	2015 to till date	Coronavirus/Bats, camels	850
COVID-19	2019 to till date	Coronavirus -Unknown (possibly pangolins)	-

Pandemics have got different symptoms and at times onset period for the disease also differs. Few details are given in table as below:

Table 2. Pandemic symptoms, onset period and deaths reported

Pandemic	Symptoms	Usual onset period	Caused by	Death
Cholera	Diarrhea, vomiting muscle cramp	2 hrs to 5 days after exposure	Bacterium vibrocholerae	1 M+
Small pox	Fever, Mouth taste soars, vomiting	1 to 3 weeks	Two viruses Variola major and Variola minor	56 M
Black death	Fever, headache, painful joints and vomiting	2 to 6 days	Bacterium Yersinia Pestis	200M
Spanish flu	Fever, fatigue	2 to 7 days	H1N1	40 to 50 M
Ebola	Fever, weakness, sore throat and muscle pain	2 to 21 days	Zaire ebolavirus	11000
Zika	Mild fever, headache	3 to 14 days	Zika virus by Aedes mosquitoes	-
HIV/AIDS	No-symptoms/headache/swollen lymph/fever	Few months may not be unaware until later stage	HIV Virus	36 M

Table 3. Penalties of pandemics (Madhav and Oppenheim et al., 2017)

Pandemic Impacts		
Health Impacts [5]	Economics Impacts	Social/Political Impacts
• Causes high morbidity and mortality.	• Direct cost: can be very high • Long term burden: can be severe • Indirect cost: can be heavy and effects GDP.	• Severe • Travel is limited • Sch/market closed • Population mobility through check points • Clashes between state and citizens.

Part 2

Machine learning has played a significant role in predicting accuracy and finding solutions to various issues related to pandemics. Few pandemics related articles which have been used to predict accuracy are given in succeeding paragraphs.

Influenza A

Through this report, a deep convolutional neural network models were designed to find host particularity for human and Influenza A viruses, based on protein supplement (Scarafoni and Telfer et al., 2019). Statistical, deep learning and conventional machine learning algorithms were applied to tropism for prediction based on the seven encoded influenza aligned protein sequences, namely these protein sequences are (HA, M, M1, NEP, PA, PB, and PB1-F2). Results obtained are given in table.

This study shows that deep Conventional neural network techniques combined with current techniques can give us even up to 99% mean accuracy on the binary prediction task while performing the prediction model's end-to-end learning. Here important is that one need not to specify handcrafted features while doing this. The findings also show that these models, combined with standard principal component analysis, can help quantifying and visualise viral strain similarity.

Table 4. Accuracy of machine learning techniques

Protein	Accuracy							
	Random Prediction	Prediction Based on Priors	Prediction Based on Strain (H+N)	Edit Distance + KNN (k = 5)	Random Forest	Baseline CNN	Tailored CNN	95% Conf. Interval for Tailored CNN
Mean	0.5	0.58	0.948	0.979	0.990	0.971	0.990	n/a
HA	0.5	0.60	0.965	0.991	0.991	0.990	0.992	(0.991,0.993)
M	0.5	0.60	0.961	0.985	0.986	0.985	0.986	(0.985,0.987)
M1	0.5	0.63	0.963	0.985	0.987	0.982	0.987	(0.986,0.988)
NEP	0.5	0.51	0.955	0.981	0.987	0.983	0.989	(0.985,0.922)
PA	0.5	0.58	0.957	0.986	0.986	0.968	0.986	(0.985,0.987)
PB	0.5	0.56	0.956	0.990	0.990	0.974	0.994	(0.993,0.995)
PB1-F2	0.5	0.62	0.875	0.938	1.0	0.917	1.0	(0.925,1.00)

Influenza A

In this paper, the skill of ANN is used for forecasting the important influenza virus antigenic types (H1, H3, and H5) and hosts (Human, Avian, and Swine), which fulfils a critical need for a computational system for influenza surveillance has been applied.

The overall experiment is performed on different k-mers and different binary encoding types in this the categorisation is done on the frequencies of k-mer nucleotide strings performed better than transformed binary data of nucleotides (Attaluri, Chen and Lu 2010). Compared to avian and swine viruses, human influenza viruses can be classified with high accuracy. Details of these studies are given in following tables:

Table 5. Computational system for influenza surveillance

Segment	Human	Avian	Swine	Mean
HA	94%	92%	90%	92%
M	95%	87%	85%	89%
NP	93%	92%	88%	91%
NA	95%	91%	87%	91%
NS	93%	87%	87%	89%
PA	94%	90%	89%	91%
PB1	97%	92%	90%	93%
PB2	95%	93%	88%	92%

Cholera

In this study ML techniques are used with the help to these techniques a cholera epidemic model was built with correlation to seasonal weather changes. Numerous studies have shown the existence of Cholera and have a strong correlation with an environmental component like geographic allocation. As we know, that in machine learning, many algorithms work differently with different parameters. Hence we can say it for sure that not only one Algorithm is good for all the difficulties as long as the data set's measurements and composition of data set are there. In this paper seven supervised ML algorithms were estimated according to their execution (Leo, Luhanga and Michael 2019). After that, the finest algorithm was selected to organize this examination based on seasonal changes and effects for the Cholera epidemic. Algorithms: Decision Tree, XG Boost,

Random Forest, K Nearest Neighbors (KNN), Extra Tree Ada Boost and Linear Discriminant Analysis (LDA). These are seven algorithms, based on principal purpose and characterstics of top-performing algorithms X.G Boost classifier gives the highest accuracy i-e up to 77% and is the best classifier. X.G. Boost algorithm executes gradient boosted decision trees that are flexible and well organized to increase the model speed.

Cholera

According to this study, In Iran a rural area of Chabahar was affected by Cholera and a prediction model was developed to analyze Cholera (Pezeshiki and Shadpour 2016). For this study, facts were collected from 465 villages and 104 villages were affected with Cholera in ten years of the study period. For this study, to get the feasible predictive model logistic regression modelling and correlate bivariate were used to determine the uncertain components. ANN with back propagation algorithm and sigmoid activation function was trained and tested on two hidden-layer perception neural network with back propagation training algorithm. The sigmoid activation function was trained and tested on two groups infected vs non infected villages; it also comprises the climate and geographical features. The analysis found out that ANN could predict Cholera with 80% of accuracy.

HIV/AIDS

A examination carried out in China at Xinjiang Area using data miming algorithms to setup a model and analyze the performances. Statistics were taken from the three groups under the high risk groups, the first group was I.D.U. (injecting drug users), second was M.S.M. (men who had sex with men) and third was FSW (Female sex workers) from 2009 to 2015 in Uramqi (Tang and Zhang 2018). The statistics also include the sex behaviour, demographic charactersitcs and serological detection output. Results showed that Random forest gets better accuracy on diagnosis on M.S.M. dataset, it got the 94.4821% and on FSW its 97.51% and on FSW it is 94.63%.

Zika

To overcome an epidemic like zika, in this paper early prognosis for observing the virus was performed with the help of Multilayer Perceptron N.N classifier to find out the Zika virus (Mahalakshmi and Suseendran 2019). In the study M.P.N.N got the accuracy level of 97%, It shows that the model using cloud computing with multilayer perceptron neural network classifier gave the best prediction accuracy so far.

Ebola

In this study EBOLA data regarding Ebola patients was used to create an app named as "Ebola Care Guidelines" at the general area Sierra Leone (Colubri and Hartley et al., 2019). Here dataset from two independent datasets was validated. The data used for this study belonged to the same area of Sierra Leone. The accuracy achieved was 64% to 74% for prediction of diseases. In conjunction with health tools, machine learning models have got vast potential to improve the standards of care in low resource settings/emergency scenario.

Now we will discuss few papers, wherein machine learning techniques have been effectively used in finding answers to various Pandemic related issues other than that of accurate prediction.

Ebola

This study used machine learning and introduced an app framework; it was introduced to predict the outcome of EBOLA patients. The app was named Miradoor and MINE (Colubri and Silver et al., 2016). This app minimised gap in data or took care of missing data to a large extent. For this purpose various algorithm like ANN, SVM and Decision Tree was used.

HIV/AIDS

In this study ML techniques and drug delivery methods are combined as these arithmetic procedure are very beneficial for increasing H.I.V. infected individuals (Dubey 2018). The entanglement of HIV/AIDS advanced ML technologies is applied for medicine expansion.

Cholera

This paper is one of its kind as it used machine learning algorithms to check and compare data statically, evaluate Cholera infections across 10 African countries. These machine learning classifiers were applied on 30 socio-economic indicators (Lei and Ganjeizadeh et al., 2017). This paper further reveals that out of these 30 indicators only two benchmark show the most acceptable output and affirm that purified water plays an influential role in reducing the expansion of the bacteria found in Cholera.

Zika

This article describes a screening strategy by applying high-resolution mass spectrometry (HRMS) to assess Z.I.K.A Virus (Z.I.K.V) infection using Random Forest classifier (Melo and Navarro et al., 2018). As based on 42 features detected by Random Forest as it picked up 12 of these features based on spectral signature identification in the sample of blood of a patient because of Z.I.K.V infection. This paper explains that by merging HRMS and the Random Forest algorithm it is a robust platform that can be implemented in big laboratories to detect ZIKA virus.

Ebola

In this study, first time to predict expected spread of pandemic an artificial Beijing named geographical location was assumed and recreated based on Geodemographics after that ML was used to enhance individual's behaviours (Zhang and Chen et al., 2015).

VARIOUS MACHINE LEARNING APPROACHES

Various ML approaches are used by different researchers about their respective papers on various pandemics. When we want to stop the spread of any pandemic than the prediction of accuracy is the most essential tool for getting the best results.

Machine Learning techniques are a significant advantage for medical science as it helps in many ways, even in Pandemics. The table mentioned below specifies the various other uses of Machine learning.

The role of Machine learning in today's world can neither be underestimated nor overlooked. As we are aware machine learning help us find the Risk of Pandemics, predicts the spread of the disease, and helps us develop drugs faster. Also machine learning can helps us find existing drugs that can help understand the diseases better and even predict the next pandemics. Even machine learning techniques can help us predicting Pandemics based on social media platforms.

Table 6. Accuracy of various ML algorithm over pandemics

Diseases	Algorithm	Accuracy
Influenza A	CNN	99%
Influenza A	ANN	98%
Cholera	XG Boost	77%
Cholera	ANN	80%
HIV	RF	94 to 97%
ZIKA	ANN	85%
ZIKA	CNN	97%
Ebola	App based on Machine learmimg	64% to 74%

Table 7. Various ML methods implemented on pandemic (Chaupis 2019, Merzouki and Estill et al., 2019)

Diseases	Methods used	Findings
Influenza A	ANN Multiple Regression Model	For monitoring or surviallances about propagation of influenza.
A (HINI) Flu	Winer Series Model	Minimizes undesired errors and optimized resources of Public Health.
HIV	Used Unsupervised Machine Learning, Cluster Analysis	Identified variables which accounted for most social behavioural variance and its use.
Ebola	ANN, SVM & DECISION Tree	Apps Miradoor & Mine minimised gaps in data
HIV	Machine Learning	Reviewed drug delivery methods with the help of machine learning and computational methods.
Cholera	Machine Learning classifiers applied on 30 socio- economic indicators	Out of given 30 indicators, 02 indicators gave best results and proved that water quality if improved can reduce spread of the disease.
Pandemic	SVM, Decision Tree and Naïve Bayes	Features from tweetsextracted and data is modeled by binary classification for pandemic prediction.

Outlook for Future

In recent studies, machine learning is used to find out the hidden patterns from a large amount of data, better predictions can be made with the help of ML. Similarly Artificial Intelligence (AI), when used during research, offers us the possibility to work speedily and productively on Pandemic (Wilson 2019). Speed in research work is the most critical factor, especially when finding the solution to any Pandemic. As faster as the research is done on this on Pandemic with the help of ML, there will be better opportunities for us as human being to control the spread of this disease. The potential of Machine Learning and A.I. as a whole is immense. Hence there is a need to make coordinate computer- based technologies in conjunction with various where machine learning should play a pioneering role to ensure that world does not face havoc Pandemic like corona (Chaupis 2019). We have a full probability wherein all future pandemics like COVID-19 can be prepared timely to minimize loss of human lives with the help of automated machine learning methods.

References

Ardabili, S. F., Mosavi A., et al., (2020). "*COVID-19 Outbreak Prediction with Machine Learning.*" March, doi: 10.20944.

Attluri, P. K., Chen, Z. and Lu, G. (2010). *"Applying neural network to classify influenza virus antigenic types and hosts."* Institute of Electrical and Electronics Engineer.

Chamola, V., Hassija, V., et al., (2020). *"Disasteer and Pandemic Management using Machine Learing: A Survey,"* Institute of Electrical and Electronics Engineer.

Chaupis, H. N., (2019). "Face to falce with Next Flu Pandemic with a wiener-series-Based Machine Learning: Fast Decision to Tackle Rapid Spread", 9th Annual Computing and Communication workship and Conference, *IEEE.*

Colubri, A., Hartley, M. A. et al., (2019). *"Machine learning Prognostic Models from the 2014-2016 Ebola Outbreak: Data-harmonization challenges, Validation Strategies and mHealth Applications."* Vol 11:54-64.

Colubri, A., Silver T. et al., (2016). *"Transforming Clinical Data into Actionable Prognosis Models: Machine-Learning Framework and Field-Deployable App to Predict outcome of Ebola Patients."* March 18; 10(3).

Damir, H. (2019). "Brief History of Pandemics (Pandemics Throughout History)." *Psychiatry of Pandemics:* 7-35.

Dubey, A. (2018). *"Machine-learning approaches in drug development of HIV/AIDS."* 3(1) 23-25.

Lei, H., Ganjezadeh F., et al., (2017). "Developing an Early warning system for Cholera in African Countries using Socio-Economic Indicators and Statistical methods." *Journal of Supply Chain and Operations Management,* Vol 15.

Leo, J., Luhanga, E. and Michael, K. (2019). "Machine learning Model for Imbalanced Cholera Dataset in Tanzania." *The Scientific World Journal Article* ID9397578.

Lepan, N., (2020). *"Visualizing the History of Pandemics."* www. visualcapatalist.com.

Madhav, N., Oppenbeim, B. et al., (2017). "Chapter 17 Pandemics: Risks, Impactsand Mitigation." In *Disease Control Priorities: Improving Health and Reducing Poverty* 3rd edition.

Mahalakshmi, B. and Suseendran, G. (2019). "Predicition of Zika Virus by Multilayer Perceptron Neural Network (MLPNN) using cloud." *IJRTE* Vol-8, Issue-2S11.

Melo, C. F. O. R., Navarro, L. C. et al., (2018), *"A Machine learning Application Based in Random Forest for Integrating Mass Spectrometry-Based Metabolomic Data: A Simple Screening Method for Patients With Zika Virus."* Apr 11; 6:31.

Merzouki, A., Estill J. et al. (2019), *"Sociobehavioural charactersistics and HIV incidence in 29 subsaharan African Countries: Unsupervised machine learning analysis using the Demographic and Health Survey."* April, doi: https://10.1101/620450.

Pezeshiki, Z., Shadpour, M. et al., (2016). *"Model of Cholera Forecasting Using Artifical Neural Network in Chabahar city Iran."* 4(1).

Qiu, W., Rutherford S. et al., (2016-2017). "The Pandemic and its impacts." *Health, Culture and Society* Vol 9-10.

Quinn, S. A. and Kumar S. (2014). "Health Inequalities and Infectious Diseases Epidemics: A Challenge for Global Health Security" *Biosecur Bioterro* 12(5):263-273.

Tang, D., Zhang M. et al., (2018). "Application of Data Mining Technology on Surveillance Report Data of HIV/AIDS High Rise Groupin Uramqi from 2009-2015." *Complexity in Medical Informatics* Vol 2018 Article ID 9193248.

"What is the difference between a pandemic, an epidemic, endemic, and an outbread?" *Inter mountain Health care:* Apr 2, 2020.

Wilson, J., (2019) "How to survive a plague-Why AI is key to fighting the next major pandemic." *Elesevier* March 2019.

Zhang, P., Chen B. et al., (2015). "The Large Scale Machine Learing in an Artifical Society: Prediction of the Ebola Outbreak in Beijing." *Computer Intelligence and Neuro Science* Vol 2015, Article ID 531650.

In: Mobile Health
Editors: G. Gupta, N. Kumar et al.
ISBN: 978-1-53619-420-3

Chapter 9

COMPUTATIONAL APPROACHES FOR MALARIA DIAGNOSIS USING MACHINE LEARNING: A REVIEW

Vandana[1]***, Kapil Sethi***[1,*] ***and Ankit Gupta***[2]
[1]School of Electrical and Computer Science,
Shoolini University of Biotechnology and Management Sciences,
Solan, Himachal Pradesh, India
[2]Interactive Technologies Institute (ITI/LARSyS) and M-ITI,
Funchal, Portugal

ABSTRACT

Computational assistance is reducing human intervention in almost every domain. Machine learning techniques are kind of computational assistance which deals with the ability to automatically learn and enhance with the experience, without being explicitly programmed. Machine learning is pivotal in terms of delivering high output, competence, reduction in cost and time necessity in approximately all fields such as electrical, medical, bioinformatics, chemistry and information

* Corresponding Author's Email: kapil.7sethi@gmail.com.

technology. Malaria is a life-threatening disease and causes a huge burden on humans. There were 212 million cases of malaria in 2015and 429 000 deaths were reported due to it. It is a widespread disease found in Asia, Europe, and America. But there is no vaccines available for malaria parasites which can be used widely despite of several efforts to develop it. The condition has become worst as all available drugs have shown resistance in some cases. Lots of research has been carried out and genomes of different pathogenic 'Plasmodium' species are now available. Image analysis software and machine learning methods are used to diagnose 'parasitemia' in microscopic blood slides. According to the literature, special techniques are used for image preprocessing, parasite detection, cell segmentation, feature computation and automatic cell classification. Molecular-biological techniques are used to classify the growth of drug-resistance, species identification and enumerating parasite density with low parasitemia. Finally, the stage of malaria endemicity, the insistence of analysis, the incident of the physician, the efficiency of health framework workers and resources are all the factors which influence the choice of malaria-diagnostic method.

INTRODUCTION

Computational assistance has transformed the world in nearly every new domain (McNamara 2019). The computational methods have benefited the multifaceted problems through monitoring, decision making and evaluation.COmputational assistance along with Machine learning techniques have delivered high output in terms of efficiency, reduction in cost and time requirement (Bartek et al., 2019) in different fields such as electrical, medical (Salehi, Baglat et al. 2020), biological (Singh, Kiran et al.), chemistry, physics, social science, information technology, health, transportation, and education (Ahmad, Eckert et al. 2018; Sethi, Jaiswal et al. 2020).

Medical technology is a significant part of the life of people globally (Morrish, 2019). In the current scenario of advancement in technology, huge data is associated with medical field and then the generation, storage and analysis of these data is now possible for making better decision in this field (Pentland 2004). There are numerous challenges in the medical field, which are multifaceted and can be benefited from the applications of machine learning methods (Sethi, Gupta et al. 2019).

Machine Learning

Machine learning (ML) is a part of Artificial intelligence (AI) that provides frameworks with the ability to automatically learn and enhance the experience without being explicitly programmed (Michie, Spiegelhalter et al. 1994). The procedure of learning from data such as, through experiences or training (instruction), in order to look for patterns in data creates enhanced decisions in the future which are based on the examples. The most important aim is to assign the computers to learn automatically without human participation or support as well as regulate the actions accordingly. ML focuses on the innovation of advanced computer programs that learn by itself (Williams and Hill 2005). ML enables the investigation of huge quantities of data. While it usually delivers earlierwith more precise results to recognize cost-effective opportunities or dangerous risks. It may also need additional time and resources to train it appropriately. Combining ML and AI can make it even more efficient in processing huge volumes of evidence (Libbrecht and Noble 2015). Most of the organizations uses ML techniques for different purposes like, Google map for guiding/finding the path, automatic friends and tag suggestion on Facebook (Wu, Brooks et al. 2019), Uber cab booking, adds recommendation on Amazon, facial recommendation on iPhone (Apple), self-driving car by Tesla, recommendation system by Netflix (Low, Gonzalez et al. 2012), Moley the robotic chef and Google translate efficiently (Lv and Tang 2011).

Machine learning comes under the broad umbrella of data mining (Mitchell 1999). Data mining (DM) has a variety of techniques that are commonly used in ML-such as classification, clustering, regression, association rules, sequential patterns, and prediction (Mosavi, Ozturk et al. 2018, Shah, Patel et al. 2020) Data mining is the computational process of discovering new patterns in large data sets, in order to drag out the information (sequence) from it and switch it into an explicable structure for future use. Since the Machine learning process is more accurate and less error-prone when compared to other DM techniques and it is much more capable of taking its own decision and resolving the issues (Gaba 2000). The different area has opted for DM and ML (Witten et al., 2016) for the betterment of their functions and outcomeses. However, the limited application of machine learning has been explored in the health care sector, despite its importance. The health care sector can be improved by using machine learning and deep learning (DL) techniques in different associated issues. Deep learning allows computational models that are composed of multiple processing layers to learn representations of data with multiple levels of abstraction. Deep learning is a subset of Machine learning and inspired by the formation of the human brain.

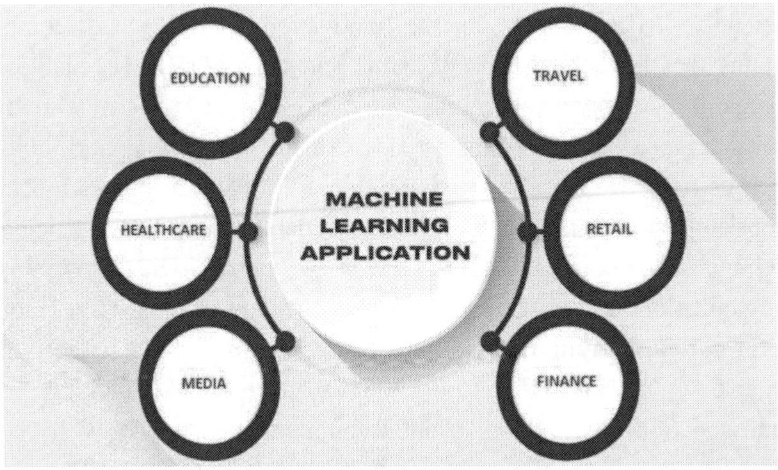

Figure 1. Areas where machine learning is used.

According to the Deng, Deep learning seeks to exploit the unknown structure in the input distribution in order to discover good representations often at multiple levels, with higher-level learned features defined in terms of lower-level features (Deng 2014). Now, deep learning is commonly used for different purposes like face recognition, automatic translation of text from images, visual recognition, healthcare (medical imaging analysis)

(Giger 2018), colorization of black & white images, natural language processing, and many more. There are different areas in medical field where machine learning and deep learning can be applied (Suzuki 2017; Nakaura, Higaki et al. 2020).

DL includes a convolution neural network (CNNs) (Kayalibay, Jensen et al. 2017), recurrent neural, and networks (RNNs) (Banerjee, Ling et al. 2019), which are commonly used algorithms. Within ML, deep learning can be the better option for classification of images as the tenser which auto feature extraction.

Machine Learning (ML) in Healthcare

It's safe to say that there are too many manual processes in medicine. Since, the progression in electronically clinical records are exceptional, however the data they give isn't obviously superior to the old paper diagrams they replaced. If technology innovation is to recover and improve the care in future, at that point the electronic data given to the doctors (specialists) requirements should be upgraded by the intensity of analytics and ML.

The importance of ML in healthcare is its ability to handle immense datasets outside the possibility of human ability, and then the consistent conversion and exploration of that data into scientific insights that will assist the doctor in arranging and giving consideration, eventually by prompting better results, lower expenses of care and expanded patient satisfaction. In the modern world, machine learning and deep learning algorithms are useful in complicated domains where human effort is insufficient, and it takes more time or automation is required (Khan and Yairi 2018). Machine learning and deep learning algorithms have the abilities to be utilized in different applications with different aims (Table 1) (Zhang, Tan et al. 2017). Medical care needs to be moved from considering machine learning as a modern idea (innovative concept) towards considering it to be a real-life tool that can be organized today and should adopt as an incremental approach (Wang and Summers 2012).

Examination discovers specific use cases in which machine learning abilities delivers some motivation from a particular innovative application (e.g., Google and Stanford).This will be a boost to incorporate more analytics, ML, and analytical algorithms into everyday clinical exercise. Preparing an ML algorithm to recognize or classify skin disease from an enormous set pictures of skin disease is something that most people recognize. Radiologists won't get outdatedwith old techniques, however radiologists of the future will supervise and evaluate the analysis that have been primarily read by a machine (Manogaran and Lopez 2017). They will utilize ML like a communitarian accomplice that recognizes particular areas of concentration, illumines noise, and helps emphasis on high possibility areas of concern

Table 1. Machine learning techniques for diagnosis of various diseases (Shailaja, Seetharamulu et al. 2018)

S.No	Reference	ML Techniques	Diseases	Dataset	Accuracy
1	(Chaurasia and Pal 2014)	J48 SVM	Heart Disease	UCI	84.35% 85.03%
2	(Vembandasamy, Sasipriya et al. 2015)	Naïve Bayes	Heart Disease	Diabetic Research Institute in Chennai	86.41%
3	(Kumari and Chitra 2013)	SVM	Diabetic Disease	UCI	78%
4	(Shailaja, Seetharamulu et al. 2018)	Naive Bayes	Diabetes type-2	Different Sectors Of Society in India	95%
5	(Shrivastavat, Sant et al. 2013)	J48	Breast Cancer	UCI Machine Learning Repository	98.14%
6	(Gayathri and Sumathi 2016)	Decision Tree	Breast Cancer	Swami Vivekan-anda Diagnostic Centre Hospital	97%
7	(Sivakami and Saraswathi 2015)	DT+SVM	Breast Cancer	UCI Machine Learning Repository	91%
8	(Shajahaan, Shanthi et al. 2013)	CART Naïve Bayes	Breast Cancer	University of Wiscons in hospitals	92.42% 97.42%
9	(Kousarrizi, Seiti et al. 2012)	SVM	Thyroid Disease	UCI	98.62%

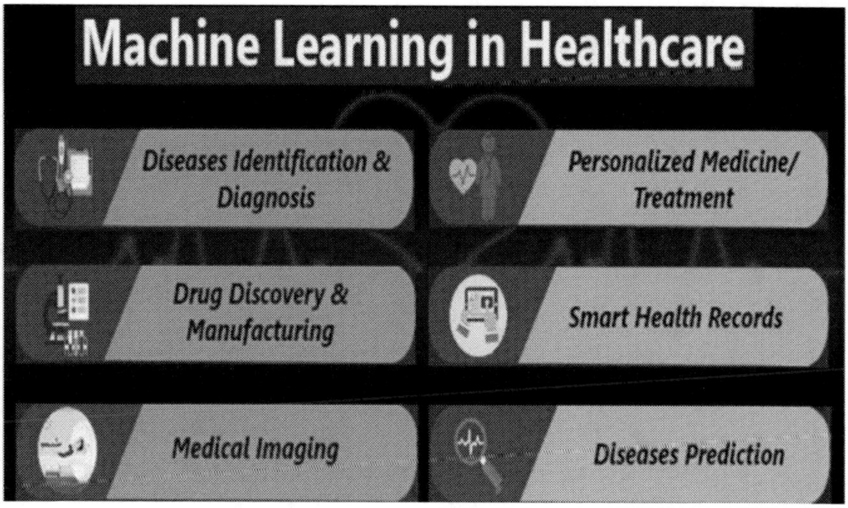

Figure 2. Use of machine learning in healthcare.

Limitless Opportunities for ML in Healthcare

Some may find out if this will provide true benefits in medical services. Wellbeing Catalyst accepts that the introduction and extensive utilization of ML in medical services will be one of the most essential, life-saving advancements ever presented. We accept the opportunities are practically limitless and proposes boundless for the technology to improve and accelerate clinical, work process, and economic results (Loftus, Tighe et al. 2020). Coming up next are only a few examples:

- Decrease readmissions: ML can reduce readmissions in a, productive, and patient tolerant focused way. Clinicians can gather every day direction regarding which patients are destined to be readmitted and how they may have the option to decrease that risk.
- Prevent clinic procured diseases (HAIs): Health frameworks can reduce HAIs, for example, focal line related bloodstream infections (CLABSIs) 40% of CLABSI patients pass away anticipating to which patients with a focal line will build up a

CLABSI. Clinicians can observer high-chance patients and intervene to decrease that hazard by concentrating on patient-explicit danger factors.

- Decrease clinic Length-of-Stay (LOS): Health frameworks can decrease LOS and improve different results like patient satisfaction by recognizing patients that are probably going to have an expanded LOS and afterward certify that best procedures are followed.
- Predict long-lasting (constant) disease: ML can help clinic frameworks recognize patients with undiscovered or misdiagnosed long-lasting sickness, forecast the likelihood that patients will develop long-lasting sickness, and existing patient-specific prevention interventions.
- Decrease 1-year mortality: Health frameworks can lessen 1-year death rates by foreseeing the probability of death in one year of discharge and afterward coordinate patients with suitable interventions, care providers, and support.
- Forecast propensity-to-pay: Health frameworks can figure out who needs updates or a reminder, who needs monetary help, and how the probability of installment (payment) changes over time and after specific occasions.
- Predict flake outs: Health frameworks can make precise predictive models to evaluate, with each planned arrangement and the danger of a flake-out, at last improving patient's consideration and the effective utilization of resources.

Malaria Disease

Malaria remains a major burden on global health, with roughly 200 million cases worldwide and more than 400,000 deaths per year. Besides biomedical research and political efforts, modern information technology is playing a key role in many attempts at fighting the disease. One of the barriers toward a successful mortality reduction has been inadequate malaria diagnosis in particular (Laishram, Sutton et al. 2012). To improve diagnosis, image analysis software and ML methods have been used to enumerate parasitemia in microscopic blood slides. The authors give an overview of these techniques and discusses the current developments in image analysis and ML for microscopic malaria diagnosis (Das, Ghosh et al. 2013). Malaria is an infectious disease which causes huge morbidity and mortality. More than one third population of the world in 107 countries is troubled due to the malaria. The malaria disease is caused by Plasmodium species, which affects people in tropical and subtropical regions of the world (Plewes, Leopold et al. 2019). It is generally present in the South American, Amazon Region and Southeast Asia including India. The maximum frequency of the disease is reported in the South Saharan region of Africa (Tauil 2006). Brazil has leading number of malarial cases in the American continent with an estimated 300,000 yearly cases (Reiners, de Souza Azevedo et al. 2010). In Brazil, malaria is found to be present in the Legal Amazon Region, which includes the Brazilian states of Acre, Amapa, Amazon, Rondonia, Roraima and Tocantins (Reiners, de Souza Azevedo et al. 2010).

Malaria leading to nearly one million losses their life's every year, is generally found in children below five years of age (Roberts and Matthews 2016).The malaria parasites are transmitted during the bites of infected female Anopheles mosquito. In humans malaria is caused by five species of Plasmodium i.e., P. falciparum, P. vivax, P. ovale, P. malariae and P. knowlesi. Although P. falciparum is responsible for a majority of mortality due to infection. P. vivax has similar infection rates with less mortality (Bousema and Drakeley 2011). Other species of protozoa and plasmodia infect reptiles, birds and mammalsProtozoans are single-celled organisms and can be seen only under a microscope. The most important diseases caused by protozoans are Amebiasis, African Trypanosomiasis, Toxoplasmosis and Malaria. One of the most efficient ways to control malaria infection is a vector control. The most important vector-borne protozoans diseases of public health in the tropical regions are caused by protozoans such as Rhizopoda, Sporozoa, Ciliates, and Flagellates (Zofou, Nyasa et al. 2014). Malaria parasites have a very complex lifecycle which depends upon specialized protein expression. Malaria host resolve the intra and extra-cellular parasite survival with the incursion of numerous types of cells and they have the capability to evade the host's immune response (Kosek, Bern et al. 2003).

SIGNS AND SYMPTOMS OF MALARIA

Malaria commonly begins within 8-25 days of infection (Krause et al., 1998) (Figure 3). The symptoms of malaria infection may contain fever, vomiting, headache, shivering, joint pain, hemolytic anemia, jaundice, hemoglobin in the urine, retinal damage and convulsions (Grewal 1981). Malaria may cause anemia and jaundice (yellow coloring of the skin and eyes) because of the loss of red blood cells. Symptoms generally show between 10 and 15 days after the mosquito bite. However, symptoms may occur later in those who have taken antimalarial medications as prevention (Nadjm and Behrens 2012).

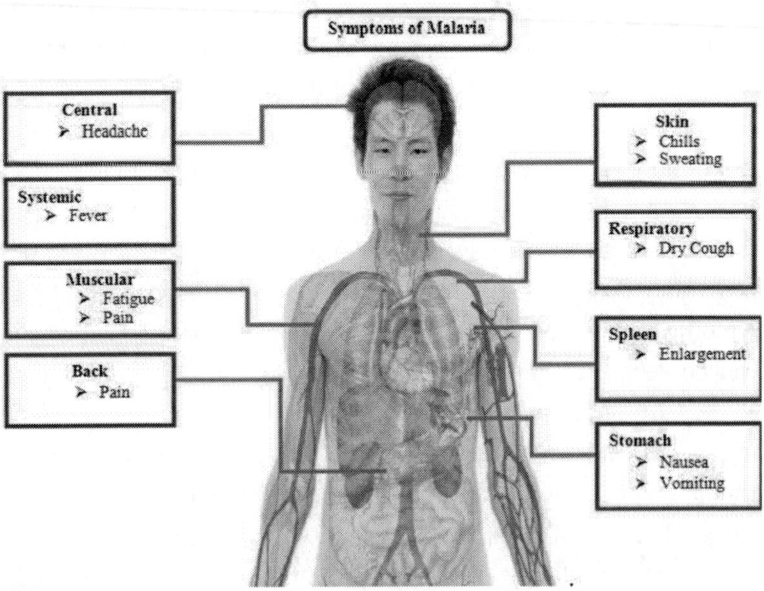

Figure 3. Main symptoms of malaria.

Initial appearances of the disease are common to all malarial species having flu-like symptoms and they can be associated to other situation such as sepsis, gastroenteritis and viral diseases (Nadjm and Behrens 2012). In human being, malaria infection can be affected by the dissimilar species of Plasmodium which contain vivax, ovale, malariae, knowlesi and falciparum, among them the most dangerous and unsafe, Plasmodium falciparum which has a 90% humanity rate cause of death due to malaria infection in young children are (Samba 1997 acute infection which normally occurs in seizures or coma, repeated malaria infections affecting less birth weight and severe anemia infections frequently occuring in pregnant women.

Diagnosis of Malaria

Malaria is a potential medical emergency and it must be treated because its delay in identification are the most common reasons of death in several nations (Organization 2015). The main protocol of malaria infection is a medical identification and it is based on signs and symptoms of malaria patients which were most commonly capable contain weakness, myalgia, chills, dizziness, abdominal pain and pruritus (Murray, Pépin et al. 2000). But, a clinical diagnosis of malaria patients depends on viral, bacterial infections and other febrile illnesses (Reyburn, Mbatia et al. 2004; Mwangi, Mohammed et al. 2005). Recently malaria infections is diagnosed through two techniques first is the microscopic diagnosis by the gold standard technique which is the streak of thin and thick side-line blood smears (Ngasala, Mubi et al. 2008), and second is the quantitative buffy coat (QBC) techniques (Bhandari, Raghuveer et al. 2008). And another method is the rapid diagnostic test (RDT) this methods detects malaria antigens in a small amount of blood by immunochromato graphic assay impregnated on a test strip (Wongsrichanalai, Barcus et al. 2007) (Figure 4).

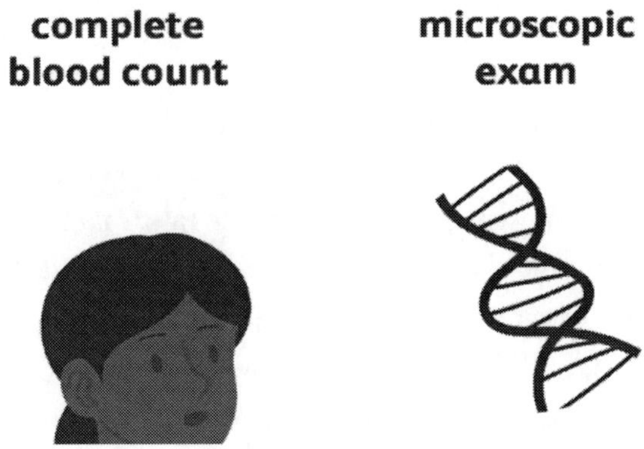

Figure 4. Diagnosis of malaria.

Malaria infection is a speedily successive disease, with a severe risk of rising and cerebral malaria with neurologic symptoms for P. falciparum infections. Hence, a suitable diagnosis of malaria is very necessary. There is room for development for current malaria diagnostic tests including reduced cost, increasing specificity and simplicity of use. The main topic of this survey is the computerized malaria diagnosis for resource-poor setting. We have devoted 2 subsections to light microscopy and RDTs. We also provisionally talk about the extra options for malaria diagnosis, while they are probably less appropriate for the conditions in remote malaria regions. For more information about malaria diagnosis, we refer readers to the surveys in (Tangpukdee, Duangdee et al. 2009; Lee, Leitao et al. 2011). As well as parasites for formative the level of parasitemia is not only important for recognize an infection and measure its severity, it also allocate observing patients by computing drug efficacy and potential drug resistance.

Light Microscopy

For malaria diagnosis the current gold-standard method is light microscopy of blood films (Pluta and Maksymilian 1988). Although other procedures of malaria analysis are being present and have developed and accepted in current years. In resource-poor settings the RDTs, microscopy are the most trendy diagnostic tool. All parasite species can be easily detected with microscopy method. It allows computing the level of parasitemia, clearing a patient after a successful treatment, and monitoring drug resistance. In addition, this method is very less restricted than other existing methods. However, its major disadvantages are that an extensive training is necessary for a microscopist to become a talented malaria slide reader,

Under a microscope to diagnosis malaria, through a droplet of the patient's blood is applied on a glass slide, which is then absorbed in a stain solution to make parasites more easily visible under a conventional light microscope, usually with a 100× oil objective. Thick and thin blood smears are used for malaria diagnosis: (Dowling and Shute 1966). A thick smear is used to identify the presence of parasites in a drop of blood and thick smears allocate a more proficient detection of parasites than thin smears, with compare to 11 times higher sensitivity (Jan, Khan et al. 2018). On the other side the advantages of thin smears, which are the result of distribution the drop of blood across the glass slide and they allow the assessor to classify malaria species and distinguish parasite stages more easily. The real microscopic examination of a single blood slide, counting quantitative parasite detection and species identification, takes a trained microscopist 15–30 minutes. Allowing for that thousands of blood slides are hand inspected for malaria every year, this adds to a huge economic effort required for malaria diagnosis.

Rapid Diagnostic Tests

Microscopic malaria diagnosis have a main advantage lies in its low cost, which gives it a dissimilar benefit in resource-poor settings (Organization 2016). Other accessible diagnostic methods have to show same ease of utilization and cost point as microscopy specified the incomplete financial funds typically obtainable in malaria-prone regions. Possibly the main participant in this sense are RDTs. They detect indication of malaria parasites (antigens) in 10–15 minutes of development. But their detection sensitivity is lower than with manual microscopy; they do not need any extraordinary equipment and need only nominal training. In high-burden areas RDTs are presently cheaper than microscopy.

According to WHO (Organization 2016) in most of the countries, microscopy method is used as comparable to ssRDTs (Organization 2016). RDTs methods are used in rural areas where the microscopy method is not available. In malaria endemic countries about 47% of malaria tests were made by RDT in worldwide (Organization 2016).. The major disadvantage of RDTs method that they do not provide quantification of the results and these methods complement each other than one replacing the other.

Other Tests

For malaria infection different type of methods are available for the diagnoses. Important criteria for this method i.e., cost per test, sensitivity, time per test, specificity and necessary the skill level of the user. Additionally, quantification of the quantity of contaminated red blood cells is essential as a prognostic indicator (Vink, Laubscher et al. 2013). Polymerase chain reaction method called as PCR has shown higher sensitivity and specificity than predictable microscopic test of stained peripheral blood smears (Tangpukdee, Duangdee et al. 2009). This method is most accurate among all other tests. Although, PCR method is very complex high-cost technology that takes many hours to process. According to (Tangpukdee, Duangdee et al. 2009) PCR is not constantly implemented in rising countries because of the complexity of the taxing and be short of possessions to execute these tests adequately and frequently. Quality control and apparatus security are also essential for the PCR technique.

Fluorescent Microscopy

Fluorescent microscopy is a laboratory test to notice malaria infection or other blood parasites. Fluorescent dye makes parasites detectable less than ultraviolet light. (Adeoye and Nga 2007) this test is more responsive than the predictable thick spread according to Adeoye and Nga.

At present, portable fluorescent microscopes with fluorescent reagent to marker parasites. This technique is very simple, reliable and responsive. This is more expensive than conventional light microscopy and is poor at determining species of parasites (Tangpukdee, Duangdee et al. 2009).

Flow Cytometry

This is a laser-based cell counting and detection technique that allows profiling thousands of cells per second. Whereas flow cytometry offer computerized parasitemia counts and low sensitivity. Flow cytometry is a smaller quantity appropriate and a diagnostic technique. However, in urban countries this technique can be helpful in the medical situation for correct counting of parasite numbers, for example in the review of drug treatment (Janse and Van Vianen 1994).

Staining Methods

The diagnosis of malaria was applied for the first time more than 100 years ago by Giemsas stain (1902). It is broadly used due to its low cost, high sensitivity, specificity and microscopical malaria examination (Keiser, Utzinger et al. 2002). However, Giemsa staining require multiple reagents, experienced personal, labor-intensive and time-consuming. Field stain that considerably reduces the staining time, necessitate drying of samples before and throughout staining (Houwen 2002). These can frequently cause false-positive readings. Another stain is Leishman's stain (1901); this stain is very high sensitive, cheap and simple to complete. The other stains are used for example Wright-Giemsa stain, is a combination of Wright and Giemsa stain, and where the previous helps in the intolerance of blood cell types.

In 1970s, (Shute and Sodeman 1973) investigate the effect of fluorochrome staining in identifying the malaria parasites at low-level infection. It has been shown that fluorochrome staining is more liable and faster than Romanowsky and Giemsa staining methods (Kawamoto 1991; Suwalka, Sanadhya et al. 2012; Wongsrichanalai and Kawamoto 2014) but involves significant performance and preparation, and suffers from artifact counting photo bleaching and phototoxicity. (Diaspro, Chirico et al. 2006). Moreover, fluorescence microscopes are more limited than standard light microscopes.

Automated Diagnosis of Malaria

For malaria diagnosis, automated microscopy equipment is a key sequence of exemption steps. The first step is regularly accomplish digital images of blood smears, which frequently depends on the apparatus. The Image acquisition part breaks down into dissimilar approaches i.e., microscopy, blood slides (thin or thick) and staining. Subsequent image achievement method performs one or many preprocessing method. This method to eliminate noise, standardize lighting, color variation and staining process. The next step commonly engage the detection and segmentation of individual blood cells and other substance that can be detectable in a blood slide image i.e., parasites or platelets. For microscopic malaria diagnosis, the Red blood cell detection and segmentation methods have been used. Cell segmentation method is followed by the computation of features. This method explains the outer shell of the segmented substance in a mathematical way. In the last step, a mathematical discrimination technique is used that classifies the segmented matter into a variety of education based on the computed features. For example, it classifies each red blood cell as infected or uninfected. The part titled Parasite classification and category, lists all the association technique used in the writing for malaria diagnosis.

MOBILE SMARTPHONES FOR MALARIA DIAGNOSIS

For microscopic malaria diagnosis, the mobile hardware solution is a small transportable slide reader into which a blood slide might be inserted. This would then produce the parasitemia. In demand, the moderately high optical magnification solution (up to 1000×) is used for malaria diagnosis in combination with oil immersion. The next most excellent way out for malaria diagnosis are small camera-equipped computing devices i.e., smartphones. This method can be attached to a magnifying device and compute the parasitemia mechanically through image analysis and machine knowledge. Modern smartphones are computing devices and their cameras give sufficient declaration for malaria diagnosis Also, Android phones developed cheap and are often formerly in the control of health-care workers.

Small magnifying devices that can be close to a smartphone's camera, allow true optical magnification compared with mere digital zooming, are commercially accessible. However, these devices are silent in the image quality provided. Therefore, a more sensible approach is to simply fix the smartphone to the eyepiece of a normal microscope with an adapter so that blood slide can be filled with the smartphone's camera.

In (Pirnstill and Coté 2015) Pirnstill and Cote present a cost-effective, optical cellphone-based transmission polarized light microscope scheme for imaging the malaria pigment known as hemozoin. Its good to find the survival of the pigment from surroundings and other artifact. The pigment is easier to observe via polarized light microscopy. However, completion of polarized light microscopy lacks extensive implementation because the available profitable plans have tricky designs and would need re-training for obtainable microscopy technicians.

The cellphone-based polarimetric microscopy plan by Pirnstill and Cote demonstrate the potential to have both the declaration and the specificity to notice malaria in a low-cost, easy-touse and modular platform. Rosado et al. 2016 obtained an image processing and analysis method supervise association to assess the attendance of P. falciparum trophozoites and white blood cells in Giemsa-stained thick blood smears (Rosado, Da Costa et al. 2016). Using a support vector machine the merge of geometric color texture, and their automatic detection of trophozoites achieved 80.5% sensitivity and of 93.8% specificity whereas their white blood cell detection achieved 98.2% sensitivity and 72.1% specificity. In (Quinn, Andama et al. 2014) accessible their 3-dimensional printable plan of an adapter to connect a smartphone to a microscope, even though all images for their trial were used with a devoted microscopic camera, available in higher pixel resolution than their smartphone camera. They obtain a workflow for mechanical analysis of thick blood smears, which is concerned with the calculation of morphologic and immediate skin.

The appearance reported 97% area under the handset operational quality curve. Skandarajah et al. 2014 built an organization mobile phone microscope that is well-matched with phones from numerous manufacturers (Skandarajah, Reber et al. 2014). They recognized that quantitative microscopy with micron-scale spatial resolution can be determined out with multiple phones and that image linearity, deformation and color can be corrected as desired. Mainly, they show that phones with greater than 5 megapixel cameras are able of approximately diffraction-limited declaration over a broad range of magnification including those suitable for single cell imaging. Furthermore, they staedt that mechanical focus, contact and color gain is normal on mobile phones with image resolution and reduces accurateness of color capture if uncorrected, and they sketch actions to avoid this wall for quantitative imaging.

References

Adeoye, G. and I. Nga (2007). "Comparison of Quantitative Buffy Coat technique (QBC) with Giemsa-stained Thick Film (GTF) for diagnosis of malaria." *Parasitology international* 56(4): 308-312.

Ahmad, M. A., C. Eckert, et al. (2018). Interpretable machine learning in healthcare. *Proceedings of the 2018 ACM international conference on bioinformatics, computational biology, and health informatics.*

Banerjee, I., Y. Ling, et al. (2019). "Comparative effectiveness of convolutional neural network (CNN) and recurrent neural network (RNN) architectures for radiology text report classification." *Artificial intelligence in medicine* 97: 79-88.

Bhandari, P., C. Raghuveer, et al. (2008). "Comparative study of peripheral blood smear, quantitative buffy coat and modified centrifuged blood smear in malaria diagnosis." *Indian Journal of Pathology and Microbiology* 51(1): 108.

Bousema, T. and C. Drakeley (2011). "Epidemiology and infectivity of Plasmodium falciparum and Plasmodium vivax gametocytes in relation to malaria control and elimination." *Clinical microbiology reviews* 24(2): 377-410.

Chaurasia, V. and S. Pal (2014). "Data mining approach to detect heart diseases." *International Journal of Advanced Computer Science and Information Technology (IJACSIT)* Vol 2: 56-66.

Das, D. K., M. Ghosh, et al. (2013). "Machine learning approach for automated screening of malaria parasite using light microscopic images." *Micron* 45: 97-106.

Deng, L. (2014). "A tutorial survey of architectures, algorithms, and applications for deep learning." *APSIPA Transactions on Signal and Information Processing 3.*

Diaspro, A., G. Chirico, et al. (2006). Photobleaching. *Handbook of biological confocal microscopy*, Springer: 690-702.

Dowling, M. and G. Shute (1966). "A comparative study of thick and thin blood films in the diagnosis of scanty malaria parasitaemia." *Bulletin of the world health organization* 34(2): 249.

Grewal, R. (1981). "Pharmacology of 8-aminoquinolines." *Bulletin of the world health organization* 59(3): 397.

Gaba, D. M. (2000). "Anaesthesiology as a model for patient safety in health care." *BMJ* 320(7237): 785-788.

Gayathri, B. and C. Sumathi (2016). Comparative study of relevance vector machine with various machine learning techniques used for detecting breast cancer. *2016 IEEE International Conference on Computational Intelligence and Computing Research (ICCIC),* IEEE.

Giger, M. L. (2018). "Machine learning in medical imaging." *Journal of the American College of Radiology* 15(3): 512-520.

Houwen, B. (2002). "Blood film preparation and staining procedures." *Clinics in laboratory medicine* 22(1): 1-14.

Jan, Z., A. Khan, et al. (2018). "A review on automated diagnosis of malaria parasite in microscopic blood smears images." *Multimedia Tools and Applications* 77(8): 9801-9826.

Janse, C. J. and P. H. Van Vianen (1994). Flow cytometry in malaria detection. *Methods in cell biology,* Elsevier. 42: 295-318.

Kawamoto, F. (1991). "Rapid diagnosis of malaria by fluorescence microscopy with light microscope and interference filter." *The Lancet* 337(8735): 200-202.

Kayalibay, B., G. Jensen, et al. (2017). *"CNN-based segmentation of medical imaging data."* arXiv preprint arXiv:1701.03056.

Keiser, J., J. Utzinger, et al. (2002). "Acridine Orange for malaria diagnosis: its diagnostic performance, its promotion and implementation in Tanzania, and the implications for malaria control." *Annals of Tropical Medicine & Parasitology* 96(7): 643-654.

Khan, S. and T. Yairi (2018). "A review on the application of deep learning in system health management." *Mechanical Systems and Signal Processing* 107: 241-265.

Kosek, M., C. Bern, et al. (2003). "The global burden of diarrhoeal disease, as estimated from studies published between 1992 and 2000." *Bulletin of the world health organization* 81: 197-204.

Kousarrizi, M. N., F. Seiti, et al. (2012). "An experimental comparative study on thyroid disease diagnosis based on feature subset selection and classification." *International Journal of Electrical & Computer Sciences IJECS-IJENS* 12(01): 13-20.

Kumari, V. A. and R. Chitra (2013). "Classification of diabetes disease using support vector machine." *International Journal of Engineering Research and Applications* 3(2): 1797-1801.

Laishram, D. D., P. L. Sutton, et al. (2012). "The complexities of malaria disease manifestations with a focus on asymptomatic malaria." *Malaria journal* 11(1): 1-15.

Lee, S. A., R. Leitao, et al. (2011). "Color capable sub-pixel resolving optofluidic microscope and its application to blood cell imaging for malaria diagnosis." *PloS one* 6(10): e26127.

Libbrecht, M. W. and W. S. Noble (2015). "Machine learning applications in genetics and genomics." *Nature Reviews Genetics* 16(6): 321-332.

Loftus, T. J., P. J. Tighe, et al. (2020). "Opportunities for machine learning to improve surgical ward safety." *The American Journal of Surgery.*

Low, Y., J. Gonzalez, et al. (2012). *"Distributed graphlab: A framework for machine learning in the cloud."* arXiv preprint arXiv: 1204.6078.

Lv, H. and H. Tang (2011). Machine learning methods and their application research. *2011 2nd International Symposium on Intelligence Information Processing and Trusted Computing,* IEEE.

Manogaran, G. and D. Lopez (2017). "A survey of big data architectures and machine learning algorithms in healthcare." *International Journal of Biomedical Engineering and Technology* 25(2-4): 182-211.

Michie, D., D. J. Spiegelhalter, et al. (1994). "Machine learning." *Neural and Statistical Classification* 13(1994): 1-298.

Mitchell, T. M. (1999). "Machine learning and data mining." *Communications of the ACM* 42(11): 30-36.

Mosavi, A., P. Ozturk, et al. (2018). "Flood prediction using machine learning models: Literature review." *Water* 10(11): 1536.

Murray, H. W., J. Pépin, et al. (2000). "Tropical medicine." *BMJ* 320(7233): 490-494.

Mwangi, T. W., M. Mohammed, et al. (2005). "Clinical algorithms for malaria diagnosis lack utility among people of different age groups." *Tropical Medicine & International Health* 10(6): 530-536.

Nadjm, B. and R. H. Behrens (2012). "Malaria: An update for physicians." *Infectious Disease Clinics* 26(2): 243-259.

Nakaura, T., T. Higaki, et al. (2020). "A primer for understanding radiology articles about machine learning and deep learning." *Diagnostic and Interventional Imaging.*

Ngasala, B., M. Mubi, et al. (2008). "Impact of training in clinical and microscopy diagnosis of childhood malaria on antimalarial drug prescription and health outcome at primary health care level in Tanzania: a randomized controlled trial." *Malaria journal* 7(1): 1-11.

Organization, W. H. (2009). *Global health risks: mortality and burden of disease attributable to selected major risks,* World Health Organization.

Organization, W. H. (2015). *Guidelines for the treatment of malaria,* World Health Organization.

Organization, W. H. (2016). *Malaria microscopy quality assurance manual-version 2,* World Health Organization.

Organization, W. H. (2016). *World malaria report 2015,* World Health Organization.

Pentland, A. (2004). "Healthwear: medical technology becomes wearable." *Computer* 37(5): 42-49.

Pirnstill, C. W. and G. L. Coté (2015). "Malaria diagnosis using a mobile phone polarized microscope." *Scientific reports* 5: 13368.

Plewes, K., S. J. Leopold, et al. (2019). "Malaria: what's new in the management of malaria?" *Infectious Disease Clinics* 33(1): 39-60.

Pluta, M. and P. Maksymilian (1988). *Advanced light microscopy*, Elsevier Amsterdam.

Quinn, J. A., A. Andama, et al. (2014). "Automated blood smear analysis for mobile malaria diagnosis." *Mobile Point-of-Care Monitors and Diagnostic Device Design* 31: 115-132.

Reiners, A. A. O., R. C. de Souza Azevedo, et al. (2010). "Adesão E Reações De Usuários Ao Tratamento Da Malária: Implicações Para A Educação Em Saúde [User Adherence and Reactions to Malaria Treatment: Implications for Health Education]." *Texto & Contexto Enfermagem* 19(3).

Reyburn, H., R. Mbatia, et al. (2004). "Overdiagnosis of malaria in patients with severe febrile illness in Tanzania: a prospective study." *BMJ* 329(7476): 1212.

Roberts, D. and G. Matthews (2016). "Risk factors of malaria in children under the age of five years old in Uganda." *Malaria journal* 15(1): 1-11.

Rosado, L., J. M. C. Da Costa, et al. (2016). "Automated detection of malaria parasites on thick blood smears via mobile devices." *Procedia Computer Science* 90: 138-144.

Salehi, A. W., P. Baglat, et al. (2020). A CNN Model: Earlier Diagnosis and Classification of Alzheimer Disease using MRI. *2020 International Conference on Smart Electronics and Communication (ICOSEC),* IEEE.

Samba, E. (1997). "The burden of malaria in Africa." *Africa health* 19(2): 17.

Sethi, K., A. Gupta, et al. (2019). Comparative Analysis of Machine Learning Algorithms on Different Datasets. *Circulation in Computer Science International Conference on Innovations in Computing (ICIC 2017),* 87.

Sethi, K., V. Jaiswal, et al. (2020). "Machine learning based support system for students to select stream (subject)." *Recent Advances in Computer Science and Communications (Formerly: Recent Patents on Computer Science)* 13(3): 336-344.

Shah, K., H. Patel, et al. (2020). "A comparative analysis of logistic regression, random Forest and KNN models for the text classification." *Augmented Human Research* 5(1): 1-16.

Shailaja, K., B. Seetharamulu, et al. (2018). Machine Learning in Healthcare: A Review. *2018 Second International Conference on Electronics, Communication and Aerospace Technology (ICECA), IEEE.*

Shajahaan, S. S., S. Shanthi, et al. (2013). "Application of data mining techniques to model breast cancer data." *International Journal of Emerging Technology and Advanced Engineering* 3(11): 362-369.

Shrivastavat, S. S., A. Sant, et al. (2013). "An overview on data mining approach on breast cancer data." *International Journal of Advanced Computer Research* 3(4): 256.

Shute, G. and T. Sodeman (1973). "Identification of malaria parasites by fluorescence microscopy and acridine orange staining." *Bulletin of the world health organization* 48(5): 591.

Singh, S., V. Kiran, et al. *"Application of Proline and Mannitol On Lepidium Sativum L. Under Abiotic Stress Condition (Heavy Metal Stress)."*

Sivakami, K. and N. Saraswathi (2015). "Mining big data: breast cancer prediction using DT-SVM hybrid model." *International Journal of Scientific Engineering and Applied Science* (IJSEAS) 1(5): 418-429.

Skandarajah, A., C. D. Reber, et al. (2014). "Quantitative imaging with a mobile phone microscope." *PloS one* 9(5): e96906.

Suwalka, I., A. Sanadhya, et al. (2012). Identify malaria parasite using pattern recognition technique. *2012 International Conference on Computing, Communication and Applications, IEEE.*

Suzuki, K. (2017). "Overview of deep learning in medical imaging." *Radiological physics and technology* 10(3): 257-273.

Tangpukdee, N., C. Duangdee, et al. (2009). "Malaria diagnosis: a brief review." *The Korean journal of parasitology* 47(2): 93.

Tauil, P. L. (2006). "Perspectivas de controle de doenças transmitidas por vetores no Brasil [Perspectives for vector-borne disease control in Brazil]." *Revista da sociedade brasileira de medicina tropical* 39(3): 275-277.

Vembandasamy, K., R. Sasipriya, et al. (2015). "Heart diseases detection using Naive Bayes algorithm." *International Journal of Innovative Science, Engineering & Technology* 2(9): 441-444.

Vink, J., M. Laubscher, et al. (2013). "An automatic vision-based malaria diagnosis system." *Journal of microscopy* 250(3): 166-178.

Wang, S. and R. M. Summers (2012). "Machine learning and radiology." *Medical image analysis* 16(5): 933-951.

Williams, D. and J. Hill (2005). *Machine learning,* Google Patents.

Wongsrichanalai, C., M. J. Barcus, et al. (2007). "A review of malaria diagnostic tools: microscopy and rapid diagnostic test (RDT)." *The American journal of tropical medicine and hygiene* 77(6_Suppl): 119-127.

Wongsrichanalai, C. and F. Kawamoto (2014). "Fluorescent microscopy and fluorescent labelling for malaria diagnosis." *Encyclopedia of Malaria* 2021.

Wu, C.-J., D. Brooks, et al. (2019). Machine learning at facebook: Understanding inference at the edge. *2019 IEEE International Symposium on High Performance Computer Architecture (HPCA),* IEEE.

Zhang, L., J. Tan, et al. (2017). "From machine learning to deep learning: progress in machine intelligence for rational drug discovery." *Drug discovery today* 22(11): 1680-1685.

Zofou, D., R. B. Nyasa, et al. (2014). "Control of malaria and other vector-borne protozoan diseases in the tropics: enduring challenges despite considerable progress and achievements." *Infectious diseases of poverty* 3(1): 1.

In: Mobile Health
Editors: G. Gupta, N. Kumar et al.
ISBN: 978-1-53619-420-3

Chapter 10

Can Mobile Health Technology Improve Health Related Quality of Life of Chronic Disease Patients in Emerging Economies?: "Happy Heart" A Randomized Controlled Trial in India

Yojna Sah Jain[1,*], Vaishali M. Patil[2], Praful Jain[3] and Omar Nada[4]

[1]School of Medical and Allied Sciences, K.R. Mangalam University, Gurugram, Haryana, India
[2]Department of Pharmaceutical Chemistry, KIET School of Pharmacy, KIET Group of Institutions, Delhi-NCR, Ghaziabad, India
[3]Department of Engineering, Zalando SE, Berlin, Germany
[4]Department of Computer Science, University of Freiburg, Fahnenbergplatz, Freiburg, Germany

[*] Corresponding Author's Email: yojna.jain@gmail.com.

ABSTRACT

Background. With widespread and ever-growing cell phone penetration and rapid developments in mobile technology, the prominence of mobile health (m-health) tools has increased as a valuable strategy for secondary prevention and management of chronic disease conditions. Due to an increasing aging population in India, along with a substantial rise in chronic disease and multimorbidity, the topic of health-related quality of life (HRQOL) has become more relevant than ever. Many trials have been performed globally to evaluate the effect of m-health tools on the quality of life of a wide range of population. However, there is dearth of scientific data on the impact of these tools on the HRQOL of chronic disease patients from emerging economies like India.

Objective. To evaluate the effect of an indigenous bilingual m-health education program on the health-related quality of life (HRQOL) of Coronary Artery Disease (CAD) patients.

Methodology. This was an open label, randomized, experimental clinical study conducted in medically managed stable CAD patients in a reputed hospital in North India. For this study a m-health based educational program comprising of a mobile application and SMS program was developed. Expert evaluation of the mobile application was conducted using Mobile Application Rating Scale (MARS) followed by a pilot user satisfaction survey done with 35 CAD patients. Thereafter a randomized clinical study using this m-health program was conducted in 312 CAD patients. HRQOL was the primary endpoint assessed using validated RAND-36 self-reported questionnaire. The statistical analysis was carried out using R Statistical Software, version 3.6.1. Happy heart program was administered to experimental group patients along with usual medical care for a period of 6 months. ANOVA and Kruskal Wallis tests were performed to determine the impact of the intervention on the comparative HRQOL scores of experimental versus non-experimental groups at baseline, at 6 months and at 9 months.

Results. The study intervention namely "Happy Heart Program" comprising of an Android^{TM} based bilingual mobile phone application along with a short message service (SMS) program was developed to deliver educational/informative/reminder content to patients in the experimental group. The mean MARS rating for the mobile application was 3.60 ± 0.86 and average user satisfaction score was 4.09 ± 0.75. The randomized controlled trial ($n = 312$) was conducted for 6 months with a 9-month final follow up and data collection time point. Statistical analysis done using ANOVA and Kruskal Wallis tests showed significant improvement in the experimental group for most of the HRQOL domain scores from baseline to 6 months and overall study duration from baseline to 9 months' time point ($p < 0.05$).

Conclusion. Present m-health study showed positive impact and effectiveness of this indigenous m-Health based education program on the HRQOL of patients who received the intervention.

Keywords: m-health, coronary artery disease, health-related quality of life, HRQOL, RAND-36

1. Introduction

1.1. What Is Mobile-Health (m-Health)

Mobile health (m-health), e-health, or telemedicine are the trend-setting developments that contribute to a gradual and steady digital transformation of the health sector (Fatehi and Wootton 2012). m-Health refers to the application of telecommunications and information technologies in the field of healthcare. Global e-Health Observatory of the World Health Organization (WHO) describes m-health as: *"Health and public health research assisted by electronic technologies such as smart phones, systems for patient tracking, personal digital assistants and other wearable applications"*.

Most m-health innovations, such as online appoinment scheduling, electronic health data sharing, e-commerce, health apps, wellness apps that we now consider to be a normal part of our everyday lives, were almost inconceivable a few years ago. But with the proliferation of smartphones, easy connectivity and availability around the globe, there is a drastic shift towards smart technology-based interventions. Today m-health delivers a vast range of services, from treatment compliance and data analysis and supply chain monitoring to patient support.

As per Telecom Regulatory Authority of India (TRAI), by Dec 2019, total telephone subscribers in India had reached 1.1 Billion mark *("Telecom Subscriptions Reports" n.d.)*. According to Statista, by Feb 2020 there are more than 3.5 billion smartphone users in the world. This widespread adoption of mobile phone technologies offers researchers and clinicians a unique opportunity to use m-health as a means of delivering healthcare in an automated, personalized, and cost-effective manner. m-Health devices may effectively reduce the pressure on health services and enable patients to effectively manage self-care and chronic diseases (Rozental et al. 2014; Vis et al. 2015; Mohr et al. 2013; Baumeister et al. 2014).

Several reports have shown the efficacy of technology-based interventions in chronic disease management (Arora et al. 2014; Capozza et al. 2015; Holtz and Lauckner 2012). Intense penetration of mobile devices and technology is certainly a positive encouragement and catalyst for increasing mobile health application and resources to be created. Particularly with regard to patient education, and therapeutic behavior change interventions mobile application are gaining growing popularity. At present there are a variety of mobile health tools available with different types of features and functionalities like:

- To collect and store health data;
- Improve medication adherence;
- Help in diet control and weight management;
- Record physical activity;
- Record disease symptoms;
- Improve Patient provider communication;
- Educational and motivational tools to promote healthy behaviors.

Out of all one of the notable focus areas of m-health technology have been in the area of *"Patient education and awareness"*. Studies conducted in various parts of the world have shown progress in the quality of treatment and awareness levels among general populations using m-health-based various resources such as short message service, and a range of mobile application etc. In India, shortage of trained healthcare professionals is one of the main reasons for health education and literacy deficits that lead to negative impact on patient-based health decisions and actions motivated by knowledge. m-Health technologies may play an important supportive role here due to easy accessibility and reach to even disadvantaged communities and geographically difficult to access areas. These tools at least theoretically show promising role in chronic disease management, home-based self-care management, and promoting changes in healthy lifestyle. This theory is driven by rapid mobile technology advancements and growing opportunities for m-health integration into existing healthcare infrastructure, as well as steady growth in mobile network coverage.

Many mobile applications are already being launched in the market and are currently operating in various countries at different scales. In view of such an increasing trend in the development and use of these instruments, m-health requires ongoing evaluation. Despite the need for assessment, the evaluation of m-health solutions based on results is not routinely carried out. This shows a research gap that needs to be addressed with more m-health related assessments to be carried out in various countries, especially developing economies like India.

1.2. Health-Related Quality of Life (HRQOL)

The World Health Organization (WHO) defines:

> "Health as not merely the absence of disease or infirmity, but a state of complete psychical, mental and social well-being." (World Health Organisation. The First Ten Years. The Health Organization. Geneva 1958)

> "Quality of Life (QoL) is individuals' perceptions of their position in life in the context of the culture and value systems in which they live and in relation to their goals, expectations, standards and concerns." (*World Health Organisation. Programme on Mental Health. Geneva* 1996)

Patrick and Erickson (1993) define health related quality of life (HRQOL) as:

> "the value assigned to duration of life as modified by the impairments, functional states, perceptions and social opportunities that are influenced by disease, injury, treatment or policy" (Patrick DL 1993).

Since the 1980s, the concept of HRQOL and its determinants has grown to incorporate several aspects of the overall quality of life that can be specifically seen to have an effect on wellbeing- physical as well as mental. As described in today's world, HRQOL now concerns the effect of health on the functional capacity of a person and on his or her sense of well-being in the physical, mental, and social realms of existence. The HRQOL model helps government agencies to effectively tackle wider areas of public health policy through a shared framework in partnership with a wider variety of healthcare stakeholders. HRQOL is increasingly gaining recognition as a measurable outcome and allowing for scientific proof of the effect of quality of life on health. It is a broad multidimensional term that usually involves self-reported measurements of functional ability, psychological state, social function, and individual health perception. HRQOL has been well known to align with the real health and status outcomes (Blaum, C. S., Ofstedal, M. B., Langa, K. M., &Wray 2003). Focusing on HRQOL as an outcome could resolve the gap between the disciplines and the social, emotional and medical services.

As obvious any illness or condition has an effect on the HRQOL of a person. Particularly chronic conditions have long-term effects on HRQOL for people. HRQOL is related to both chronic diseases (diabetes, breast cancer, arthritis and hypertension) and to their risk factors (body mass index, physical inactivity and smoking status). During the past decades due to increasing prevalence of chronic disorders, HRQOL of people worldwide have been negatively impacted. The concept of HRQOL thus has been widely accepted and promoted. The term HRQOL is also used interchangeably with other terms like self-reported health, patient-assessed outcomes, patient-reported outcomes etc. HRQOL metrics serve as useful survey instruments to classify potential health issues in a particular population; assess different facets of public health programs; assess emerging technologies; and determine cost-benefit reasoning for promoting decision-making in the economic assessment of health care.

Summarily, HRQOL analysis and evaluation may:

- Assist in calculating the burden of preventable disease, illness and disability;
- Provide valuable new insights into the relationship between risk factors and HRQOL;
- Help track progress towards health targets in a country/region;
- Make a distinction between fairly poor perceived health subgroups;
- Interpretation and dissemination of such data can help to define gaps in health policy and legislation;
- Assist to allocate resources based on needs not met;
- Develop and document effectiveness of strategic plan directly

Evaluations of HRQOL have long been regarded as useful for offering knowledge on the functioning and well-being of individuals and populations, thereby leading to effective decision-making for community based public health programs. HRQOL assessments offer useful contextual knowledge on the well-being of the person alongside the valuable information obtained from clinical and laboratory evaluations of the condition. Mostly HRQOL is expressed by generic measures. This is because generic metrics may be used in different ways and across illness and across severities of medical disorders. In addition, standardized HRQOL tests have often proved effective in measuring patient outcomes across various multiple health care delivery systems. Based on the requirement various tools are available to calculate HRQOL. It is often calculated in the form of questionnaires. These instruments are used widely because their findings can be translated to numerical values that allow researchers to equate improvements in one form of HRQOL with those in other types of patient. Some of the commonly used generic HRQOL measurement tools are:

- Short-Form (SF-36 ®) Survey
- EuroQoL Domain (EQ-5D)
- WHOQOL-100
- WHOQOL-BREF

HRQOL evaluation with SF-36 and RAND-36 are two standardized HRQOL measurements most commonly used worldwide to assess the overall burden of illness with people with various forms of illness. There are currently two similar variants of the questionnaire: the RAND-36 Item Health Survey, a public domain format, and the SF-36 Item Health Survey, a proprietary, commercially distributed type. Minor variations in rating procedures for two of the eight subscales occur between RAND-36 and SF-36. The RAND-36 is a 36-item questionnaire designed to be used as a standardized HRQOL test (https:/www.rand.org/health/surveys tools/mos/ 36-item-short). They are approved for use in assessments of health policies, general public studies, scientific study and clinical practice. These approaches are widely used in economic evaluation, as their findings can be converted into quantitative values. This helps researchers to compare improvements in HRQOL in one category of patient to those in other types of patients, and to draw concrete principles from evaluations that aid in decision making.

Overview of m-Health over the Past Decade

Mobile health (m-health) technologies, including Integrated Voice Response (IVR), Short Message Service (SMS) or Text Messaging (SMS) and Smartphones, have been researched worldwide for their effects on changing healthy habits and controlling CVDs (Burke et al. 2015; Shan et al. 2019; Rowland et al. 2020). In Table 1 and Table 2 we have summarized key randomized controlled trials that examined a number of m-Health approaches to improve lifestyle and/or avoid and handle CVDs in low-and middle-income countries.

Table 1. Key examples of m-Health tools developed worldwide for therapeutic behavioral modification

m-Health Tool	Characteristics	Intervention components	Country	Ref.
IVR	Weekly	-Patient education -Nurse phone counseling	USA	Handley, Shumway, and Schillinger 2008
IVR	32 weekly counseling sessions	- Collection of patient health information using study-issued home measurement devices.. - Behavior change and motivational messages targeting compliance to medication, physical activity and diet.	USA	Migneault et al. 2012
Website learning module & E-mail	Website learning module - weekly; E-mail - monthly	-Website based learning modules -Self-monitoring of body-weight, diet, physical activity -E-mail- progress summary	USA	Appel et al. 2011
IVR	10 weekly counseling sessions	-Customized messages to change home environment to promote physical activity and healthy diet	USA	Estabrooks et al. 2009
IVR	Counseling sessions (approx. 15 in a year)	-Instructions to improve cognitive and behavioral skills. -Motivation for improvement in physical activity	USA	King et al. 2014
SMS	2-5 SMS per day or customized	-Tips, suggestions, prompts, reminders for diet, physical activity, weight management behaviors	USA	Norman et al. 2013
SMS, MMS	4 times per day	-Behavior change strategies to target weight loss	USA	Shapiro et al. 2012
Group Teleconference	6 weekly 1-hour	-Lifestyle counseling sessions	Canada	Nolan et al. 2011
IVR	Post-hospital discharge calls on day 3, 14 and 30	-Questions related to smoking status, use of pharmacotherapy, self-help information	Canada	Reid et al. 2007
SMS	4 messages for 24 weeks	- motivation for smoking cessation, healthy diet and physical activity	Australia	Handley, Shumway, and Schillinger 2008

m-Health Tool	Characteristics	Intervention components	Country	Ref.
SMS	Weekly messages	-Motivational reminder messages to wear pedometer and maintain activity	New Zealand	Newton, Wiltshire, and Elley 2009
SMS	3 times per week for 3 months; followed by weekly and then monthly	-Information on diabetes and lifestyle modification	Hong Kong	Wong et al. 2013
SMS and internet messages	3 SMS per week, 3rd message via internet	-Step 1- collect feedback from participants through a website (self-measured waist circumference, body weight, BP, diet, exercise). -Step 2- SMS and internet messages to participant about diet and exercise recommendations based on website posting	South Korea	Shapiro et al. 2012

Table 2. Example of key m-health tools developed worldwide for prevention and management of CVDs

m-Health Tool	Characteristics	Intervention components	Country	Ref.
IVR	Weekly patient-initiated calls	-IVR reported BP, medication, adherence, and symptoms. -IVR based education, motivational messages	USA	Friedman et al. 1996
IVR	Weekly	-Self-reported home BP monitoring, pharmacist follow-up	USA	Magid et al. 2011
Telemonitoring (TM) website	6 times per week -BP	-Home based BP telemonitoring. -Transmit BP readings to pharmacist for medication adjustment as needed.	USA	Margolis et al. 2013
SMS	Daily messages	-Messages and reminders to educate and motivate.	USA	Arora et al. 2014
IVR	3 reminders	-Two-way communication with patients and healthcare providers. -Automated patient reminders to send health data to healthcare professionals .	USA	Homko et al. 2012

Table 2. (Continued)

m-Health Tool	Characteristics	Intervention components	Country	Ref.
IVR	monthly	-Reinforcement calls to patients. -Self-management support program.	USA	Lorig et al. 2008
SMS	2-6 messages per day	-Self-management support through SMS. -Monthly nurse calls.	USA	Nundy et al. 2014
IVR	Bi-weekly	-Assessment of behavior and symptom assessment. -Customized patient feedback. -Nurse care manager for telephone follow-up.	USA	J D Piette, Weinberger, and McPhee 2000
IVR	Weekly	-Assessment and self-care education. -Nurse care manager for follow-up.	USA	J D Piette et al. 2001
Cell phone transmission via WellDoc	Monthly	-Real time feedback on HbA1c levels.	USA	Quinn et al. 2008
Mobile coaching and web portal	Automated communication as per patient and provider interactions	-Messages in response to patient-reported blood glucose values like automated medication management, lifestyle behavior	USA	Quinn et al., 2011
IVR	Weekly	-IVR and monthly Group Medical Visit groups for evaluation of self-management support	USA	Schillinger et al. 2008
IVR	3 calls	-Reminders to encourage for dilated eye exam and lab tests. -Token gifts	USA	Simon et al. 2010
IVR	Weekly for 30 days	-Geisinger Monitoring Program -IVR Protocol to reduce transmission rate and improve management	USA	Graham et al. 2012
SMS	Daily or 3 times per week	-Educational messages (1-way). -Messages to improve adherence to medications (2-way)	USA	Park et al. 2014

m-Health Tool	Characteristics	Intervention components	Country	Ref.
Remote monitoring with alters triggered by device	Remote monitoring for customized duration	-Remote follow-up and wireless auto alerts to clinic nurses or physicians	France, Hungary, Israel, Italy, Spain, Switzerland	Boriani et al. 2013
IVR	Weekly	-Home based self-care support calls. -Forwarding of patient reports to respective clinics.	Honduras	John D Piette et al., 2011
IVR	Weekly	-Automated monitoring, behavior-change reminders, home-based BP monitoring	Honduras Mexico	John D Piette et al., 2012
Internet-based CBT	Weekly	-Internet-based E-coaching and online attention control (Health Watch)	Australia	Glozier et al. 2013
IVR call-in	Weekly	-Evaluation of patient's health and self-care with customised feedback, email alerts	Australia	Williams et al. 2012
Smartphone (Hactive application)	Customized	-Use to collect, store, analyze and visualize heart rate profile of an individual	Australia	Goldberg and Ho 2020
SMS, Phone call	28 SMS to each participant in the duration of 7 months	-SMS related to health education. -Phone call to every 40th participant to check authenticity of response.	India	Mohan et al. 2017

Table 3. m-Health services for prevention and management of CVDs

Type of Prevention	IVR	SMS/Text	Smartphone
Primordial prevention	Information about access to resources to promote CVD health. Testimonials from others about use of these services.	Messages - to promote knowledge and demand for community-based programs for promotion of healthy lifestyle. Used by Public fitness centers	GPS - for locating sources of healthy food, bike/walking paths, and nearby places of exercise
Primary prevention	Goal setting and monitoring for diet, physical activity, weight management; customized reminders and reinforcement related to behavioral goals	Frequent reminders, encouragement and advice for prevention of CVDs. Some examples include smoking cessation and activity promotion	Risk calculators and applications to track efforts toward behavior change goals. Feedback on dietary choices and weight changes.
Secondary prevention	To monitor health and self-care with the help of validated scales. Customized behavior changes messages using the recorded voice to present complex messages.	SMS requests - to report blood pressure. Reminders - adherence and encouragement reinforcing behavior change.	Dashboards for tracking indicators of CVD like adherence, BP. Peer support from social media. Online information about self-care.

The purpose of these investigational studies was to understand CVDs and their risk factors. The role of m-health technology in improving prevention and control of CVDs has been actively tracked in order to overcome shortcomings and enhance implementations. The key factors to be considered are patient costs, literacy needs, interaction complexity, patient needs, future scope and evidence of efficacy. Selection of the right m-health instrument depends on the illness and the clinical state of the patient.

The m-health services for prevention and management of CVDs can be categorized based on the level of clinical condition of the patient (Allida et al. 2020; Burke et al. 2015; (Shan et al. 2019) Villarreal and Berbey-Alvarez 2020). The three major categories namely, IVR, SMS/Text messages and smartphone along with their features are elaborated in Table 3.

For HRQOL measurements, tools like RAND 36 Item Short-Form (SF-36®) survey, EuroQoL 5 Domain (EQ-5D) tool, WHO-QOL BREF questionnaire are being routinely used to investigate or monitor the patient's quality of life (Ray et al. 2006; Haroon et al. 2007; Bedi et al. 2005; R M Kohli et al. 2005; Rewa M Kohli et al. 2005; Wig et al. 2006; Rajeswari et al. 2005; Muniyandi et al. 2007; Birrell et al. 2000; Anchah et al. 2017; Sinha, Van Den Heuvel, and Arokiasamy 2013; Bullinger et al. 1998; Gandek et al. 1998; Wagner et al. 1998).

Indian studies have well utilized the RAND-36 and SF-36 tools for HRQOL measurements in some clinical conditions including CVDs (Medhi GK, Sarma J, Pala S, Bhattacharya H, Bora PJ 2019; Shivaprasad et al. 2018; Shah, Rashmi, and Nanjundappa 2018; Pius, Mini, and Thankappan 2019; Singh et al. 2013; Babu et al. 2011; Gupta, Kant, and Mishra 2014; Varma, Kusuma, and Babu 2010; Villarreal and Berbey-Alvarez 2020).

Studies report application of HRQOL measurements for understanding the prevention and control measures of chronic and/or acute clinical pathologies to current pandemic COVID19 (Chen et al. 2020).

With the growing elderly population in India, as well as significant rise in chronic disease conditions and multimorbidity, the issue of health-related quality of life (HRQOL) is assuming greater relevance because people with poor functional health are also likely to have poor HRQOL. Data on the impact of chronic diseases, CAD in particular on Indian patient's HRQOL are lacking. Therefore, the primary objective of this study was to explore the functional status and its relationship with various dimensions of HRQOL among CAD patients in an outpatient clinical setting of Gurugram, Haryana, India.

2. METHODOLOGY

2.1. Development and Pilot Testing of M-Health (Happy Heart) Program

Present work aimed to develop a bilingual mobile phone application to educate heart patients about heart diseases and their management. The target user group for this mobile application were diagnosed cases of CAD visiting Cardiology Outpatient Clinic at a reputed hospital in Gurugram, Haryana. However, the usability of this program applies not only to patients with CAD, but also to other chronic disease patients who may benefit from positive changes in lifestyle. This program consisted of Two Components (Figure 1):

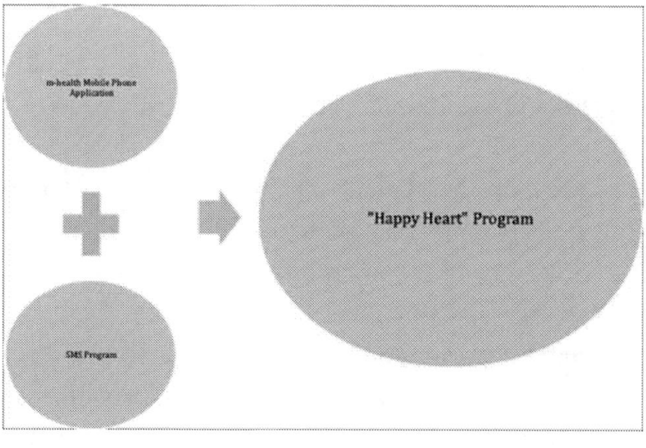

Figure 1. Happy Heart Program composition.

- *A Mobile Phone Application:* A bilingual educational mobile phone application for heart patients,
- *A short message service (SMS) program:* A SMS program to deliver Text messages to patients in experimental group to provide education; referral to patient education material on mobile application and reinforcement of positive lifestyle changes.

Content Development

The content creation for the mobile application and the Short Message Service (SMS) software was focused on the Behavior Change strategies which included:

- the provision of information,
- the provision of encouragement,
- prompting about consequences,
- monitoring self-behavior,
- advice about setting graded tasks;
- time spaced reminders for healthy behaviors e.g., physical activity and diet.

Abraham and Michie integrate these approaches in their taxonomy with a variety of fundamental psychological frameworks such as the concept of information-motivation-behavioral abilities, logical philosophy of action, structured behavioral theory, relational cognitive theory, regulation theory and operational conditioning (Michalos, Zumbo, and Hubley 2000).

In order to develop the content for this education program we did a detailed review of the health and disease related education requirements for our target group followed by comprehensive examination of the relevant literature, and current instructional brochures and leaflets. We also collected and synthesized appropriate information from books, journals, and internet sources. Interviews were performed with cardiologists, surgeons, physiotherapists, dietitians, and nurses. After thorough literature review a content structure comprising of 6 modules was finalised for development of this program. Script was written following the principles of good scientific literature, and medical writing. Content was scientific but language was kept simple and easy to comprehend.

Other than the basic information related to heart and heart diseases, specific and systematic focus was put on the significance of healthy eating, stress control and physical exercise in the prevention and management of heart diseases. Throughout the study material there was intentional repetition of diet and physical activity related information in order to encourage lifestyle improvement among the users. Throughout the content we conformed to, the "Question-Answer" and "Simple Statement" format so that information is delivered in a straightforward manner. We also included a few video messages like "Message from Cardiologists, Yoga expert and Physiotherapist" to bring variety in content and improve user engagement and interest. A self-help BMI calculator was also included in the mobile application.

Software Development

We developed Happy Heart mobile application based on the systematic instructional design model (Hilgart et al. 2012). The architecture and layout of the mobile application were determined based on the purpose, scope, and content structure of the program. Since the majority of target market patients were Android™ phone users, considering the time and budget constraints we created this smartphone application for Android™ only. We used a built-in Java SE development kit 8 and Android Studio for software development. Testing of the mobile application was done on various Android™ based phone models. Iterations were made so that the content look and appear alike regardless of phone model changes. Based on the content menu, the data was added to the smartphone application using the slide-show format due to increased readability, simple organization of content and the ability to deliver information in a controlled manner. We also included pictures, videos and graphics as appropriate to increase the appeal of the application and ensure better engagement of the users. After multiple rounds of review by experts and iterations as per feedback the first version of the mobile application was released for user satisfaction testing.

Expert Assessment of Mobile Application

Pilot testing of this application consisted of an expert assessment followed by a User satisfaction survey among the target population. Expert evaluation of Happy Heart mobile application was done by 3 software engineers and two healthcare professionals. We used a peer-reviewed, objective, multidimensional measure called Mobile Application Rating Scale (MARS) for this assessment (Hilgart et al. 2012). MARS assesses mobile application quality on a 5-point scale (1-Inadequate to 5-Excellent) across 5 core criteria: engagement, functionality, aesthetics, information quality, and subjective quality.

User Satisfaction Evaluation

The user satisfaction survey was carried out at the study site, Paras Hospital Gurugram, India. Hospital's Independent Ethics Committee gave approval to conduct this study. In a random fashion we identified, requested and enrolled 35 CAD patients who were visiting the cardiology OPD at Paras Hospital Gurugram and consented to participate in the survey. These patients were given access to the test version of the software and we helped them install the mobile application on their mobiles. The feedback was obtained using a structured questionnaire designed to assess the level of satisfaction with multimedia education content. This was a 14-item questionnaire assessing opinions on a 5-point scale (1 = Poor/Strongly Disagree to 5 = Excellent/Strongly Agree) on the overall experience, quality of content, usefulness, design and functionality of the mobile application.

Development of SMS Program

One of the greatest constraints of mobile device efficacy testing is if the device is not accessed by experimental group patients and therefore, they actually don't use it as specified in the study protocol. This could impede the impact of the intervention on the patient population and influence the outcomes. Human intervention should not be implemented, e.g., contacting patients individually time and time again and asking them to use the program during the research duration. It is not feasible in the setting of real life. Therefore, we approached patients only for research briefing and later for data collection at defined time points to closely replicate real-life scenarios.

Several trials have shown effective therapeutic behavior changes and health results with utilization of SMS programs as a single m-health technique. Therefore, in this educational program we incorporated an SMS program along with the mobile application to cover those patients who may not open the application as desired and designed in the protocol. This SMS program therefore was a six-month program to be administered alongside the smartphone application to the experimental group patients. This comprised a pool of 61 short text messages.

The purpose of this SMS program was to:

- Increase patient's probability of utilizing this mobile application as needed for this study.
- Cover all patients who switched off mobile phone automatic notification feature.
- Act as an extra remembering and behavioral change mechanism for patients in study community.

Broadly three types of messages were developed in both Hindi and English. Study subjects were asked about their preferred language and based on that the messages were sent in either Hindi or English.

- General Messages Like Welcome Message; And Information About Study.
- Reminder Messages Related to Exercise, Diet, Tracking Progress etc.
- Disease Knowledge Related Messages.

Most of the messages had a link to a relevant module or section within the mobile application that contained detailed information on the topic. All SMSs were kept short and straight forward referring to details in the mobile applications if needed.

2.2. HRQOL Study Tool

We used RAND 36-Item Health Survey (Version 1.0) in our study as it was freely available for both use and analysis. RAND-36 comprises 36 items that evaluate eight health concepts. These eight domains are enlisted below:

- 10 item Physical functioning
- 4 item Role limitations caused by physical health problems
- 3 item Role limitations caused by emotional problems
- 2 item Social functioning
- 5 item Emotional well- being
- 4 item Energy/fatigue
- 2 item Pain, and
- 5 items General health perceptions.

To self-administer RAND-36 it takes about 7-10 minutes. Additionally, administering RAND-36 by telephone or in person is also possible. In addition to the 8 domain scales, component summary scores for physical and mental health can also be calculated. The reliability and validity of the tool has been tested in multiple languages, including in elderly populations (Hays and Morales 2001).

While there is no "gold standard" in the field of QoL science, the SF-36 has gained such a high reputation among researchers that it is often referred to as the "gold standard" for health status instruments (Michalos, Zumbo, and Hubley 2000). Despite small variations, SF-36 and RAND-36 have been shown to be strongly correlated in studies previously performed (Hays and Morales 2001; Orwelius et al. 2018). RAND-36 questionnaire is also demonstrated to be suitable for and comprehensible to lay persons in the Indian population (Sinha, Van Den Heuvel, and Arokiasamy 2013).

RAND-36 was assessed using the score guidelines on their website https://www.rand.org/health-care/surveys_tools/mos/36-item-short-form/scoring.html

2.3. m-Health Study Details

- *Study Design:* Open label, randomized, experimental clinical study in CAD patients. Study population was divided into two categories: Experimental group received Happy heart program along with ongoing hospital medical care compared against a Non-experimental group received the usual pharmacological medical care only.
- *Study Site:* Cardiology outpatient department (OPD) of Paras Hospitals, Gurugram, Haryana, India. This is a reputed tertiary care hospital located in the heart of Gurugram, Haryana.
- *Study Duration:* The study was conducted for a period of 6 months with a follow up at 9 months from enrollment in the study.
- *Sample Size*: A total of 312 patients were enrolled in the study.

  Inclusion Criteria:

  - Patients above 18 years and below 75 years of age
  - Patients of both sexes
  - Patients diagnosed of Coronary artery disease
  - Patients who owned an android based smartphone and were comfortable using it
  - Patients attending cardiology outpatient department (OPD)
  - Patients who consented to participate in the study.

  Exclusion Criteria:

  - Patients below 18 years, and elderly patients more than 75 years of age
  - Pregnant and lactating women
  - Patients with malignancy

    - Patients with any debilitating, life threatening serious systemic illness.

  Based on age, we divided the patients into three groups:

  - Young age - 25-45 years
  - Middle age - 46–65 years
  - Elderly - 65-75 years.

- *Ethical Considerations:* This research was carried out in accordance with the Basic Principles defined in US 21 CFR Part 312.20 and ICH (09 May 1997) 'Guidance for Good Clinical Practice' and the principles enunciated in the Declaration of Helsinki (Edinburgh, October 2000).
- *Institutional Review Board:* Study was commenced after obtaining approval from Independent Ethics Committee (IEC) of Paras Hospital, Gurgaon.
- *Confidentiality of Data:* The data identifying each study subject by name will be kept confidential and used only for research purposes.
- *Study Conduction Description:* Figure 2 gives an overall process flow for the conduction of this study.

All patients who were recruited were randomized into experimental or non-experimental categories. Data was collected by both groups at three time points. The baseline data assessment was donc for the experimental group, then a 6-month trial was made, and then once again the data was obtained. After 6 months the experiment was stopped, and the data was collected again, 3 months later. Data was obtained 3 times at baseline, 6- and 9- months for the non-experimental group, without any intervention.

The overall intervention programme was a structured systematic program, administered in a phase-wise fashion to patients in experimental group. Patients were able to see a limited content after installing the smartphone application. New content was introduced each week. The SMS delivered to the same patients synced with the progress of their mobile application thus ensuring that SMS reminders are matching with the relevant content available to the patient at a particular stage of the overall program.

Rationale for structured approach was:

- To improve user's engagement by providing new content every week.
- To ensure users get sufficient time to go through a small piece of content rather than giving a big amount of information together.
- To build on the patient's education level in a phase wise gradual manner.

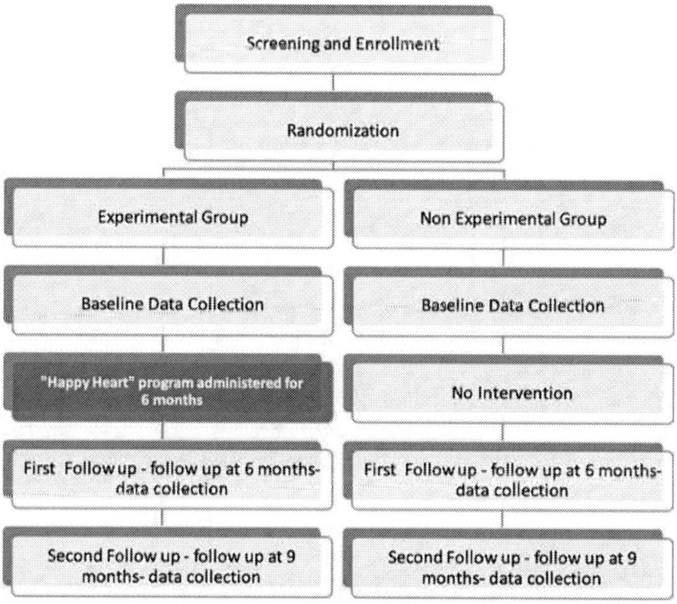

Figure 2. Study conduction process flow.

Statistical Analysis

A socio-demographic and disease characteristic analysis of the study sample was done. The general health status analysis of the entire study population was performed at the baseline to assess the homogeneity of the sample. We used MS Excel™ for the descriptive analysis and statistical analysis was done using R Statistical Software, version 3.6.1. Post scoring of RAND-36 domain and component summary scores both parametric and non-parametric tests were done to analyze the impact of our study intervention on the health status of study population. ANOVA test were done on the final HRQOL scores obtained for all subjects at all time points. We also summarized the score into two summary components, one for physical (PCS) and one for Mental components (MCS). ANOVA tests were carried out to test our study hypotheses as under:

$H0_1$: There is no significant positive effect of the m-health education program on the HRQOL of patients in the experimental group as compared to the non-experimental group.

OR

There is no significant difference between the HRQOL scores of experimental versus non-experimental groups at baseline,6 and 9 months.

$H1_1$: There is a significant positive effect of the m-health education program on the HRQOL of patients in the experimental group as compared to the non-experimental group.

OR

There is a significant difference between the HRQOL scores of experimental versus non-experimental groups at baseline,6 and 9 months.

RESULTS

Development of Mobile Application

A mobile application based on Android™ named Happy Heart was designed and developed. This application is available at the Google Play store on https://play.google.com/store/applications/details?id = com. consultancy.adsam.happyheart.happyheart.

The content of the application was finalized and arranged in 6 modules as summarized in Figure 3.

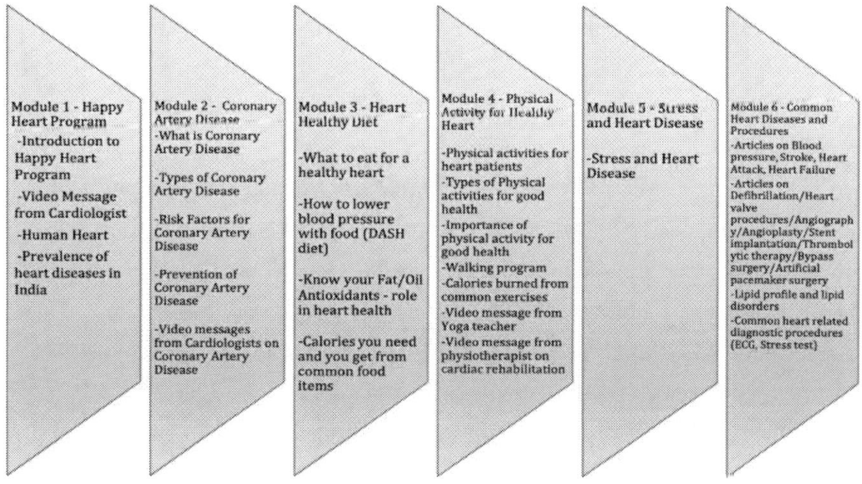

Figure 3. Happy Heart mobile application module wise content composition.

Expert Assessment Using MARS Tool

MARS tool was used by 3 software engineers and 2 healthcare providers to rate this application. Happy Heart mobile application scored a mean MARS score of 3.60 ± 0.86. This was above average as rated by the experts. The subjectivity score for the app was 3.30 ± 1.03. Engagement score was (2.84 ± 0.80), the lowest among all. Functionality score was (4.05 ± 0.68), highest of all assessed parameters. The descriptive statistics for this analysis is plotted in Table 4.

Table 4. MARS core criteria assessment for Happy Heart mobile application

Domain	Mean	SD	Max	Min
Engagement	2,84	0,80	5,00	2,00
Functionality	4,05	0,69	5,00	3,00
Aesthetics	3,67	0,72	5,00	2,00
Information	3,86	0,69	5,00	3,00
Application subjective quality	3,30	1,03	5,00	1,00

Note: MARS = Mobile Application Rating Scale.

User Satisfaction Evaluation

Table 5 summarizes the user feedback survey done for our mobile application.

Thirty-five CAD patients participated in this survey (Mean age 54, 22.86% female; 77.14% male). A total of 57.14% were from urban regions while 42.86% patients belonged to rural areas. Majority of the patients (54.28%) were graduate or above.

A total of 97% users agreed that *"This application is a useful tool to improve knowledge & awareness about heart diseases"* and *"The application was a useful tool for self-learning"*. Majority (95%) of the users were satisfied with the usefulness of the program. A total of 94% participants agreed that *"This application is a useful tool to help in prevention and management of heart diseases"*. More than 91% agreed that *"Applying the given information can lead to a healthy lifestyle". A total of* 89% reported that *"Content structure is appropriate for the purpose of this application";* that *"Overall composition of the application is appropriate"*, and *"It is easy to use the application"*. A total of 86% users reported that *"The design, color, font size of the content is appropriate"*. In summary, 95% users were satisfied with the usefulness of the application; almost 80% were satisfied with the quality of content and 67% were satisfied with the design, layout and functionality of this application.

Table 5. Result of user satisfaction survey for "Happy Heart" mobile application

Domains (N = 35)	Mean	SD	% users who rated the application >4
Overall experience	4.09	0.70	80%
Quality of content	4.30	0.77	80.95%
Usefulness	4.44	0.59	95%
Design and functionality	4.44	0.60	67%

Demographic and Clinical Analysis of Study Population

In the present study a total of 312 diagnosed cases of Coronary artery disease (CAD) were recruited in an outpatient clinical setting of a North Indian tertiary care center. A total of 74.68% were male and 25.32% females. Mean age of the study population was 57.64 ± 10.63 years. Majority of the patients (60.90%) who participated in this study came from urban dwelling. Out of the total study population, a large percentage of patients were educated. A total of 48.4% were graduates and above, 24.68% had education up to 10th and 26.92% had completed their education until grade 12.

Risk factors were recorded at the baseline for the study population (Figure 3). A large percentage of patients had a history of smoking (74.68%) while 39.74% were smoking during the study period. Other risk factors were also found to be prevalent. 55.77% patients were hypertensive, 40.06% were diabetic, and 37.18% had dyslipidemia.

The burden of risk factors was similar in both groups at baseline. History of smoking was the most prevalent risk factor in both groups (121 in experimental vs 112 in non-experimental groups). Hypertension (91 in experimental vs 83 in non-experimental group) and diabetes (60 in experimental vs 65 in non-experimental group) were the top most comorbidities.

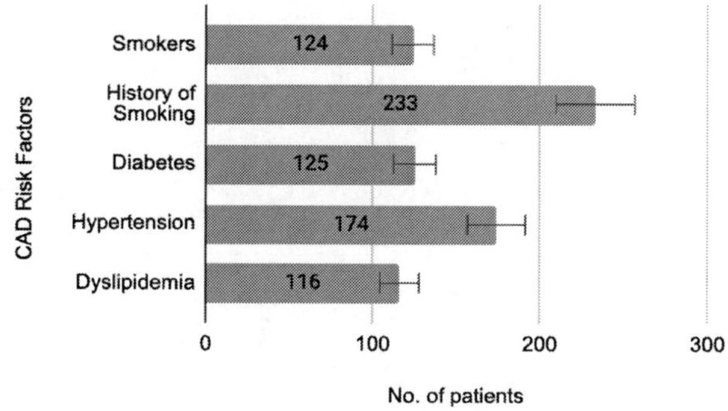

Figure 4. Risk factor characterization of study population at baseline.

HRQOL Analysis for Patient Health Status (RAND-36)

A total of 312 patients were administered the RAND-36 questionnaire. Equal number of patients were randomized to experimental and non-experimental groups (n = 156). All eight domain scores along with PCS and MCS summary scores were calculated as per RAND-36 scoring protocol for overall study population. There was a dropout of 11.22% at first follow up at 6 months and of 25% for second follow up at 9 months.

Health Status at Baseline

Firstly, we analyzed the health status of our study population at baseline. Table 6 gives Mean ± SD of overall study population for all eight HRQOL domains at the baseline.

Overall health status of the population was found to be much lower than normal. MCS was 40.27 ± 13.91, while PCS was 36.52 ± 10.32. In terms of individual domain scores, RE was highest (52.24 ± 50.03) and PF was the lowest scoring domain (40.78 ± 24.03). Table 7 summarizes component summary and individual domain scores for experimental and non-experimental groups at baseline as per age, gender, dwelling and education.

Table 6. HRQOL domain scores for overall study population at baseline

Domain	Code	Mean	SD
Physical component summary	PCS	36.52	10.32
Mental component summary	MCS	40.27	13.91
Physical functioning	PF	40.78	24.03
Role Functioning/Physical	RP	51.68	47.01
Bodily Pain	BP	48.04	32.85
Energy/Fatigue	VT	42.26	26.49
Social Functioning	SF	51.16	29.14
Role Functioning/Emotional	RE	52.24	50.03
Emotional well being	MH	49.99	22.98
General Health	GH	46.39	22.03

Table 7. Group wise HRQOL scores at baseline for different variables

Variable			PCS		MCS		PF		RP		BP		VT		SF		RE		MH		GH	
Gender		N	Mean	SD	Mean	SD	Mean	SD	Mean	SD	Mean	SD	Mean	SD	Mean	SD	Mean	SD	Mean	SD	Mean	SD
Male	Exp	116	37.40	9.52	40.50	14.59	44.35	22.72	56.68	46.20	45.65	31.09	42.87	26.16	51.40	30.52	54.31	50.03	51.17	24.22	48.68	21.53
	NE	117	37.74	10.83	42.33	13.20	42.48	24.82	56.41	47.13	53.85	33.86	46.27	26.71	54.81	28.09	59.83	49.24	52.89	21.50	49.47	22.37
Female	Exp	40	35.07	11.14	38.01	12.37	36.88	23.71	44.38	46.85	45.38	36.52	38.67	23.88	48.13	26.64	42.50	50.06	46.20	20.83	41.50	20.98
	NE	39	31.75	8.93	35.72	14.52	29.10	22.47	30.13	43.75	40.51	29.16	32.14	27.23	42.63	29.49	33.33	47.76	41.64	23.92	35.38	19.88
Age (yrs)																						
25-45	Exp	23	43.03	8.24	41.20	15.21	65.87	16.49	66.30	43.70	51.20	32.01	48.12	25.82	58.70	30.49	60.87	49.90	55.48	24.87	54.78	21.08
	NE	15	47.04	8.04	48.39	10.42	74.33	15.22	86.67	35.19	68.50	28.20	59.56	22.88	70.00	21.55	86.67	35.19	68.53	18.01	62.67	19.72
46-65	Exp	92	37.88	9.47	40.90	14.20	44.51	19.87	58.70	46.06	48.70	32.55	44.28	25.61	52.31	30.33	56.52	49.84	51.39	23.37	48.42	21.21
	NE	85	36.93	10.62	39.21	13.43	41.88	22.28	50.00	49.85	50.06	33.61	42.04	26.92	49.71	27.82	50.59	50.29	48.05	21.70	44.56	22.33
66-75	Exp	41	30.89	9.11	36.77	12.91	24.62	19.34	34.76	44.68	35.43	30.98	32.68	23.56	42.07	25.58	34.15	48.01	43.41	21.88	38.82	20.60
	NE	56	32.30	9.18	40.84	14.61	25.54	19.69	39.73	42.31	46.38	32.65	39.29	28.16	50.00	30.71	48.21	50.42	48.21	23.09	43.57	22.09
Locality																						
Urban	Exp	96	38.84	9.46	41.54	14.10	47.37	22.34	63.02	43.83	49.74	30.99	45.00	25.74	53.91	29.54	59.38	49.37	53.21	22.80	50.23	21.35
	NE	94	37.45	10.60	41.91	13.76	42.82	24.40	55.05	47.32	52.39	33.67	45.46	28.15	54.26	27.28	58.51	49.53	52.26	22.73	48.16	22.68
Rural	Exp	60	33.54	9.99	37.17	13.68	34.54	22.34	38.33	47.05	38.92	33.85	36.67	24.69	45.21	28.94	38.33	49.03	44.60	23.65	41.42	20.93
	NE	62	34.41	10.63	38.81	13.74	33.55	24.72	41.94	47.21	47.66	32.45	38.60	26.03	47.98	30.88	45.16	50.17	46.77	22.14	42.58	22.12
Education																						
Till 10th	Exp	34	33.09	9.84	36.32	13.64	33.45	21.60	35.29	46.10	38.01	35.40	35.29	23.70	44.49	30.49	35.29	48.51	42.82	24.03	39.85	19.98
	NE	43	34.23	10.20	39.32	14.10	31.16	22.49	41.28	45.61	51.57	33.96	39.53	25.63	48.55	29.28	46.51	50.47	46.98	23.50	41.74	22.49
Till 12th	Exp	39	37.50	10.45	40.63	13.97	44.10	25.13	55.77	47.80	48.21	31.94	42.74	24.98	50.96	30.54	53.85	50.50	52.31	23.52	48.72	22.73
	NE	45	35.38	10.66	39.62	14.02	37.67	24.56	45.56	47.76	46.11	32.74	39.41	29.50	50.28	29.97	48.89	50.55	48.53	21.57	46.33	22.06
Above Grad	Exp	83	38.00	9.54	40.95	14.19	45.33	22.08	59.94	44.68	47.44	31.34	44.02	26.44	52.86	28.65	56.63	49.86	51.66	22.81	48.82	21.27
	NE	68	38.08	10.84	42.24	13.50	45.15	25.27	58.09	47.99	52.76	33.15	46.96	26.97	54.78	27.91	60.29	49.29	53.06	22.56	48.35	22.86

Note: Exp = Experimental; NE = Non-experimental; PCS = Physical component summary; MCS = Mental component summary; PF = Physical functioning; RP = Role Functioning/Physical; BP = Bodily Pain; VT = Energy/Fatigue; SF = Social Functioning; RE = Role Functioning/Emotional; MH = Emotional well-being; GH = General Health.

Table 8. Group wise HRQOL scores at first follow up for different variables

Variable			PCS		MCS		PF		RP		BP		VT		SF		RE		MH		GH	
Gender		N	Mean	SD	Mean	SD	Mean	SD	Mean	SD	Mean	SD	Mean	SD	Mean	SD	Mean	SD	Mean	SD	Mean	SD
Male	Exp	102	45.51	9.47	49.36	12.69	63.31	22.06	82.35	38.31	68.36	29.62	62.42	27.20	71.08	28.36	82.35	38.31	67.98	23.57	67.66	23.56
	NE	102	43.84	10.97	48.14	11.65	57.45	24.40	78.43	41.33	68.63	32.32	58.82	26.09	67.65	27.66	78.43	41.33	65.57	20.82	62.03	25.72
Female	Exp	38	42.98	12.97	45.96	13.22	55.92	29.38	68.42	47.11	65.79	37.20	55.61	28.80	64.47	31.51	68.42	47.11	62.74	24.66	61.64	27.56
	NE	35	36.76	9.96	40.00	14.57	41.86	21.59	54.29	50.54	49.86	31.86	40.00	27.10	49.29	27.94	54.29	50.54	50.74	25.68	44.43	23.00
Age (yrs)																						
25-45	Exp	19	47.84	8.80	46.69	11.82	76.45	18.55	84.21	37.46	66.84	25.29	60.35	23.67	68.42	25.47	84.21	37.46	64.05	21.36	64.08	24.14
	NE	15	48.53	8.85	49.64	10.91	77.67	19.44	86.67	35.19	73.00	28.46	63.56	25.43	74.17	22.39	86.67	35.19	71.73	19.91	67.67	21.62
45-65	Exp	87	45.23	10.51	48.92	13.02	61.81	23.31	79.31	40.74	68.62	32.01	62.07	27.92	70.40	30.63	79.31	40.74	67.37	23.74	67.89	25.09
	NE	74	42.66	10.98	46.10	12.82	56.22	22.54	72.97	44.71	64.19	33.06	55.31	27.18	63.85	28.71	72.97	44.71	61.84	22.33	57.79	26.94
65-75	Exp	34	42.10	11.17	48.16	13.34	51.55	25.85	73.53	44.78	65.66	34.88	56.86	29.60	66.91	28.35	73.53	44.78	65.88	26.11	62.35	24.43
	NE	48	39.02	11.14	44.87	13.63	41.67	22.56	66.67	47.64	60.42	34.61	49.03	28.17	58.07	30.01	66.67	47.64	58.58	24.41	53.96	25.76
Locality																						
Urban	Exp	85	45.56	10.26	49.05	12.87	63.44	22.92	80.00	40.24	70.09	30.54	62.12	28.08	71.03	29.64	80.00	40.24	68.11	23.18	67.04	25.33
	NE	82	43.26	11.11	46.83	13.12	57.26	24.42	74.39	43.92	66.16	33.52	56.34	28.98	65.55	27.33	74.39	43.92	63.61	23.94	60.08	26.41
Rural	Exp	55	43.68	10.97	47.48	12.94	58.01	26.34	76.36	42.88	63.91	33.44	58.18	27.20	66.59	28.77	76.36	42.88	64.16	25.00	64.45	23.97
	NE	55	40.20	10.99	44.91	12.61	47.82	23.99	69.09	46.64	60.36	32.52	50.54	25.03	59.09	30.66	69.09	46.64	59.05	21.44	53.73	25.48
Education																						
Till 10th	Exp	31	41.60	12.40	44.87	13.38	52.60	27.92	67.74	47.52	58.79	38.54	54.19	28.01	61.29	32.65	67.74	47.52	58.58	24.97	59.31	24.96
	NE	37	40.98	10.31	45.91	12.63	46.49	22.11	72.97	45.02	66.55	32.96	53.69	23.57	60.14	29.73	72.97	45.02	60.11	22.10	54.59	23.40
Till 12th	Exp	33	47.58	7.34	51.20	10.50	67.35	18.83	90.91	29.19	74.09	21.87	65.45	22.26	73.48	25.34	90.91	29.19	72.00	19.97	72.69	19.17
	NE	40	40.65	11.81	44.66	12.93	51.13	25.51	67.50	47.43	58.19	33.82	48.83	28.42	61.25	29.66	67.50	47.43	59.40	22.38	56.00	27.20
Above Grad	Exp	76	44.93	10.67	48.69	13.42	62.23	24.28	77.63	41.95	68.49	31.89	61.05	29.50	70.72	29.19	77.63	41.95	67.45	24.47	65.87	26.29
	NE	60	43.59	11.12	47.09	13.18	59.33	24.45	75.00	43.67	65.92	32.86	57.67	28.99	65.83	27.80	75.00	43.67	64.40	24.03	60.36	27.12

Note: Exp = Experimental; NE = Non-experimental; PCS = Physical component summary; MCS = Mental component summary; PF = Physical functioning; RP = Role Functioning/Physical; BP = Bodily Pain; VT = Energy/Fatigue; SF = Social Functioning; RE = Role Functioning/Emotional; MH = Emotional well-being; GH = General Health.

Table 9. Group wise HRQOL scores at second follow up for different variables

Variable			PCS		MCS		PF		RP		BP		VT		SF		RE		MH		GH	
Gender		N	Mean	SD	Mean	SD	Mean	SD	Mean	SD	Mean	SD	Mean	SD	Mean	SD	Mean	SD	Mean	SD	Mean	SD
Male	Exp	86	40.79	12.03	43.69	14.26	50.91	29.01	73.26	44.52	57.24	34.87	49.77	31.89	56.40	33.36	73.26	44.52	55.21	23.50	51.93	32.29
	NE	84	39.70	12.67	44.06	13.61	46.79	28.56	72.62	44.86	57.74	37.51	49.60	31.12	56.25	34.08	72.62	44.86	55.43	27.18	49.21	33.70
Female	Exp	34	36.24	12.85	37.98	14.34	39.40	30.72	52.94	50.66	47.21	36.28	38.63	29.76	45.22	33.71	52.94	50.66	44.71	27.67	41.40	29.92
	NE	30	33.53	10.40	37.06	15.47	29.83	22.95	53.33	50.74	45.25	32.73	32.44	29.44	40.00	34.49	53.33	50.74	42.00	28.82	33.67	28.34
Age (Yrs)																						
25-45	Exp	17	41.38	12.03	40.84	13.39	59.35	28.59	70.59	46.97	51.03	33.03	44.71	28.94	56.62	29.69	70.59	46.97	49.65	26.31	46.91	33.85
	NE	14	38.20	10.92	39.21	12.78	48.93	27.75	71.43	46.88	45.36	31.47	39.05	26.13	49.11	33.42	71.43	46.88	44.00	26.16	37.50	31.42
45-65	Exp	72	40.01	11.98	43.16	14.11	47.65	26.78	72.22	45.10	55.52	35.51	48.98	31.19	55.03	33.48	72.22	45.10	53.06	27.59	50.68	31.66
	NE	59	38.95	12.98	43.13	14.89	44.75	29.12	69.49	46.44	57.54	37.97	47.12	34.22	53.60	36.63	69.49	46.44	54.44	28.65	46.78	34.28
66-75	Exp	31	37.29	13.55	40.20	15.97	41.22	35.74	54.84	50.59	53.63	37.39	42.15	34.23	47.18	36.47	54.84	50.59	51.74	32.51	46.05	32.06
	NE	41	36.78	12.10	41.94	14.34	36.59	26.37	63.41	48.77	53.11	36.40	44.23	29.35	50.61	33.18	63.41	48.77	50.93	28.10	45.34	31.99
Locality																						
Urban	Exp	73	40.64	12.23	43.21	14.14	50.85	28.65	73.97	44.18	56.23	35.95	48.95	31.80	55.31	33.78	73.97	44.18	53.81	28.14	50.29	32.87
	NE	66	37.80	12.24	40.74	14.53	42.80	27.15	63.64	48.47	52.16	35.94	43.54	31.69	49.62	34.25	63.64	48.47	49.27	28.09	43.64	32.74
Rural	Exp	47	37.74	12.55	40.29	14.91	42.66	31.24	57.45	49.98	51.54	34.76	42.98	31.23	50.00	33.68	57.45	49.98	49.79	29.31	46.86	30.49
	NE	48	38.45	12.67	44.25	14.08	41.67	29.67	72.92	44.91	57.60	37.61	47.22	31.42	55.21	35.62	72.92	44.91	55.50	28.06	47.16	33.54
Education																						
Till 10th	Exp	27	34.26	12.13	36.04	15.07	33.89	27.57	40.74	50.07	43.52	36.08	36.30	31.07	38.89	34.38	40.74	50.07	42.96	27.68	40.51	28.91
	NE	32	38.44	12.33	43.96	13.41	40.16	27.10	75.00	43.99	57.81	38.66	46.88	29.89	54.69	34.45	75.00	43.99	53.50	25.98	46.37	31.75
Till 12th	Exp	31	43.44	11.03	45.92	12.37	56.25	27.06	83.87	37.39	63.71	32.70	54.19	27.90	62.50	29.40	83.87	37.39	58.32	27.82	57.18	31.31
	NE	34	36.82	12.07	40.88	14.28	40.44	28.24	61.76	49.33	51.10	35.88	41.37	29.85	48.16	34.83	61.76	49.33	50.94	27.44	42.94	31.31
Above Grad	Exp	62	39.81	12.51	42.77	14.54	49.33	30.46	70.97	45.76	54.48	35.63	47.31	32.79	54.84	33.90	70.97	45.76	53.23	28.72	48.51	32.82
	NE	48	38.72	12.79	42.01	15.25	45.10	29.02	66.67	47.64	54.58	36.24	46.53	33.98	52.86	35.47	66.67	47.64	51.50	30.43	45.83	35.45

Note: Exp = Experimental; NE = Non-experimental; PCS = Physical component summary; MCS = Mental component summary; PF = Physical functioning; RP = Role Functioning/Physical; BP = Bodily Pain; VT = Energy/Fatigue; SF = Social Functioning; RE = Role Functioning/Emotional; MH = Emotional well-being; GH = General Health.

Health Status at First Follow Up (6 Months)

Table 8 summarizes component summary and individual domain scores at 6-months follow up as per age, gender, dwelling and education divided for experimental and non-experimental groups. This was the first and primary follow up time point for data collection. Intervention given to experimental group patients was stopped after 6 months. A total of 277 patients completed the survey and gave data at this time point.

Health Status at Second Follow Up (9 Months)

Table 9 summarizes component summary and individual domain scores at 9-months follow up as per age, gender, dwelling and education divided for experimental and non-experimental groups. This was the second follow up time point for data collection. A total of 234 patients completed the survey and gave data at this time point.

Comparative Analysis of RAND-36 Scores

To understand the impact of our study intervention on the health status of our patient population, we conducted One-way Analysis of Variance (ANOVA) and Kruskal Wallis tests on the results of the RAND-36 survey done at baseline, first and second follow up.

Figure 5 illustrates the HRQOL scores at all the three time points for overall study population.

Figure 6 and Figure 7 compile the comparative HRQOL scores at study time points for experimental and non-experimental groups respectively. The results in both groups follow the similar trend but the amount of improvement in the experimental group was found to be higher than non-experimental group.

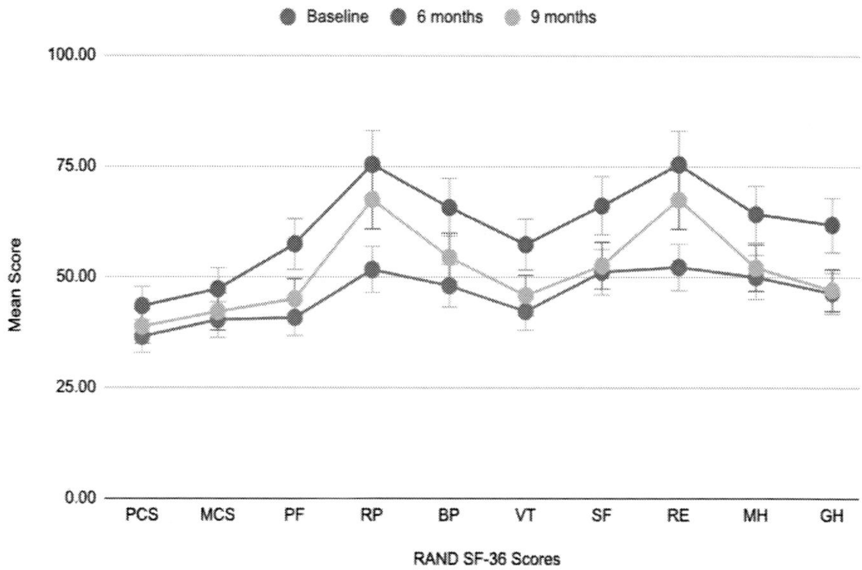

Figure 5. HRQOL scores at baseline, first and second follow up for overall population.

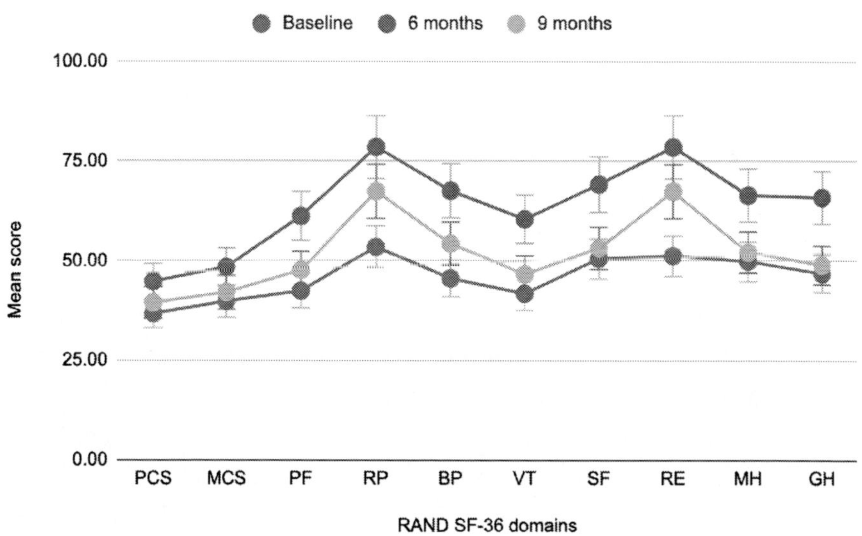

Figure 6. HRQOL scores at baseline, first and second follow up for experimental group.

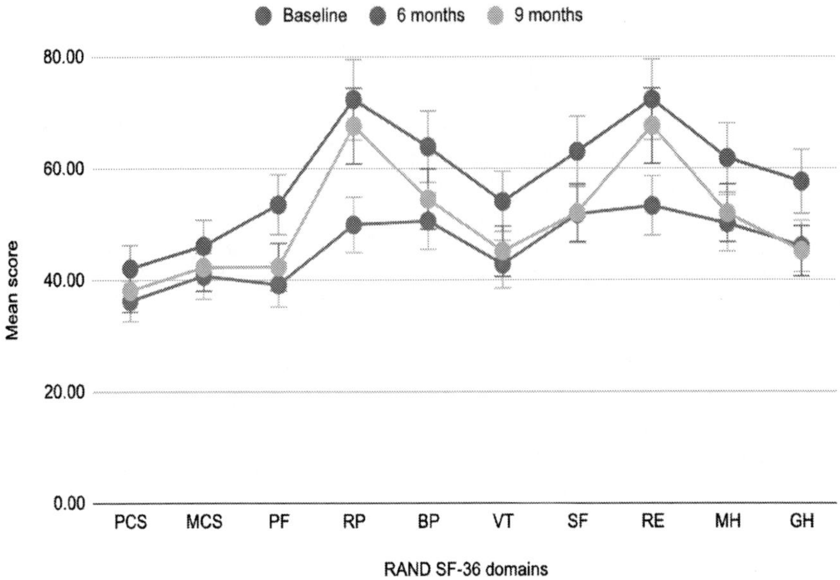

Figure 7. HRQOL scores at baseline, first and second follow up for non-experimental group.

Results from One-Way Analysis of Variance (ANOVA) for HRQOL

ANOVA tests compared the changes in RAND-36 scores individually for each group from Baseline to first follow up, from first to second follow up, and for overall study period from baseline to second follow up. Table 10 summarizes the level of significance (p and t values) obtained from ANOVA analysis to compare HRQOL score for overall study population at all three time points. Results show that there was a significant improvement in all HRQOL parameters in both the groups from baseline to first follow up ($p < 0.005$). At baseline PCS score was 36.80 ± 10.32 that changed to 43.44 ± 10.91 at first follow up. At baseline MCS score was 40.27 ± 13.91 that changed to 47.26 ± 12.92 at first follow up. The percentage change for PCS was 21.78%; and for MCS was 21.51% from baseline to first follow up.

Table 10. ANOVA for HRQOL of overall study population at baseline, first and second follow up

Domain	Group	Baseline to Fu1		Fu1 to Fu2		Baseline to Fu2		DF
		T value	P value	T value	P value	T value	P value	
MCS	Exp	29.72	0.00*	14.09	0.00*	1.64	0.20	274
	NE	11.78	0.00*	4.95	0.03*	0.79	0.37	268
PCS	Exp	45.16	0.00*	14.01	0.00*	4.01	0.05*	274
	NE	20.61	0.00*	7.10	0.01*	1.70	0.19	268
GH	Exp	50.82	0.00*	23.60	0.00*	0.43	0.51	274
	NE	16.59	0.00*	11.06	0.00*	0.06	0.81	268
RP	Exp	23.82	0.00*	4.10	0.04*	6.06	0.01*	274
	NE	17.07	0.00*	0.66	0.42	9.21	0.00*	268
BP	Exp	34.90	0.00*	10.14	0.00*	4.63	0.03*	274
	NE	11.78	0.00*	4.54	0.03*	0.85	0.36	268
PF	Exp	46.69	0.00*	16.51	0.00*	2.67	0.10	274
	NE	24.47	0.00*	11.21	0.00*	0.97	0.33	268
VT	Exp	36.74	0.00*	14.41	0.00*	1.96	0.16	274
	NE	12.29	0.00*	5.74	0.02*	0.43	0.51	268
SF	Exp	29.91	0.00*	16.90	0.00*	0.49	0.48	274
	NE	11.01	0.00*	7.49	0.01*	0.00	0.96	268
RE	Exp	25.83	0.00*	4.10	0.04	7.49	0.01*	274
	NE	11.63	0.00*	0.66	0.42	5.69	0.02*	268
MH	Exp	36.60	0.00*	19.39	0.00*	0.56	0.46	274
	NE	19.25	0.00*	9.39	0.00*	0.35	0.56	268

Note: * signifies statistically significant difference ($p < 0.05$); Exp = Experimental; FU1 = First Follow up; FU2 = Second Follow up; NE = Non-experimental; PCS = Physical component summary; MCS = Mental component summary; PF = Physical functioning; RP = Role Functioning/Physical; BP = Bodily Pain; VT = Energy/Fatigue; SF = Social Functioning; RE = Role Functioning/Emotional; MH = Emotional well-being; GH = General Health

Comparing study results for 6- and 9-months' time points illustrate a drop in all HRQOL scores in both groups. This shows that the improvement observed in the experimental group that may be attributed to the study intervention didn't sustain for next 3 months once the intervention was stopped. At first follow up, PCS score was 43.44 ± 10.91 that decreased to 38.81 ± 12.37 at second follow up. At first follow up MCS score was 47.26 ± 12.92 that changed to 42.14 ± 14.39 at second follow up. For both the groups we saw a statistically significant decline in scores from first follow up to second follow up. The only exception was RP and RE scores for non-experimental groups that didn't show any significant difference when measured at these two time points. If we look at overall study duration from baseline to second follow up, for most of the components there was no statistically significant difference in the final scores when compared to baseline. There was statistically significant improvement in PCS score exclusively in the experimental group. This indicates that the physical health status of the experimental group improved during the study period indicating that physical health ability of the participants in the experimental group improved. An exclusive improvement was also seen in BP scores of experimental groups. Statistically significant improvement in both the groups were noted for RP, and RE scores as well.

Results from Kruskal Wallis Analysis

We used Kruskal Wallis test to compare the results of the experimental group to those of non-experimental groups at different time points. In this analysis we first calculated the difference in mean between the results of experimental and non-experimental groups separately from baseline to first follow up, first to second follow up and baseline to second follow up. Then we applied Kruskal Wallis test to determine if there was a statistically significant difference between these changes or not. This specifically tests our hypothesis to determine if our m-health intervention had any impact on the study results or not.

Table 11 demonstrates changes in domain and summary scores for all groups at baseline, first and second follow-up. As noted, the ‘p’ values are above 0.05 for all scores calculated at the baseline for both groups. This suggests that the HRQOL of both groups was equivalent at the baseline level. In other words, we should conclude that there was no statistically significant difference between the HRQOL of both groups when we started the experiment.

Table 11. Kruskal Wallis test to compare HRQOL scores between experimental and non-experimental groups

Domain	Baseline		FU1		p value (Baseline)	Change (Baseline - FU1)		P value (FU1)	FU 2		Change-(FU1-FU2)		Change (Baseline-FU2)		p value (FU2)	DF
	Exp	NE	Exp	NE		Exp	NE		Exp	NE	Exp	NE	Exp	NE		
PCS	36.80±9.97	36.24±10.68	44.821±10.54	42.02±11.12	0.47	8.02	5.79	0.01*	39.49±12.38	38.07±12.37	-5.32	-3.95	2.70	1.83	0.00*	268.00
MCS	39.85±14.05	40.67±13.79	48.43±12.87	46.05±12.90	0.57	8.57	5.38	0.09	42.06±14.45	42.22±14.38	-6.36	-3.84	2.21	1.54	0.01*	268.00
PF	42.43±23.13	39.12±24.86	61.30±24.37	53.46±24.60	0.18	18.87	14.33	0.00*	47.64±29.83	42.32±28.11	-13.66	-11.14	5.21	3.19	0.00*	268.00
RP	53.52±46.52	49.83±47.56	78.57±41.17	72.26±44.93	0.14	25.05	22.42	0.22	67.5±47.03	67.54±47.02	-11.07	-4.72	13.97	17.70	0.99	268.00
BP	45.57±32.44	50.51±33.16	67.66±31.73	63.83±33.12	0.17	22.08	13.32	0.37	54.39±35.41	54.45±36.58	-13.26	-9.38	8.82	3.94	0.99	268.00
VT	41.79±25.58	42.73±27.44	60.57±27.7	54.01±27.5	0.74	18.78	11.28	0.02*	46.61±31.58	45.08±31.48	-13.96	-8.93	4.82	2.35	0.01*	268.00
SF	50.56±29.52	51.76±28.83	69.28±29.28	62.95±28.77	0.90	18.72	11.19	0.04*	53.22±33.70	51.97±34.78	-16.06	-10.98	2.67	0.21	0.01*	268.00
RE	51.28±50.14	53.20±50.05	78.57±41.17	72.26±44.93	0.73	27.29	19.06	0.22	67.5±47.03	67.54±47.02	-11.07	-4.72	16.22	14.34	0.99	268.00
MH	49.89±23.43	50.07±22.58	66.55±23.89	61.78±22.99	0.84	16.66	11.70	0.09	52.23±28.55	51.89±28.12	-14.32	-9.89	2.34	1.82	0.01*	268.00
GH	46.83±21.55	45.94±22.55	66.02±24.75	57.53±26.13	0.69	19.19	11.58	0.00*	48.94±31.87	45.12±32.97	-17.08	-12.41	2.11	-0.82	0.02*	268.00

Note: All values presented as Mean ± SD; * signifies statistically significant difference ($p < 0.05$); Exp = Experimental; FU1 = First Follow up; FU2 = Second Follow up; NE = Non-experimental; PCS = Physical component summary; MCS = Mental component summary; PF = Physical functioning; RP = Role Functioning/Physical; BP = Bodily Pain; VT = Energy/Fatigue; SF = Social Functioning; RE = Role Functioning/Emotional; MH = Emotional well-being; GH = General Health.

Looking at the transition from baseline to the first follow-up for both groups, as seen in the ANOVA study, there has been a significant increase in both groups' ratings. However, in the experimental group, we saw a small improvement in the PCS summary score ($p = 0.01$) compared to the non-experimental group. For MCS the p value was 0.09, which is significant but at the borderline. Out of the domain scores we found that the experimental group showed statistically significant improvement in the scores for PF ($p = 0.00$), VT ($p = 0.02$), SF ($p = 0.04$), MH ($p = 0.09$) and GH ($p = 0.00$) when compared to the non-experimental group. Similarly, from first to second follow up there was a decline in scores for all domains and summary components in both the groups as shown in ANOVA analysis as well. When we look at the overall change from baseline to second follow up in both groups, we saw that overall health status of both the groups improved. However, Kruskal Wallis test results infer that the change was statistically significantly more in experimental group versus non-experimental group with regard to most of the domains. Changes in the PCS ($p = 0.09$), MCS ($p = 0.09$), PF ($p = 0.00$), VT ($p = 0.01$), SF ($p = 0.01$), MH ($p = 0.01$) and GH ($p = 0.02$) scores were found to be significantly more in the experimental group versus non-experimental group when measured from baseline to second follow up. However, the between group difference was not significant for RP, BP and RE ($p = 0.99$) domains.

DISCUSSION

m-Health technology has become widely popular as an innovative, cost effective, and extensible means of delivering patient knowledge and resources beyond the conventional health care system. Use of m-health technology in chronic disease management especially CVDs has been studied in many countries. Interventions ranged from text message alerts for drug compliance, behavioral intervention training programs, biosensors for monitoring and communication of vital factors such as blood pressure, temperature, etc. (Rehman et al. 2017; Varnfield et al. 2014; Frederix et al.

2015; Blasco et al. 2012). However, scientific studies in general have lagged behind in line with trends, leaving a large gap between hypothesis and proof about efficacy, safety and sustainability of efficacy, if any. Moreover, there is considerable potential for exploring the use of m-health services and strategies in developing economy like India. This is all the more important because, amid increasing internet and smartphone penetration, low internet self-efficacy and lack of quality health education material in local languages are India's key formidable barriers to the development and growth of m-health resources. Present project was intended to develop and test a new educational strategy that can create and distribute learning content in a convenient and inexpensive way for even less skilled smartphone users. In this study, we assessed the effects of such a mobile health-based education program on Indian CAD patients in terms of its effect on their health-related quality of life (HRQOL). The inspiration behind the creation of the Happy Heart mobile application was to meet the basic needs of our target patient population, which included primarily patients with low internet self-efficacy in Hindi-speaking, Elderly, Rural North Indian CAD.

Based on the findings of the pilot customer satisfaction survey, the Happy heart mobile application satisfied the majority of users. The findings of this analysis on customer satisfaction are close to those of Min Jung Cho in Korea (Cho, Sim, and Hwang 2014). The findings of this customer satisfaction study are promising in limited sample size, as they reflect a high degree of patient interest. This paves path for adoption and implementation of new strategies and digital tools for dissemination of disease related education and self-care for the management of chronic diseases in Indian population.

With regard to the randomized controlled trial conducted using this Happy Heart Education Program, out of 312 patients enrolled in the randomized control trial, 88.78% patients completed the study till first follow up while 75% completed the study till the second follow up at 9 months post recruitment. Almost 77% of the subjects entering the experimental arm completed the study. These results indicate that patients appreciated involvement and reflected their passion and interest for discovering new ways of learning and the associated advantages of accessing health-related knowledge. Knowing the material is available in Hindi has improved the desire to engage.

The risk factors in this population were similar to the established global CAD risk factors. A total of 57.7% of the sample population had elevated blood pressure; more than 40% had diabetes and 37% had dyslipidemia. Particularly after diagnosis of CAD, only 40 percent of patients were still smoking, but 74.7 percent of the population had a history of moderate to heavy smoking. Females from rural areas were also smoking bidi, hookah, or had exposure to smoke from cooking stove heated by burning wood, charcoal, animal dung or crop residue in rural areas. At baseline the risk factors were comparable in both groups. As reported in several other previous studies, hypertension and diabetes were the most common comorbidities in this study population.

We measured the HRQOL in our chosen sample population as the primary endpoint for this research using the widely accepted RAND-36 as our measurement tool. There is only limited data on HRQOL in rural India, and for elderly population. Our study covers both types of patients.

At baseline the HRQOL as assessed in this population was much lower than the normative values in the healthy population for both physical and mental components and all eight domain scales of the RAND-36 in this study population. This indicates a poor health status of people with CAD in India. This is consistent with all previous research in this field in various countries. PCS score was 36.52 ± 10.32 and MCS score was slightly better (40.27 ± 13.91). The mean scores of RAND-36 subscales ranged from 40.78 for physical functioning to 52.24 for RE. Results show that mental and social domain scores were better than physical capability related domains like physical functioning, energy, and general health perception. This shows that the most affected health domain among this population was the physical component. These scores indicating very low health status of individuals were similar to the ones observed in several other studies that showed markedly decreased HRQOL in chronic disease conditions (Bardage and Isacson 2001; Lam and Lauder 2000).

The mean PCS score of 36.52 in our study was way less than the PCS of 55.0 reported from Tehran (Pius, Mini, and Thankappan 2019) and from the Andhra Pradesh in India (49.0) (Varma, Kusuma, and Babu 2010) among older adults. Our PCS score was similar to the PCS value of 41.0 in the United States (Mishra and Schofield 1998). The lowest mean score of 40.78 in our study was for physical functioning. In our study, RE had the highest mean score of 52.24. A study done in Brazil also reported the highest mean score for RE (86.1) amongst all subscales. But all the subscales were much higher in this study than ours indicating comparatively poorer health status in Indian population (Lima et al. 2009). The poorer HRQOL among women in our study was similar to that reported by Ghosh in India (Ghosh 2015).

Our mean MCS score was 40.27. This was much lower than the mean MCS score (63.8) reported in a study conducted in Tehran (Tajvar, Arab, and Montazeri 2008). It was also lesser than MCS score of 52.0 reported in another similar study done in India (Varma, Kusuma, and Babu 2010). MCS score in our study was also lower than the normative MCS score of 51.0 in the USA. Mean PCS and MCS score in our study decreased with age as reported from a study done in Australia (Mishra and Schofield 1998). Highest subscale score was for RE that is one of the psychological subscales in RAND-36. This may be attributed to various underlying factors such as low self-esteem, low perception of body image and appearance, low life satisfaction, etc. However, overall psychological scores were found to be better than scores for physical subscales.

Thus, overall, we found that CAD not only adversely influences physical dimensions of RAND-36 but also the other dimensions such as MH, RE, SF, and GH. This was consistent with previous studies (Lin et al. 2011; Loos-Ayav et al. 2007). The general perception of health indicated by GH component was also found to be significantly lower than functionally normal individuals indicating that perception of general health deteriorates with declining levels of functional status (Lin et al. 2011). Social aspects were also found to be negatively impacted due to CAD in this patient population. In line with previous studies this indicates a link between functional disability and social well-being (Tough, Siegrist, and Fekete 2017).

When we compared the results of RAND-36 between both groups at baseline the p value was >0.05 for all the domains. This shows that there was no statistically significant difference between the health status of both groups at baseline before starting the intervention.

Present study was a longitudinal study. We recorded our end points at baseline, 6 months and then 9 months post recruitment. Many studies in the past have studied the impact of different interventions by observing change in HRQOL from baseline to a certain time point (3 or 6 months). Our rationale for keeping a third data collection time point was to test the long-term effect of a m-health tool even after discontinuation of the program. In this project we studied this effect at 9 months i.e., 3 months after intervention completion. This adds on value to study results as it provides evidence and data on sustainability of the results of m-health tools for a long period of time.

Statistical analysis using both parametric and non-parametric tests showed that there was an improvement in most of the HRQOL parameters from baseline to first follow up at 6 months. ANOVA test was done on the change from baseline to each time point for both groups independently. This showed improvement in both groups. One reason for positive changes in health status even in non-experimental groups may be a natural course of health improvement in most of the patients after CAD treatment. Tofighi S et al. in an Iranian study assessed HRQOL in CAD patients for 3 years. The mental health score improved while physical score decreased in this study (Tofighi et al. 2012). Similar results were observed in certain previous studies as well (Hlatky et al. 2002; 2004). Thus, these findings indicate that timely treatment of CAD with therapeutic and surgical interventions positively impacts the quality of life of individuals over time.

Current research was designed to test HRQOL in Indian CAD patients in order to identify some of its key contributors. Understanding the conditions that lead to HRQOL is essential to the creation of the most effective treatments to enhance or sustain the quality of life. In this study, it was found that not only physical but also social and emotional well-being in CAD patients was very poor relative to typical healthy individuals. This should be taken seriously as, considering the socioeconomic and family context, the physical and emotional well-being of these patients was not assumed to be very poor. This suggests that chronic conditions not only hinder patients physically, but also affect their emotional and social well-being. Family and society should pay attention to this aspect and establish policies to enhance the quality of life of their family members suffering from chronic diseases such as CAD by providing them with more social and emotional care, particularly for the elderly.

We also conducted Kruksal Wallis tests to compare the result of both groups to each other at baseline, first and second follow up. This helped to assess the impact of our study intervention. As results demonstrate there was significant improvement in the RAND-36 domain and summary component scores of experimental groups as compared to non-experimental groups for baseline to first follow up change and also in overall study duration. This test was supplementary to the ANOVA analysis. Purpose of ANOVA was to check whether HRQOL domain scores changed significantly or not for each of the groups when compared from baseline to first, first to second and baseline to second follow up. Kruskal Wallis test determined if the degree/extent of changes between two groups at each time point were significant or not. The ANOVA and Kruskal Wallis methodological analysis indicate that the quality of life of patients improved from baseline to first follow-up for both groups.

The second 9-month follow-up showed a decrease in all subscale domain scores in both groups. For the entire population, PCS decreased from 43.44 at first follow up to 38.81 at second follow up. MCS declined from 47.26 to 42.14 at the second follow-up. In both male and female patients in all categories, RP and RE ranked the highest; the lowest among both genders in the experimental group was the VT score, while PF was the lowest among both genders in the non-experimental group. The VT scale reflects the energy/fatigue level of the individual. The VT domain can be more seriously impacted because people with physical disabilities suffer from elevated levels of exhaustion and decreased levels of energy relative to individuals without disabilities.

Interestingly the net change in non-experimental group from first to second follow up was more than experimental group for all the scales. With regard to the result interpretation for the experimental group, we saw a large decline in the scores for all domains. Highest decline of 17.08 was for GH, followed by 16.06 points for SF domain, and 14.32 for MH domain. This raises concerns about sustainability and the positive effects of m-health tools on HRQOL. This also indicates that imparting education and awareness to patients is important but one-time effort may not be sufficient. A continuous reinforcement plays a critical role to ensure sustainability of lifestyle changes and maintenance of positive health outcomes. This is doable if such programs are administered to patients for long-term using cost effective strategies like m-health educational programs and other tools.

Analyses of overall study results from baseline to second follow up for HRQOL in this population revealed an improvement in both the groups. This can be attributed to the impact of continuous medical care given to both groups resulting in better HRQOL over time for the majority of the patient population. However, ANOVA and Kruskal Wallis tests reveal that the changes were significantly better in the experimental group as compared to non-experimental groups for most of the domains. Only for RP, BP and RE subscales the comparative difference between experimental and non-experimental groups was not found to be significant ($p = 0.99$). Among experimental group patients highest change from baseline to second follow up was found for RE (16.22) followed by RP (13.97) and BP (8.82). Among non-experimental groups the highest change from baseline to second follow up was found for RP (17.70) followed by RE (14.34).

Overall results from this study suggest positive impact of our study intervention that was a m-health based patient education program on the HRQOL of CAD patients from North India.

CONCLUSION

Digital technologies have rapidly been used worldwide to strengthen public health services. Mobile telephones and SMS are highly attractive options to use as a tool for self-help interventions for public health benefits, particularly for chronic disease management in resource-constrained emerging economies. m-Health could be a viable way to address the evolving problems of inadequate health and patient education related concerns in India. Increased m-health programs in this setting could mitigate the incidence of high-risk factors by promoting HRQOL and enhancing primary prevention measures. Possible advantages of m-health include improved follow-up visits and better prescription adherence in the prevention of primary and secondary CVD. Current research findings indicate impact of m-health-based education initiative on positive behavior improvements and quality of life of patients undergoing the intervention. This provides promising support for the growth and leveraging of m-health in India to strengthen healthcare facilities. The data synthesized through this study demonstrates how a basic mobile-based platform can provide relevant health knowledge and positive reinforcement towards healthy lifestyle changes to patients from diverse demographic backgrounds.

In conclusion, innovations through the use of cell phone applications will potentially inspire, promote and enable care processes and improve healthcare delivery. Therefore, research in innovative solutions is a need of the hour. Given the resource constraints in Indian healthcare system, Indian public health policy should increase its focus on secondary prevention of CVD. As worldwide research has demonstrated, m-health instruments can successfully support the mainstream health care system to improve disease related education, awareness and encourage healthier behavior among patients. These techniques, unlike traditional approaches, offer various advantages including cost-effectiveness and scalability. The future work should focus on identification and mitigation of the obstacles to acceptability, engagement and sustainability of the m-health tools and techniques for meaningful long-term effects. For addressing these obstacles, more concentrated and inclusive collaboration is advocated between government agencies and private players working in this domain.

REFERENCES

Allida, Sabine, Huiyun Du, Xiaoyue Xu, Roslyn Prichard, Sungwon Chang, Louise D Hickman, Patricia M Davidson, and Sally C Inglis. "MHealth Education Interventions in Heart Failure." *The Cochrane Database of Systematic Reviews* 7, no. 7 (July 2020): CD011845. https://doi.org/10.1002/14651858.CD011845.pub2.

Anchah, Lawrence, Mohamed Azmi Hassali, Melissa Siaw Han Lim, Mohamed Izham Mohamed Ibrahim, Kui Hian Sim, and Tiong Kiam Ong. "Health Related Quality of Life Assessment in Acute Coronary Syndrome Patients: The Effectiveness of Early Phase I Cardiac Rehabilitation." *Health and Quality of Life Outcomes* 15, no. 1 (2017): 1–14. https://doi.org/10.1186/s12955-016-0583-7.

Appel, Lawrence J, Jeanne M Clark, Hsin-Chieh Yeh, Nae-Yuh Wang, Janelle W Coughlin, Gail Daumit, Edgar R 3rd Miller, et al. "Comparative Effectiveness of Weight-Loss Interventions in Clinical Practice." *The New England Journal of Medicine* 365, no. 21 (November 2011): 1959–68. https://doi.org/10.1056/NEJMoa1108660.

Arora, Sanjay, Anne L Peters, Elizabeth Burner, Chun Nok Lam, and Michael Menchine. "Trial to Examine Text Message-Based MHealth in Emergency Department Patients with Diabetes (TExT-MED): A Randomized Controlled Trial." *Annals of Emergency Medicine* 63, no. 6 (June 2014): 745-54.e6. https://doi.org/10.1016/j.annemergmed.2013.10.012.

Babu, Abraham Samuel, Arun G Maiya, M Milton George, Ramachandran Padmakumar, and Vasudeva Guddattu. *"Effects of Combined Early In-Patient Cardiac Rehabilitation and Structured Home-Based Program on Function among Patients with Congestive Heart Failure: A Randomized Controlled Trial"* 12, no. 3 (2011): 99–103.

Bardage, C, and D G Isacson. "Hypertension and Health-Related Quality of Life. An Epidemiological Study in Sweden." *Journal of Clinical Epidemiology* 54, no. 2 (February 2001): 172–81. https://doi.org/10.1016/s0895-4356(00)00293-6.

Baumeister, H, L Reichler, M Munzinger, and J Lin. "The Impact of Guidance on Internet-Based Mental Health Interventions - A Systematic Review." *Internet Interventions* 1, no. 4 (2014): 205–15. https://doi.org/10.1016/j.invent.2014.08.003.

Bedi, Gurdesh S, Nikhil Gupta, Rohini Handa, Hemraj Pal, and R M Pandey. "Quality of Life in Indian Patients with Rheumatoid Arthritis." *Quality of Life Research: An International Journal of Quality of Life Aspects of Treatment, Care and Rehabilitation* 14, no. 8 (October 2005): 1953–58. https://doi.org/10.1007/s11136-005-4540-x.

Birrell, F N, A B Hassell, P W Jones, and P T Dawes. "How Does the Short Form 36 Health Questionnaire (SF-36) in Rheumatoid Arthritis (RA) Relate to RA Outcome Measures and SF-36 Population Values? A Cross-Sectional Study." *Clinical Rheumatology* 19, no. 3 (2000): 195–99. https://doi.org/10.1007/s100670050155.

Blasco, Ana, Montserrat Carmona, Ignacio Fernandez-Lozano, Carlos H Salvador, Mario Pascual, Pilar G Sagredo, Roberto Somolinos, et al. "Evaluation of a Telemedicine Service for the Secondary Prevention of Coronary Artery Disease." *Journal of Cardiopulmonary Rehabilitation and Prevention* 32, no. 1 (2012): 25–31. https://doi.org/10.1097/HCR.0b013e3182343aa7.

Blaum, C S, Ofstedal, M B, Langa, K M, &Wray, L A. "Functional Status and Health Outcomes in Older Americans with Diabetes Mellitus." *Journal of the American Geriatrics Society* 51, no. 6 (2003): 745–753.

Boriani, Giuseppe, Antoine Da Costa, Renato Pietro Ricci, Aurelio Quesada, Stefano Favale, Saverio Iacopino, Francesco Romeo, et al. "The MOnitoring Resynchronization DEvices and CARdiac PatiEnts (MORE-CARE) Randomized Controlled Trial: Phase 1 Results on Dynamics of Early Intervention with Remote Monitoring." *Journal of Medical Internet Research* 15, no. 8 (August 2013): e167. https://doi.org/10.2196/jmir.2608.

Bullinger, M, J Alonso, G Apolone, A Leplege, M Sullivan, S Wood-Dauphinee, B Gandek, et al. "Translating Health Status Questionnaires and Evaluating Their Quality: The IQOLA Project Approach. International Quality of Life Assessment." *Journal of Clinical Epidemiology* 51, no. 11 (November 1998): 913–23. https://doi.org/10.1016/s0895-4356(98)00082-1.

Burke, Lora E, Jun Ma, Kristen M J Azar, Gary G Bennett, Eric D Peterson, Yaguang Zheng, William Riley, et al. "Current Science on Consumer Use of Mobile Health for Cardiovascular Disease Prevention: A Scientific Statement From the American Heart Association." *Circulation* 132, no. 12 (September 2015): 1157–1213. https://doi.org/10.1161/CIR.0000000000000232.

Capozza, Korey, Sarah Woolsey, Mattias Georgsson, Jeff Black, Nelly Bello, Clare Lence, Steve Oostema, and Christie North. "Going Mobile with Diabetes Support: A Randomized Study of a Text Message-Based Personalized Behavioral Intervention for Type 2 Diabetes Self-Care." *Diabetes Spectrum* 28, no. 2 (2015): 83–91. https://doi.org/10.2337/diaspect.28.2.83.

Chen, Ke-Yang, Ting Li, Fang-Hua Gong, Jin-San Zhang, and Xiao-Kun Li. "Predictors of Health-Related Quality of Life and Influencing Factors for COVID-19 Patients, a Follow-Up at One Month." *Frontiers in Psychiatry* 11 (2020): 668. https://doi.org/10.3389/fpsyt.2020.00668.

Cho, Min Jung, Jae Lan Sim, and Seon Young Hwang. "Development of Smartphone Educational Application for Patients with Coronary Artery Disease." *Healthcare Informatics Research* 20, no. 2 (2014): 117–24. https://doi.org/10.4258/hir.2014.20.2.117.

Estabrooks, Paul A, Jo Ann Shoup, Michelle Gattshall, Padma Dandamudi, Susan Shetterly, and Stan Xu. "Automated Telephone Counseling for Parents of Overweight Children: A Randomized Controlled Trial." *American Journal of Preventive Medicine* 36, no. 1 (January 2009): 35–42. https://doi.org/10.1016/j.amepre.2008.09.024.

Fatehi, Farhad, and Richard Wootton. "Telemedicine, Telehealth or e-Health? A Bibliometric Analysis of the Trends in the Use of These

Terms." *Journal of Telemedicine and Telecare* 18, no. 8 (December 2012): 460–64. https://doi.org/10.1258/jtt.2012.gth108.

"Final Report on the Aspirin Component of the Ongoing Physicians' Health Study." *The New England Journal of Medicine* 321, no. 3 (July 1989): 129–35. https://doi.org/10.1056/NEJM198907203210301.

Frederix, Ines, Dominique Hansen, Karin Coninx, Pieter Vandervoort, Dominique Vandijck, Niel Hens, Emeline Van Craenenbroeck, Niels Van Driessche, and Paul Dendale. "Medium-Term Effectiveness of a Comprehensive Internet-Based and Patient-Specific Telerehabilitation Program With Text Messaging Support for Cardiac Patients: Randomized Controlled Trial." *Journal of Medical Internet Research* 17, no. 7 (July 23, 2015): e185–e185. https://doi.org/10.2196/jmir.4799.

Friedman, R H, L E Kazis, A Jette, M B Smith, J Stollerman, J Torgerson, and K Carey. "A Telecommunications System for Monitoring and Counseling Patients with Hypertension. Impact on Medication Adherence and Blood Pressure Control." *American Journal of Hypertension* 9, no. 4 Pt 1 (April 1996): 285–92. https://doi.org/10.1016/0895-7061(95)00353-3.

Gandek, B, J E Jr Ware, N K Aaronson, J Alonso, G Apolone, J Bjorner, J Brazier, et al. "Tests of Data Quality, Scaling Assumptions, and Reliability of the SF-36 in Eleven Countries: Results from the IQOLA Project. International Quality of Life Assessment." *Journal of Clinical Epidemiology* 51, no. 11 (November 1998): 1149–58. https://doi.org/10.1016/s0895-4356(98)00106-1.

Ghosh, D. "Impact of Gender Aspect on Self-Perceived Quality of Life of Elderly." In *MPRA Paper No. 66686, 14:19 UTC.*, 2015.

Glozier, Nicholas, Helen Christensen, Sharon Naismith, Nicole Cockayne, Liesje Donkin, Bruce Neal, Andrew Mackinnon, and Ian Hickie. "Internet-Delivered Cognitive Behavioural Therapy for Adults with Mild to Moderate Depression and High Cardiovascular Disease Risks: A Randomised Attention-Controlled Trial." *PloS One* 8, no. 3 (2013): e59139. https://doi.org/10.1371/journal.pone.0059139.

Goldberg, Adam, and Joshua W K Ho. "Hactive: A Smartphone Application for Heart Rate Profiling." *Biophysical Reviews* 12, no. 4 (August 2020): 777–79. https://doi.org/10.1007/s12551-020-00731-3.

Graham, Jove, Janet Tomcavage, Doreen Salek, Joann Sciandra, Duane E Davis, and Walter F Stewart. "Postdischarge Monitoring Using Interactive Voice Response System Reduces 30-Day Readmission Rates in a Case-Managed Medicare Population." *Medical Care* 50, no. 1 (January 2012): 50–57. https://doi.org/10.1097/MLR.0b013e318229433e.

Gupta, B, S Kant, and Rachna Mishra. *"Effect of Nutrition Education Intervention on Symptomatic Markers of Indian Patients with Chronic Obstructive Pulmonary Disease"* 1, no. 3 (2014): 105–14. https://doi.org/10.15406/jnhfe.2014.01.00016.

Handley, Margaret A, Martha Shumway, and Dean Schillinger. "Cost-Effectiveness of Automated Telephone Self-Management Support with Nurse Care Management among Patients with Diabetes." *Annals of Family Medicine* 6, no. 6 (2008): 512–18. https://doi.org/10.1370/afm.889.

Haroon, Nigil, Amita Aggarwal, Able Lawrence, Vikas Agarwal, and Ramnath Misra. "Impact of Rheumatoid Arthritis on Quality of Life." *Modern Rheumatology* 17, no. 4 (2007): 290–95. https://doi.org/10.1007/s10165-007-0604-9.

Hays, R D, and L S Morales. "The RAND-36 Measure of Health-Related Quality of Life." *Annals of Medicine* 33, no. 5 (2001): 350–57. https://doi.org/10.3109/07853890109002089.

Hilgart, Michelle M, Lee M Ritterband, Frances P Thorndike, and Mable B Kinzie. "Using Instructional Design Process to Improve Design and Development of Internet Interventions." *J Med Internet Res* 14, no. 3 (June 2012): e89. https://doi.org/10.2196/jmir.1890.

Hlatky, Mark A, Derek B Boothroyd, Kathryn A Melsop, Maria M Brooks, Daniel B Mark, Bertram Pitt, Guy S Reeder, et al. "Medical Costs and Quality of Life 10 to 12 Years after Randomization to Angioplasty or Bypass Surgery for Multivessel Coronary Artery Disease." *Circulation*

110, no. 14 (October 2004): 1960–66. https://doi.org/10.1161/01.CIR. 0000143379.26342.5C.

Hlatky, Mark A, Derek Boothroyd, Eric Vittinghoff, Penny Sharp, and Mary A Whooley. "Quality-of-Life and Depressive Symptoms in Postmenopausal Women after Receiving Hormone Therapy: Results from the Heart and Estrogen/Progestin Replacement Study (HERS) Trial." *JAMA* 287, no. 5 (February 2002): 591–97. https://doi.org/10. 1001/jama.287.5.591.

Holtz, Bree, and Carolyn Lauckner. "Diabetes Management via Mobile Phones: A Systematic Review." *Telemedicine Journal and E-Health: The Official Journal of the American Telemedicine Association* 18, no. 3 (April 2012): 175–84. https://doi.org/10.1089/tmj.2011.0119.

Homko, Carol J, Larry C Deeb, Kimberly Rohrbacher, Wadia Mulla, Dimtrios Mastrogiannis, John Gaughan, William P Santamore, and Alfred A Bove. "Impact of a Telemedicine System with Automated Reminders on Outcomes in Women with Gestational Diabetes Mellitus." *Diabetes Technology & Therapeutics* 14, no. 7 (July 2012): 624–29. https://doi.org/10.1089/dia.2012.0010.

King, Abby C, Eric B Hekler, Cynthia M Castro, Matthew P Buman, Bess H Marcus, Robert H Friedman, and Melissa A Napolitano. "Exercise Advice by Humans versus Computers: Maintenance Effects at 18 Months." *Health Psychology: Official Journal of the Division of Health Psychology, American Psychological Association* 33, no. 2 (February 2014): 192–96. https://doi.org/10.1037/a0030646.

Kohli, R M, Suvarna Sane, Kishore Kumar, R S Paranjape, and S M Mehendale. "Modification of Medical Outcome Study (MOS) Instrument for Quality of Life Assessment & Its Validation in HIV Infected Individuals in India." *The Indian Journal of Medical Research* 122, no. 4 (October 2005): 297–304.

Kohli, Rewa M, Suvarna Sane, Kishore Kumar, Ramesh S Paranjape, and Sanjay M Mehendale. "Assessment of Quality of Life among HIV-Infected Persons in Pune, India." *Quality of Life Research: An International Journal of Quality of Life Aspects of Treatment, Care and Rehabilitation* 14, no. 6 (August 2005): 1641–47. https://doi.org/10.1007/s11136-004-7082-8.

Lam, C L, and I J Lauder. "The Impact of Chronic Diseases on the Health-Related Quality of Life (HRQOL) of Chinese Patients in Primary Care." *Family Practice* 17, no. 2 (April 2000): 159–66. https://doi.org/10.1093/fampra/17.2.159.

Lima, Margareth Guimarães, Marilisa Berti de Azevedo Barros, Chester Luiz Gésar César, Moisés Goldbaum, Luana Carandina, and Rozana Mesquita Ciconelli. "Health Related Quality of Life among the Elderly: A Population-Based Study Using Sf-36 Survey." *Cadernos de Saude Publica* 25, no. 10 (2009): 2159–67. https://doi.org/10.1590/s0102-311x2009001000007.

Lin, Cheng-chieh, Chia-ing Li, Chiu-kai Chang, Chiu-shong Liu, Chih-hsueh Lin, Hsin Meng, Yih-dar Lee, Fei-na Chen, and Tsai-chung Li. *"Reduced Health-Related Quality of Life in Elders with Frailty: A Cross-Sectional Study of Community-Dwelling Elders in Taiwan"* 6, no. 7 (2011): 1–7. https://doi.org/10.1371/journal.pone.0021841.

Loos-Ayav, C, N Chau, C Riani, and F Guillemin. "Functional Disability in France and Its Relationship with Health-Related Quality of Life - a Population-Based Prevalence Study." *Clinical and Experimental Rheumatology* 25, no. 5 (2007): 701–8.

Lorig, Kate, Philip L Ritter, Frank Villa, and John D Piette. "Spanish Diabetes Self-Management with and without Automated Telephone Reinforcement: Two Randomized Trials." *Diabetes Care* 31, no. 3 (March 2008): 408–14. https://doi.org/10.2337/dc07-1313.

Magid, David J, P Michael Ho, Kari L Olson, David W Brand, Lesley K Welch, Karen E Snow, Anne C Lambert-Kerzner, Mary E Plomondon, and Edward P Havranek. "A Multimodal Blood Pressure Control Intervention in 3 Healthcare Systems." *The American Journal of Managed Care* 17, no. 4 (April 2011): e96-103.

Margolis, Karen L, Stephen E Asche, Anna R Bergdall, Steven P Dehmer, Sarah E Groen, Holly M Kadrmas, Tessa J Kerby, et al. "Effect of Home Blood Pressure Telemonitoring and Pharmacist Management on

Blood Pressure Control: A Cluster Randomized Clinical Trial." *JAMA* 310, no. 1 (July 2013): 46–56. https://doi.org/10.1001/jama.2013.6549.

Medhi GK, Sarma J, Pala S, Bhattacharya H, Bora P J, Visi V. "Association between Health Related Quality of Life (HRQOL) and Activity of Daily Living (ADL) among Elderly in an Urban Setting of Assam, India Introduction." *India.J Family Med Prim Care* 8, no. 5 (2019): 1760–64.

Michalos, Alex C, Bruno D Zumbo, and Anita Hubley. "Health and the Quality of Life." *Social Indicators Research* 51, no. 3 (2000): 245–86. https://doi.org/10.1023/A:1007010401301.

Migneault, Jeffrey P, Julien J Dedier, Julie A Wright, Timothy Heeren, Marci Kramish Campbell, Donald E Morisky, Peter Rudd, and Robert H Friedman. "A Culturally Adapted Telecommunication System to Improve Physical Activity, Diet Quality, and Medication Adherence among Hypertensive African-Americans: A Randomized Controlled Trial." *Annals of Behavioral Medicine: A Publication of the Society of Behavioral Medicine* 43, no. 1 (February 2012): 62–73. https://doi.org/10.1007/s12160-011-9319-4.

Mishra, G, and M J Schofield. "Norms for the Physical and Mental Health Component Summary Scores of the SF-36 for Young, Middle-Aged and Older Australian Women." *Quality of Life Research* 7, no. 3 (1998): 215–20. https://doi.org/10.1023/A:1024917510063.

Mohan, Bishav, Sarit Sharma, Shruti Sharma, Dinesh Kaushal, Bhupinder Singh, Shibba Takkar, Naved Aslam, Abhishek Goyal, and Gurpreet S Wander. "Assessment of Knowledge about Healthy Heart Habits in Urban and Rural Population of Punjab after SMS Campaign-A Cross-Sectional Study." *Indian Heart Journal* 69, no. 4 (2017): 480–84. https://doi.org/10.1016/j.ihj.2017.05.007.

Mohr, David C, Michelle Nicole Burns, Stephen M Schueller, Gregory Clarke, and Michael Klinkman. "Behavioral Intervention Technologies: Evidence Review and Recommendations for Future Research in Mental Health." *General Hospital Psychiatry* 35, no. 4 (2013): 332–38. https://doi.org/10.1016/j.genhosppsych.2013.03.008.

Muniyandi, M, R Rajeswari, R Balasubramanian, C Nirupa, P G Gopi, K Jaggarajamma, F Sheela, and P R Narayanan. "Evaluation of Post-Treatment Health-Related Quality of Life (HRQoL) among Tuberculosis Patients." *The International Journal of Tuberculosis and Lung Disease: The Official Journal of the International Union against Tuberculosis and Lung Disease* 11, no. 8 (August 2007): 887–92.

Newton, Kirsty H, Esko J Wiltshire, and C Raina Elley. "Pedometers and Text Messaging to Increase Physical Activity: Randomized Controlled Trial of Adolescents with Type 1 Diabetes." *Diabetes Care* 32, no. 5 (May 2009): 813–15. https://doi.org/10.2337/dc08-1974.

Nolan, Robert P, Ross E G Upshur, Hazel Lynn, Thomas Crichton, Ellen Rukholm, Donna E Stewart, David A Alter, et al. "Therapeutic Benefit of Preventive Telehealth Counseling in the Community Outreach Heart Health and Risk Reduction Trial." *The American Journal of Cardiology* 107, no. 5 (March 2011): 690–96. https://doi.org/10.1016/j.amjcard.2010.10.050.

Norman, Gregory J, Julia K Kolodziejczyk, Marc A Adams, Kevin Patrick, and Simon J Marshall. "Fruit and Vegetable Intake and Eating Behaviors Mediate the Effect of a Randomized Text-Message Based Weight Loss Program." *Preventive Medicine* 56, no. 1 (January 2013): 3–7. https://doi.org/10.1016/j.ypmed.2012.10.012.

Nundy, Shantanu, Jonathan J Dick, Chia-Hung Chou, Robert S Nocon, Marshall H Chin, and Monica E Peek. "Mobile Phone Diabetes Project Led to Improved Glycemic Control and Net Savings for Chicago Plan Participants." *Health Affairs (Project Hope)* 33, no. 2 (February 2014): 265–72. https://doi.org/10.1377/hlthaff.2013.0589.

Orwelius, Lotti, Mats Nilsson, Evalill Nilsson, Marika Wenemark, Ulla Walfridsson, Mats Lundström, Charles Taft, Bo Palaszewski, and Margareta Kristenson. "The Swedish RAND-36 Health Survey - Reliability and Responsiveness Assessed in Patient Populations Using Svensson's Method for Paired Ordinal Data." *Journal of Patient-Reported Outcomes* 2, no. 1 (2018): 0–9. https://doi.org/10.1186/s41687-018-0030-0.

Park, Linda G, Jill Howie-Esquivel, Misook L Chung, and Kathleen Dracup. "A Text Messaging Intervention to Promote Medication Adherence for Patients with Coronary Heart Disease: A Randomized Controlled Trial." *Patient Education and Counseling* 94, no. 2 (February 2014): 261–68. https://doi.org/10.1016/j.pec.2013.10.027.

Patrick D L, Erickson P. *Health Status and Health Policy: Quality of Life in Health Care Evaluation and Resource Allocation.* New York: New York: Oxford University Press, 1993.

Piette, J D, M Weinberger, F B Kraemer, and S J McPhee. "Impact of Automated Calls with Nurse Follow-up on Diabetes Treatment Outcomes in a Department of Veterans Affairs Health Care System: A Randomized Controlled Trial." *Diabetes Care* 24, no. 2 (February 2001): 202–8. https://doi.org/10.2337/diacare.24.2.202.

Piette, J D, M Weinberger, and S J McPhee. "The Effect of Automated Calls with Telephone Nurse Follow-up on Patient-Centered Outcomes of Diabetes Care: A Randomized, Controlled Trial." *Medical Care* 38, no. 2 (February 2000): 218–30. https://doi.org/10.1097/00005650-200002000-00011.

Piette, J D, M Weinberger, S J McPhee, C A Mah, F B Kraemer, and L M Crapo. "Do Automated Calls with Nurse Follow-up Improve Self-Care and Glycemic Control among Vulnerable Patients with Diabetes?" *The American Journal of Medicine* 108, no. 1 (January 2000): 20–27. https://doi.org/10.1016/s0002-9343(99)00298-3.

Piette, John D, Hema Datwani, Sofia Gaudioso, Stephanie M Foster, Joslyn Westphal, William Perry, Joel Rodríguez-Saldaña, Milton O Mendoza-Avelares, and Nicolle Marinec. "Hypertension Management Using Mobile Technology and Home Blood Pressure Monitoring: Results of a Randomized Trial in Two Low/Middle-Income Countries." *Telemedicine Journal and E-Health: The Official Journal of the American Telemedicine Association* 18, no. 8 (October 2012): 613–20. https://doi.org/10.1089/tmj.2011.0271.

Piette, John D, Milton O Mendoza-Avelares, Martha Ganser, Muhima Mohamed, Nicolle Marinec, and Sheila Krishnan. "A Preliminary Study of a Cloud-Computing Model for Chronic Illness Self-Care

Support in an Underdeveloped Country." *American Journal of Preventive Medicine* 40, no. 6 (June 2011): 629–32. https://doi.org/10.1016/j.amepre.2011.02.014.

Pius, Anna, G K Mini, and K R Thankappan. "Health Related Quality of Life and It's Correlates among Older Adults in Rural Pathanamthitta District, India: A Cross Sectional Study Using SF-36." *Ageing International* 44, no. 3 (2019): 271–82. https://doi.org/10.1007/s12126-018-9342-x.

Quinn, Charlene C, Suzanne Sysko Clough, James M Minor, Dan Lender, Maria C Okafor, and Ann Gruber-Baldini. "WellDoc Mobile Diabetes Management Randomized Controlled Trial: Change in Clinical and Behavioral Outcomes and Patient and Physician Satisfaction." *Diabetes Technology & Therapeutics* 10, no. 3 (June 2008): 160–68. https://doi.org/10.1089/dia.2008.0283.

Quinn, Charlene C, Michelle D Shardell, Michael L Terrin, Erik A Barr, Shoshana H Ballew, and Ann L Gruber-Baldini. "Cluster-Randomized Trial of a Mobile Phone Personalized Behavioral Intervention for Blood Glucose Control." *Diabetes Care* 34, no. 9 (September 2011): 1934–42. https://doi.org/10.2337/dc11-0366.

Rajeswari, R, M Muniyandi, R Balasubramanian, and P R Narayanan. "Perceptions of Tuberculosis Patients about Their Physical, Mental and Social Well-Being: A Field Report from South India." *Social Science & Medicine (1982)* 60, no. 8 (April 2005): 1845–53. https://doi.org/10.1016/j.socscimed.2004.08.024.

Ray, J, S K Das, P K Gangopadhya, and T Roy. "Quality of Life in Parkinson's Disease--Indian Scenario." *The Journal of the Association of Physicians of India* 54 (January 2006): 17–21.

Rehman, Hasan, Ayeesha K Kamal, Pamela B Morris, Saleem Sayani, Anwar T Merchant, and Salim S Virani. *"Mobile Health (MHealth) Technology for the Management of Hypertension and Hyperlipidemia: Slow Start but Loads of Potential,"* 2017. https://doi.org/10.1007/s11883-017-0649-y.

Reid, Robert D, Andrew L Pipe, Bonnie Quinlan, and Joanna Oda. "Interactive Voice Response Telephony to Promote Smoking

Cessation in Patients with Heart Disease: A Pilot Study." *Patient Education and Counseling* 66, no. 3 (June 2007): 319–26. https://doi.org/10.1016/j.pcc.2007.01.005.

Rowland, Simon P, J Edward Fitzgerald, Thomas Holme, John Powell, and Alison McGregor. "What Is the Clinical Value of MHealth for Patients?" *Npj Digital Medicine* 3, no. 1 (2020): 1–6. https://doi.org/10.1038/s41746-019-0206-x.

Rozental, Alexander, Gerhard Andersson, Johanna Boettcher, David Daniel Ebert, Pim Cuijpers, Christine Knaevelsrud, Brjánn Ljótsson, Viktor Kaldo, Nickolai Titov, and Per Carlbring. "Consensus Statement on Defining and Measuring Negative Effects of Internet Interventions." *Internet Interventions* 1, no. 1 (2014): 12–19. https://doi.org/10.1016/j.invent.2014.02.001.

Schillinger, Dean, Hali Hammer, Frances Wang, Jorge Palacios, Ivonne McLean, Audrey Tang, Sharon Youmans, and Margaret Handley. "Seeing in 3-D: Examining the Reach of Diabetes Self-Management Support Strategies in a Public Health Care System." *Health Education & Behavior: The Official Publication of the Society for Public Health Education* 35, no. 5 (October 2008): 664–82. https://doi.org/10.1177/1090198106296772.

Shah, Lata, Serah Rashmi, and Dhanpal Nanjundappa. "Effectiveness of Reminiscence Therapy on Health Related Quality of Life among the Old Age People Residing at a Selected Old Age Home, Bengaluru, India." *Janaki Medical College Journal of Medical Science* 6 (2018): 44–54. https://doi.org/10.3126/jmcjms.v6i02.22060.

Shan, Rongzi, Jie Ding, Timothy B Plante, and Seth S Martin. "*Mobile Health Access and Use Among Individuals With or At Risk For*," no. 1 (2019). https://doi.org/10.1161/JAHA.119.014390.

Shapiro, Jennifer R, Tina Koro, Neal Doran, Sheri Thompson, James F Sallis, Karen Calfas, and Kevin Patrick. "Text4Diet: A Randomized Controlled Study Using Text Messaging for Weight Loss Behaviors." *Preventive Medicine* 55, no. 5 (November 2012): 412–17. https://doi.org/10.1016/j.ypmed.2012.08.011.

Shivaprasad, C, Boppana Rakesh, Kolly Anish, Pullikal Annie, Goel Amit, and C S Dwarakanath. "*Impairment of Health - Related Quality of Life among Indian Patients with Hypothyroidism*," 2018, 2018–21. https://doi.org/10.4103/ijem.IJEM.

Simon, Steven R, Connie Mah Trinacty, Stephen B Soumerai, John D Piette, James B Meigs, Ping Shi, Arthur Ensroth, and Dennis Ross-Degnan. "Improving Diabetes Care among Patients Overdue for Recommended Testing: A Randomized Controlled Trial of Automated Telephone Outreach." *Diabetes Care* 33, no. 7 (July 2010): 1452–53. https://doi.org/10.2337/dc09-2332.

Singh, Harminder, Kamalpreet Kaur, Navin Dulhani, Akash Bansal, Bithika N Kumar, Vinod Kumar, and Singh Chouhan. "Assessment of Quality of Life in a Cohort of Newly Diagnosed Patients on Haart Regimen, in Resource Restricted Tribal Region of Chhattisgarh, India: A Prospective Study Full Text Introduction Discussion." *Journal of Global Infectious Diseases* 5, no. 3 (2013): 104–9.

Sinha, Richa, Wim A Van Den Heuvel, and Perianayagam Arokiasamy. "Validity and Reliability of MOS Short Form Health Survey (SF-36) for Use in India." *Indian Journal of Community Medicine* 38, no. 1 (2013): 22–26. https://doi.org/10.4103/0970-0218.106623.

Tajvar, Maryam, Mohammad Arab, and Ali Montazeri. "Determinants of Health-Related Quality of Life in Elderly in Tehran, Iran." *BMC Public Health* 8, no. 1 (2008): 323. https://doi.org/10.1186/1471-2458-8-323.

"*Telecom Subscriptions Reports.*" Accessed March 10, 2020. https://main.trai.gov.in/release-publication/reports/telecom-subscriptions-reports.

Tofighi, Shahram, Aliasghar Ahmad Kiadaliri, Jamil Sadeghifar, Mehdi Raadabadi, and Jahanara Mamikhani. "Health-Related Quality of Life among Patients with Coronary Artery Disease: A Post-Treatment Follow-up Study in Iran." *Cardiology Research and Practice* 1, no. 1 (2012). https://doi.org/10.1155/2012/973974.

Tough, Hannah, Johannes Siegrist, and Christine Fekete. "*Social Relationships, Mental Health and Wellbeing in Physical Disability: A*

Systematic Review," 2017, 1–18. https://doi.org/10.1186/s12889-017-4308-6.

Varma, G R, Y S Kusuma, and B V Babu. "Health-Related Quality of Life of Elderly Living in the Rural Community and Homes for the Elderly in a District of India. Application of the Short Form 36 (SF-36) Health Survey Questionnaire." *Zeitschrift Fur Gerontologie Und Geriatrie* 43, no. 4 (August 2010): 259–63. https://doi.org/10.1007/s00391-009-0077-x.

Varnfield, Marlien, Mohanraj Karunanithi, Chi-Keung Lee, Enone Honeyman, Desre Arnold, Hang Ding, Catherine Smith, and Darren L Walters. "Smartphone-Based Home Care Model Improved Use of Cardiac Rehabilitation in Postmyocardial Infarction Patients: Results from a Randomised Controlled Trial." *Heart (British Cardiac Society)* 100, no. 22 (November 2014): 1770–79. https://doi.org/10.1136/heartjnl-2014-305783.

Villarreal, Vladimir, and Aranzazu Berbey-Alvarez. "Evaluation of MHealth application Related to Cardiovascular Diseases: A Systematic Review." *Acta Informatica Medica: AIM: Journal of the Society for Medical Informatics of Bosnia & Herzegovina: Casopis Drustva Za Medicinsku Informatiku BiH* 28, no. 2 (June 2020): 130–37. https://doi.org/10.5455/aim.2020.28.130-137.

Vis, Christiaan, Annet Kleiboer, Reinhard Prior, Erland Bønes, Marco Cavallo, Stella Anne Clark, Els Dozeman, et al. "Implementing and Up-Scaling Evidence-Based EMental Health in Europe: The Study Protocol for the MasterMind Project." *Internet Interventions* 2, no. 4 (2015): 399–409. https://doi.org/10.1016/j.invent.2015.10.002.

Wagner, A K, B Gandek, N K Aaronson, C Acquadro, J Alonso, G Apolone, M Bullinger, et al. "Cross-Cultural Comparisons of the Content of SF-36 Translations across 10 Countries: Results from the IQOLA Project. International Quality of Life Assessment." *Journal of Clinical Epidemiology* 51, no. 11 (November 1998): 925–32. https://doi.org/10.1016/s0895-4356(98)00083-3.

Wig, Naveet, Raja Lekshmi, Hemraj Pal, Vivek Ahuja, Chander Mohan Mittal, and Sunil Kumar Agarwal. "The Impact of HIV/AIDS on the

Quality of Life: A Cross Sectional Study in North India." *Indian Journal of Medical Sciences* 60, no. 1 (January 2006): 3–12. https://doi.org/10.4103/0019-5359.19670.

Williams, Emily D, Dominique Bird, Andrew W Forbes, Anthony Russell, Susan Ash, Robert Friedman, Paul A Scuffham, and Brian Oldenburg. "Randomised Controlled Trial of an Automated, Interactive Telephone Intervention (TLC Diabetes) to Improve Type 2 Diabetes Management: Baseline Findings and Six-Month Outcomes." *BMC Public Health* 12 (August 2012): 602. https://doi.org/10.1186/1471-2458-12-602.

Wong, Carlos K H, Colman S C Fung, S C Siu, Yvonne Y C Lo, K W Wong, Daniel Y T Fong, and Cindy L K Lam. "A Short Message Service (SMS) Intervention to Prevent Diabetes in Chinese Professional Drivers with Pre-Diabetes: A Pilot Single-Blinded Randomized Controlled Trial." *Diabetes Research and Clinical Practice* 102, no. 3 (December 2013): 158–66. https://doi.org/10.1016/j.diabres.2013.10.002.

World Health Organisation. Programme on Mental Health. Geneva. World Health Organisation, 1996.

World Health Organisation. The First Ten Years. The Health Organization. Geneva. World Health Organisation, 1958.

ABOUT THE EDITORS

Dr. Gaurav Gupta
Assistant Professor
Yogananda School of AI Computers and Data Science, Shoolini University, Solan, H.P. INDIA

Dr. Gaurav Gupta received BE degree (2006) from Dr. B. R. Ambedkar University, Agra, Uttar Pradesh. He received PG (2011) and Ph.D. (2020) degree in the stream of Computer Science Engineering from KSOU-VIT, Karnataka and Shoolini University respectively. He attended number of conferences and presented papers in the field of machine learning and artificial intelligence. Roughly, he has served on 5 conference and workshop program committees and served as the session chair for INDIACom-2021 and session coordinator at IFIP WG8.6 by Indian Institute of Management Tiruchirappalli, India during December 17-19, 2020 He published about 20+ research paper in reputed journals as well as 12+ papers in conferences. He also published 12+ books with national and international publishing house. Currently he is working as an Assistant professor in School of Electrical and Computer Science Engineering, Shoolini University, Solan, Himachal Pradesh. He has guided 15 M. Tech Students and currently guiding 2 M. Tech and 3 Ph. D students. His area of interest is in the field of Machine Learning, Big data, Cloud Computing and Databases.

Dr. Nagesh Kumar
Assistant Professor
Yogananda School of AI Computers and Data Science, Shoolini University, Solan, H.P. INDIA

Dr. Nagesh Kumar Working as an Assistant Professor in Shoolini University of Biotechnology and Management Sciences, Solan (HP). Academic Qualifications are PhD (CSE) from Jaypee University of Information Technology, Waknaghat, Solan (HP) India; M. Tech (CSE) from HPU, Summerhill, Shimla (HP) India; B. Tech (CSE) from Green Hills Engineering College, Kumarhatti, Solan (HP) India. Research interests are Wireless Sensor Networks, Network Security, Cyber-physical-human systems, IoT for industries and Smart Agriculture.

Dr. Yashwant Singh
Associate Professor
Central University, Jammu. J&K INDIA

Dr. Yashwant Singh received the bachelor's degree from SLIET Longowal, the master's degree from Punjab Engineering College, Chandigarh, and the Ph.D. degree from Himachal Pradesh University, Shimla. He was with the Jaypee University of Information Technology for 10 Years. He is currently an Associate Professor and the Head of the Department of Computer Science and Information Technology, Central University of Jammu, where he has been a Faculty Member since 2017. He is also a Visiting Professor at Jan Wyzykowski University, Polkowice, Poland. He has collaborated actively with researchers in several other disciplines of computer science, particularly machine learning and electrical engineering. Roughly, he has served on 30 conference and workshop program committees and served as the General Chair for PDGC-2014, ICRIC-2018, ICRIC-2019, and ICRIC-2020. He currently serves as the Coordinator of the Kalam Centre for Science and Technology (KCST), Central University of Jammu, established by DRDO. He has published more than 70 research articles in international journals, international conferences, and book chapters of repute. He has research projects worth INR 15 Crore (Approx.) in his credit. He has guided three Ph.D. and 24 M.Tech. students. He has visited eight countries for his academic visits, i.e., U.K., Germany, Poland, Chez Republic, Hungary, Slovakia, Austria, and Romania. His research interests lie in the area of the Internet of Things, wireless sensor networks, ICS/SCADA cybersecurity, ranging from theory to design to implementation.

Dr. Varun Jaiswal

Assistant Professor

BioNano Technology, Department of Food & Nutrition Gachon University, 1342Seongnam-Daero, Sujeong-Gu, Seongnam-Si, Gyeonggi-Do, Republic of Korea

Dr. Varun Jaiswal is a researcher of Indian origin working in the area of Bioinformatics which spans from medical informatics to artificial intelligence and genomics of host and pathogens. He is presently working as Assistant Professor at Gachon University South Korea. He is an alumnus of JNU, New Delhi, and serves as Assistant Director in the National Centre of Disease Control (NCDC), New Delhi. During the COVID-19 outbreak, he played a key role in the development of testing, training, and genome sequencing facility at the NCDC. He has expertise in both dry, wet-lab experiments and administration. He has applied machine learning methods in diverse fields which include biology, chemistry, medicine, computer science, and social science. He has authored dozens of papers in reputed top-tier journals of diverse fields. Numbers of students have completed their Ph.D. and Master's degree under his able guidance. He prefers to work with new and emerging technology to answer different challenging problems of the nation and the world. He strongly believes that artificial intelligence-powered by machine learning will change the global scenario in favor of humanity in almost all fields.

INDEX

A

access, 10, 19, 35, 115, 124, 193, 195, 196, 209, 261, 269, 274
accessibility, 3, 9, 81, 206, 260
accounting, 35, 43, 73, 116
adjustment, 7, 55, 61, 146, 266
administrators, 32, 43, 71, 81, 99
adults, 28, 157, 297
advancement(s), vii, viii, 7, 11, 20, 21, 22, 35, 37, 42, 44, 49, 55, 56, 58, 59, 60, 61, 69, 78, 82, 83, 86, 168, 174, 182, 194, 195, 197, 199, 205, 206, 209, 232, 237, 261
age, 119, 136, 152, 153, 154, 175, 200, 239, 251, 253, 277, 278, 282, 283, 284, 288, 297
agriculture, 1, 15, 28
AI, 17, 18, 26, 34, 67, 82, 83, 97, 98, 108, 113, 117, 124, 125, 163, 165, 166, 167, 168, 175, 176, 183, 185, 198, 199, 200, 228, 230, 233, 317, 318
algorithm, 26, 32, 82, 86, 87, 170, 177, 178, 186, 188, 217, 220, 223, 224, 225, 226, 227, 236, 254
ANOVA, 258, 280, 288, 290, 291, 294, 298, 299, 300
arrhythmia, 176, 177, 188
artery, 259, 277, 283
artificial intelligence, vii, viii, 37, 67, 82, 87, 108, 115, 164, 165, 185, 233, 249, 317, 318
assessment, 22, 33, 50, 51, 55, 61, 70, 79, 86, 92, 206, 261, 263, 267, 274, 278, 281
assets, 50, 98, 123, 198, 199
astigmatism, 138, 145, 150
authenticity, 118, 119, 120, 122, 268
automate, 37, 38, 82, 83, 115
automation, viii, 82, 108, 175, 235
awareness, 101, 102, 260, 282, 300, 301

B

barriers, 9, 19, 29, 35, 238, 295
base, 40, 41, 74, 77, 100, 141, 163, 167, 168, 172, 175, 176, 180, 183, 194, 219, 295
behaviors, 99, 125, 168, 260, 265, 272
benefits, 6, 18, 19, 41, 91, 109, 116, 125, 130, 157, 199, 205, 237, 301

blockchain, 6, 98, 116, 117, 118, 119, 120, 121, 122, 123, 124, 126, 198
blood, 110, 116, 134, 146, 151, 207, 226, 232, 239, 241, 242, 243, 245, 246, 247, 248, 249, 250, 251, 252, 253, 267, 269, 294, 296
blood pressure, 269, 294, 296
blood smear, 241, 243, 246, 248, 249, 250, 252, 253
bloodstream, 134, 146, 237
brain, 40, 105, 111, 116, 133, 137, 171, 172, 173, 186
breast cancer, 127, 250, 253, 254, 262
breast milk, 134, 144, 146, 157, 159, 160
breastfeeding, 130, 131, 132, 133, 134, 140, 141, 142, 143, 144, 145, 146, 154, 157, 158, 159, 160, 161, 162
business model, 32, 90, 125
businesses, 118, 119, 120, 122, 124, 198
buyer(s), 118, 119, 124, 125

C

CAD, 258, 271, 274, 277, 282, 283, 295, 296, 297, 298, 300
candidates, 140, 149, 151
case study/studies, viii, 32, 85, 89, 117, 167, 192, 213
cell phones, 191, 193, 194, 195, 196, 208, 209, 210
challenges, 3, 5, 11, 13, 14, 22, 95, 110, 121, 123, 125, 166, 229, 232, 255
children, 146, 154, 157, 239, 241, 253
China, 174, 179, 220, 224
chronic diseases, 260, 262, 271, 295, 299
classes, 36, 51, 169, 176
classification, 51, 77, 83, 92, 169, 170, 172, 173, 176, 177, 178, 180, 183, 184, 227, 232, 233, 235, 247, 249, 250, 253
cleaning, 9, 84, 147
clients, 6, 37, 44, 58, 60, 62, 63, 65, 66, 69, 70, 79, 81, 192, 197, 202, 212
climate, 7, 52, 224
clinical trials, 165, 167, 185
CNN, 86, 93, 170, 172, 173, 175, 176, 178, 179, 180, 183, 184, 218, 222, 227, 249, 250, 253
cognitive impairment, 171, 172, 186
collaboration, 36, 62, 63, 64, 102, 117, 302
color, 246, 248, 282
communication, 4, 5, 11, 19, 36, 80, 94, 102, 123, 200, 266, 267, 294
community/communities, 79, 161, 178, 219, 261, 263, 269, 275
complexity, 3, 67, 104, 113, 244, 270
compliance, 259, 265, 294
complications, 122, 136, 139, 141, 153, 177
composition, 131, 223, 271, 281, 282
comprehension, 50, 57, 62, 193
computation, 166, 232, 246
computer, 2, 10, 31, 33, 35, 37, 61, 62, 68, 78, 79, 82, 94, 98, 109, 126, 165, 168, 178, 180, 228, 233, 319
computing, viii, 2, 86, 94, 95, 105, 176, 225, 242, 243, 247
conference, 249, 317, 319
consumption, 10, 113, 121, 124
convergence, viii, 98, 127
cooperation, 36, 65, 193, 200, 213
cornea, 129, 132, 136, 137, 140, 141, 143, 145, 149, 150, 151, 153, 155, 156
coronary artery disease, 259, 277, 283
cost, 3, 4, 8, 18, 55, 72, 98, 123, 206, 221, 231, 232, 233, 242, 243, 244, 245, 247, 248, 260, 263, 294, 300, 301
counseling, 192, 207, 265
COVID-19 and machine learning, vi, vii, viii, 18, 26, 32, 82, 83, 84, 85, 86, 93, 94, 95, 113, 127, 163, 164, 165, 166, 167, 168, 169, 170, 175, 176, 177, 178, 179, 180, 181, 182, 183, 184, 185, 186, 188, 195, 213, 217, 218, 219, 221, 222, 223,

225, 226, 227, 228, 229, 230, 231, 232, 233, 234, 235, 236, 237, 249, 250, 251, 252, 253, 254, 255, 304, 317, 318, 319
cure, 130, 164, 220
customers, 49, 52, 57, 71, 85, 120, 170, 201, 211
cybersecurity, 3, 13, 320
cycles, 22, 52, 59, 106, 134, 204

D

data analysis, 32, 43, 57, 86, 167, 172, 259
data collection, 1, 60, 101, 109, 110, 111, 173, 258, 275, 288, 298
data mining, 32, 75, 76, 77, 84, 85, 93, 94, 95, 98, 127, 233, 249, 251, 253, 254
data set, 56, 83, 84, 85, 223, 233
database, 36, 38, 41, 42, 44, 53, 64, 69, 72, 80, 111, 119, 121, 172, 175, 176, 179, 184
death rate, 194, 202, 238
deaths, 220, 221, 232, 238
decision support system, viii, 14, 31, 32, 34, 35, 36, 37, 38, 39, 40, 42, 43, 48, 50, 53, 58, 66, 79, 85, 86, 87, 88, 89, 90, 91, 92, 93, 94, 95
decision trees, 74, 91, 170, 224
decision-making process, 32, 33, 38, 52, 59
deep learning, viii, 32, 86, 87, 93, 126, 128, 164, 165, 166, 167, 168, 170, 171, 172, 174, 175, 176, 178, 180, 181, 183, 184, 186, 187, 188, 189, 222, 234, 235, 249, 250, 252, 254, 255
depth, 56, 138, 152
designers, 68, 79, 106, 107
detection, 86, 93, 114, 165, 167, 170, 173, 175, 176, 177, 179, 180, 183, 184, 187, 188, 224, 232, 243, 244, 245, 246, 248, 250, 253, 254
developed countries, 159, 198, 203, 213
diabetes, 131, 134, 137, 145, 151, 164, 171, 177, 178, 180, 188, 197, 236, 251, 262, 266, 283, 296, 302, 303, 304, 306, 307, 308, 310, 311, 312, 313, 314, 316
diet, 113, 197, 260, 265, 266, 269, 272, 273
digital health, 112, 192, 204, 206
digital technologies, 125, 126, 174
digital twins, v, viii, 97, 98, 99, 100, 101, 102, 104, 105, 106, 107, 108, 109, 110, 111, 112, 113, 114, 115, 116, 117, 118, 119, 121, 122, 123, 124, 125, 126, 127
discomfort, 143, 152, 160, 161
disease diagnosis, vii, 164, 178, 183, 186, 250
diseases, vii, 2, 18, 113, 131, 150, 164, 166, 172, 174, 178, 181, 183, 219, 225, 227, 236, 237, 239, 254, 255, 273, 282
distribution, 10, 87, 121, 234, 243
diversity, 12, 71, 84
doctors, 9, 10, 116, 145, 165, 167, 174, 197, 198, 213, 220, 235
drugs, 10, 100, 134, 137, 144, 146, 164, 203, 227, 232
dry eyes, 139, 146, 151

E

ECG, 26, 101, 176, 177, 179, 180, 188
ecosystem, 28, 99, 108, 122
education, 99, 103, 109, 127, 160, 194, 232, 246, 259, 260, 265, 266, 267, 272, 274, 279, 283, 284, 288, 295, 300, 301
elderly population, 270, 276, 296
electricity, 82, 116, 121
emergency, 8, 10, 18, 20, 94, 101, 102, 200, 203, 208, 209, 225, 241
employees, 32, 50, 69, 109
encouragement, 54, 157, 260, 269, 272
end-users, 61, 79, 122
energy, 11, 91, 101, 104, 121, 124, 153, 296, 299

engineering, viii, 5, 32, 34, 50, 62, 67, 68, 69, 80, 94, 98, 206, 319
environment, 9, 41, 67, 109, 111, 154, 157, 169, 199, 265
epidemic, 167, 213, 218, 219, 220, 223, 225, 230
equipment, viii, 10, 38, 39, 68, 81, 87, 244, 246
Europe, 112, 128, 218, 232, 315
evidence, 132, 159, 214, 233, 270, 298
execution, 7, 33, 61, 65, 81, 199, 203, 208, 223
exercise(s), 20, 55, 111, 114, 195, 201, 206, 208, 236, 266, 269
expertise, 35, 70, 79, 149, 318
exposure, 134, 221, 296
extraction, 151, 172, 182, 235

F

facilitators, 19, 29, 124
financial, 33, 35, 36, 52, 70, 75, 79, 105, 118, 193, 243
fluorescence, 246, 250, 254
fog computing, 2
food, 2, 114, 203, 269
forecasting, 56, 71, 170, 219, 223
France, 97, 116, 268, 303, 308

G

genomics, 127, 251, 318
Germany, 113, 257, 319
glasses, 134, 135, 137, 138, 139, 140, 142, 147, 148, 151, 152, 153, 154
glucose, 9, 207, 267
Google, 90, 91, 94, 171, 233, 236, 254, 280
GPS, 57, 113, 209, 269
growth, 12, 60, 67, 131, 140, 171, 232, 261, 295, 301
guidance, 25, 195, 205, 319
guidelines, 41, 46, 72, 132, 133, 134, 202, 204, 277

H

healing, 141, 146, 151
health, vii, viii, ix, 2, 6, 9, 11, 12, 17, 18, 20, 21, 22, 23, 26, 27, 28, 29, 86, 87, 98, 99, 108, 112, 115, 125, 126, 127, 131, 137, 142, 144, 157, 164, 166, 167, 183, 191, 192, 193, 194, 195, 196, 197, 198, 199, 200, 201, 202, 204, 205, 206, 207, 209, 210, 211, 212, 213, 214, 215, 218, 225, 232, 234, 238, 247, 249, 250, 252, 253, 254, 258, 259, 260, 261, 262, 263, 264, 265, 266, 268, 269, 270, 272, 275, 276, 277, 279, 280, 284, 288, 292, 294, 296, 297, 298, 300, 301
health care, 20, 21, 22, 28, 29, 86, 87, 164, 183, 192, 200, 209, 213, 214, 218, 234, 249, 252, 263, 294, 301
health care system, 192, 294, 301
health education, 258, 260, 268, 280, 295, 300
health information, 192, 193, 195, 204, 208, 265
health services, viii, 191, 196, 201, 213, 260, 270, 295
health status, 18, 276, 279, 284, 288, 294, 296, 297, 298
healthcare, v, vi, vii, viii, 1, 2, 3, 4, 5, 6, 7, 8, 9, 11, 12, 13, 14, 15, 17, 18, 19, 22, 26, 28, 93, 97, 98, 99, 100, 101, 102, 103, 105, 107, 119, 120, 121, 122, 128, 159, 163, 164, 165, 166, 167, 168, 170, 180, 183, 184, 185, 188, 189, 191, 192, 193, 194, 195,196, 198, 199, 204, 206, 207, 208, 209, 210, 213, 234, 235, 237, 249, 251, 253, 259, 260, 262, 266, 274, 281, 301, 304, 308

health-related quality of life, ix, 258, 259, 271, 295
heart disease, 86, 113, 249, 271, 273, 282
heart rate, 26, 112, 113, 268
history, 67, 90, 92, 93, 117, 194, 197, 201, 205, 219, 220, 283, 296
HIV/AIDS, 221, 224, 225, 227, 229, 230, 307, 315
homes, 17, 19, 121, 210
hormone(s), 131, 132, 133, 144, 145, 157
host, 222, 240, 318
HRQOL, 258, 259, 261, 262, 263, 264, 270, 271, 276, 280, 284, 285, 286, 287, 288, 289, 290, 291, 292, 293, 295, 296, 297, 298, 299, 300, 301, 308, 309
human, vii, 2, 6, 21, 32, 37, 38, 39, 41, 47, 56, 58, 67, 78, 82, 85, 97, 100, 101, 105, 111, 112, 114, 116, 131, 133, 154, 156, 157, 158, 159, 161, 163, 167, 168, 174, 175, 181, 191, 198, 222, 223, 228, 231, 233, 234, 235, 241, 318
human body, 6, 21, 100, 105, 112, 114, 116
human brain, 114, 181, 234
human milk, 131, 133, 157, 159, 161
hybrid, 78, 90, 91, 254
hypertension, 145, 262, 296
hypothesis, 35, 76, 292, 295

I

iatrogenic, 149, 150, 158
ideal(s), 46, 49, 54, 63, 70, 124, 149, 150, 151, 192, 193, 198, 212
identification, 33, 55, 61, 71, 79, 169, 176, 226, 232, 241, 243, 301
identity, 12, 119, 123, 154
image(s), 20, 33, 82, 84, 91, 101, 111, 137, 145, 163, 170, 172, 173, 174, 175, 178, 180, 187, 198, 232, 234, 235, 239, 246, 247, 248, 249, 250, 254
image analysis, 239, 247, 254
improvements, 8, 99, 107, 130, 131, 132, 133, 134, 145, 170, 263, 264, 301
income, 35, 75, 264
India, vi, 1, 17, 31, 90, 94, 97, 129, 154, 163, 191, 204, 213, 217, 220, 231, 236, 239, 257, 258, 259, 260, 261, 268, 270, 274, 277, 295, 296, 297, 300, 301, 307, 309, 312, 313, 314, 315, 316, 317, 318
individuals, 8, 25, 40, 52, 76, 109, 125, 136, 140, 145, 147, 153, 154, 194, 196, 205, 213, 225, 261, 263, 296, 297, 298, 299, 300
industry/industries, viii, 1, 3, 5, 13, 17, 19, 22, 26, 86, 109, 112, 116, 118, 120, 121, 122, 123, 124, 127, 164, 166, 185, 199, 203, 204, 210, 318
infection, 9, 174, 218, 219, 226, 239, 240, 241, 242, 244, 245, 246
influenza, 218, 223, 228
information technology, 82, 86, 232, 238
infrastructure, 108, 123, 191, 261
injury, 139, 164, 262
integration, 15, 27, 117, 261
integrity, 12, 118, 123
intelligence, vii, viii, 35, 37, 45, 47, 54, 56, 57, 66, 67, 82, 87, 90, 92, 93, 94, 108, 115, 121, 123, 164, 165, 185, 233, 249, 255, 317, 318
interface, 18, 32, 38, 52, 55, 61, 62, 63, 64, 65, 69, 91, 94
Internet of Thing(s), viii, 2, 5, 6, 8, 13, 14, 15, 17, 20, 27, 28, 165, 184, 320
intervention, 97, 165, 168, 175, 231, 258, 259, 274, 278, 280, 288, 291, 292, 294, 298, 299, 300, 301
investment(s), 49, 50, 105
IoT devices, viii, 1, 3, 5, 12, 15, 17, 110, 124, 125
Iran, 161, 224, 230, 314
issues, 3, 5, 6, 20, 24, 32, 33, 35, 37, 38, 39, 40, 44, 52, 54, 58, 67, 68, 70, 73, 78, 79, 81, 89, 94, 131, 137, 146, 148, 151, 152,

156, 164, 202, 217, 219, 222, 225, 234, 262

L

lactation, v, viii, 129, 130, 131, 132, 133, 134, 158
language processing, 126, 170, 235
lasers, 136, 146, 153
LASIK, v, 129, 130, 132, 133, 134, 135, 136, 137, 138, 140, 141, 142, 143, 144, 145, 146, 147, 148, 149, 150, 151, 152, 153, 154, 155, 156
lead, 2, 73, 98, 109, 110, 122, 149, 151, 167, 170, 193, 260, 282, 298
learning, vii, viii, 18, 32, 53, 66, 83, 84, 85, 86, 87, 88, 93, 94, 113, 114, 126, 127, 128, 164, 165, 166, 167, 168, 169, 170, 171, 172, 174, 175, 176, 177, 178, 180, 181, 182, 183, 184, 185, 186, 187, 188, 189, 195, 217, 219, 222, 223, 225, 226, 227, 228, 229, 230, 231, 232, 233, 234, 235, 236, 237, 249, 250, 251, 252, 253, 254, 255, 265, 282, 295, 296, 317, 319
lens, 137, 150, 151, 153
life cycle, 59, 91, 93
lifestyle changes, 272, 300, 301
light, 4, 13, 34, 49, 68, 79, 137, 141, 156, 219, 242, 243, 245, 246, 247, 249, 250, 252

M

machine learning, vii, viii, 18, 32, 83, 84, 85, 86, 93, 94, 113, 127, 164, 165, 166, 167, 168, 169, 170, 175, 176, 177, 178, 180, 181, 182, 183, 184, 185, 188, 217, 219, 222, 223, 225, 226, 227, 228, 229, 230, 231, 232, 233, 234, 235, 236, 237, 249, 250, 251, 252, 253, 254, 255, 317, 319
majority, 239, 273, 295, 300
malaria, viii, 128, 232, 239, 240, 241, 242, 243, 244, 245, 246, 247, 248, 249, 250, 251, 252, 253, 254, 255
management, 10, 12, 33, 36, 41, 43, 50, 51, 52, 53, 55, 57, 61, 70, 73, 75, 88, 89, 94, 95, 102, 103, 109, 169, 250, 252, 258, 260, 261, 266, 267, 269, 270, 271, 273, 282, 294, 295, 301
manufacturing, 5, 34, 36, 50, 57, 67, 71, 75, 86, 87, 91, 97, 112, 119, 120, 122, 124
measurement(s), 12, 20, 33, 104, 110, 151, 223, 262, 263, 264, 265, 270, 296
media, 98, 167, 194, 195, 209, 227, 269
medical, viii, 1, 2, 4, 6, 7, 8, 9, 11, 12, 18, 21, 22, 23, 24, 26, 27, 28, 82, 86, 89, 93, 98, 99, 100, 102, 116, 122, 123, 128, 152, 164, 166, 172, 180, 182, 183, 191, 192, 193, 194, 195, 196, 197, 198, 199, 200, 201, 202, 204, 205, 206, 207, 208, 209, 210, 211, 212, 213, 214, 226, 230, 231, 232, 234, 235, 237, 241, 245, 250, 252, 254, 257, 258, 262, 263, 267, 273, 277, 300, 303, 305, 306, 307, 311, 313, 315, 316, 318
medical care, 6, 7, 21, 22, 192, 193, 194, 195, 196, 197, 198, 199, 200, 204, 205, 207, 208, 210, 211, 212, 213, 258, 277, 300
medical science, 86, 98, 226
medication, 34, 67, 134, 193, 203, 205, 209, 260, 265, 266, 267
medicine, 1, 2, 6, 10, 29, 82, 89, 93, 100, 112, 113, 128, 136, 147, 167, 174, 200, 209, 214, 225, 235, 249, 250, 251, 255, 302, 304, 305, 306, 309, 310, 311, 312, 313, 314, 319
memory, 9, 11, 12, 57, 66, 80, 171, 209
mental health, 213, 276, 298
messages, 82, 265, 266, 267, 269, 270, 272, 273, 275, 276

methodology, 5, 7, 23, 52, 55, 58, 59, 60, 61, 62, 91, 107, 165, 204
m-health, vii, viii, 22, 28, 192, 193, 199, 201, 210, 211, 212, 214, 229, 258, 259, 260, 261, 264, 265, 266, 267, 268, 269, 270, 275, 277, 280, 292, 294, 298, 300, 301
microscope, 239, 243, 247, 248, 250, 251, 252, 254
microscopy, 242, 243, 244, 245, 246, 247, 248, 249, 250, 252, 254, 255
mobile device, vii, 176, 191, 193, 195, 206, 207, 212, 253, 260, 274
mobile health, vii, viii, ix, 20, 28, 191, 192, 193, 194, 195, 196, 197, 198, 199, 200, 205, 206, 207, 208, 209, 210, 212, 213, 214, 215, 258, 259, 260, 264, 295
mobile phone, vii, 19, 56, 248, 252, 254, 258, 259, 271, 272, 275
modelling, 40, 41, 71, 72, 89, 94, 105
models, 36, 40, 42, 43, 53, 58, 70, 72, 73, 74, 75, 76, 83, 93, 94, 111, 112, 117, 164, 166, 174, 175, 178, 180, 182, 184, 192, 208, 209, 222, 225, 234, 238, 251, 253, 273
modifications, 27, 117, 130, 132
modules, 5, 265, 272, 280
mortality, 176, 221, 238, 239, 252
motivation, 151, 236, 265, 272
MRI, 93, 101, 163, 172, 173, 179, 185, 186, 187, 253
multidimensional, 84, 262, 274
multimedia, 108, 127, 274
myopia, 138, 145, 161

N

neural network, 165, 170, 172, 173, 175, 179, 181, 182, 183, 187, 188, 222, 224, 225, 228, 235, 249
neural networks, 175, 181, 182, 187
nodes, 9, 11, 74, 169, 182
nurses, 160, 268, 272
nursing, viii, 140, 143, 192, 209, 210, 211, 212, 213, 215
nursing home, viii, 192, 209, 210, 211, 212, 213

O

operations, 34, 99, 102, 134, 152, 153
ophthalmologist, 134, 145, 175
opportunities, 5, 18, 56, 79, 103, 208, 228, 233, 237, 261, 262
optimization, 70, 75, 94
organ, 112, 113, 116
organize, 48, 201, 223
organs, 100, 105, 111, 112
outpatient, 271, 277, 283
ownership, 120, 124, 197

P

pain, 151, 221, 241
pandemic, vi, 86, 217, 218, 219, 220, 221, 225, 226, 227, 228, 230, 270
parasite(s), 128, 232, 239, 240, 242, 243, 244, 245, 246, 249, 250, 253, 254
participants, 124, 266, 282, 292
pattern recognition, 128, 168, 254
permit, 45, 57, 192, 208
photorefractive keratectomy, 134, 161, 162
physical activity, 29, 113, 260, 265, 269, 272, 273
physicians, 142, 143, 147, 168, 251, 268
physics, 128, 232, 254
platform, vii, 4, 5, 19, 26, 55, 62, 108, 109, 117, 120, 123, 126, 226, 248, 301
plausibility, 59, 60, 193
playing, 1, 87, 165, 238
policy, 262, 263, 301

population, vii, 2, 9, 99, 166, 218, 239, 258, 262, 274, 277, 279, 283, 284, 288, 289, 290, 291, 295, 296, 297, 299, 300
prediction, viii, 41, 93, 95, 98, 163, 165, 166, 167, 168, 170, 171, 172, 173, 174, 177, 178, 180, 183, 184, 188, 219, 222, 224, 225, 226, 227, 228, 230, 233, 251, 254
pregnancy, viii, 129, 130, 131, 132, 134, 135, 141, 142, 144, 145, 146, 147, 154, 158, 159, 161
pregnancy and lactation-associated osteoporosis, 130
premenopausal osteoporosis, 130
preparation, 39, 73, 116, 150, 200, 246, 250
prevention, vii, 238, 240, 258, 266, 269, 270, 273, 282, 301
principles, 74, 90, 127, 204, 206, 264, 273, 278
probability, 58, 138, 228, 238, 275
problem-solving, 38, 44, 45, 52
producers, 121, 203, 204
professionals, viii, 26, 44, 122, 164, 193, 196, 260, 266, 274
prognosis, 169, 171, 225
programming, 38, 39, 42, 44, 55, 56, 60, 61, 62, 64, 68, 75, 76, 80, 81, 201
project, 69, 82, 110, 111, 214, 295, 298
protection, 7, 146, 147, 193, 203
public health, 174, 198, 239, 259, 262, 263, 301

Q

quality of life, ix, 114, 258, 259, 261, 262, 270, 271, 295, 298, 299, 301
questionnaire, 258, 264, 270, 274, 276, 284

R

RAND-36, 258, 259, 264, 270, 276, 277, 280, 284, 288, 290, 296, 297, 298, 299, 306, 310
reading, 12, 103, 136, 138, 149, 151, 153
reality, 47, 75, 134, 205
reasoning, 76, 144, 263
recall, 34, 67, 167
recognition, 33, 169, 170, 234, 262
recommendations, iv, 50, 113, 114, 115, 122, 162, 266
regression, 75, 77, 83, 132, 142, 169, 224, 233, 253
reinforcement, 83, 168, 183, 269, 272
relevance, 98, 250, 271
reliability, 20, 21, 27, 120, 276
reproduction, 7, 23, 73
requirement(s), 12, 37, 43, 45, 48, 55, 58, 60, 61, 70, 78, 79, 81, 87, 92, 103, 106, 121, 132, 205, 212, 232, 235, 263, 272
researchers, viii, 2, 69, 84, 87, 116, 172, 178, 220, 226, 259, 263, 264, 276, 319
resources, 3, 11, 33, 75, 78, 79, 87, 169, 180, 197, 227, 232, 233, 238, 260, 263, 269, 294
response, 111, 113, 267, 268
restrictions, 48, 70, 193
retail, 32, 33, 119, 209
retina, 134, 136, 137, 141
revenue, 104, 118, 125
risk(s), 9, 10, 71, 72, 91, 95, 98, 100, 103, 113, 134, 136, 139, 142, 146, 151, 167, 172, 197, 224, 233, 237, 242, 252, 262, 263, 270, 283, 296, 301
risk factors, 113, 262, 263, 270, 283, 296, 301
rules, 22, 40, 41, 44, 46, 63, 65, 69, 72, 74, 141, 154, 169, 203, 204
rural areas, 3, 244, 282, 296

S

safety, 9, 117, 127, 146, 147, 249, 251, 295
science, viii, 35, 40, 62, 86, 92, 98, 174, 226, 232, 276, 319
scope, 36, 52, 123, 125, 200, 202, 210, 270, 273
security, 6, 7, 10, 12, 20, 34, 67, 68, 82, 92, 94, 101, 117, 118, 119, 123, 126, 194, 202, 244
self-efficacy, 160, 161, 295
sensitivity, 141, 172, 173, 217, 243, 244, 245, 248
sensor(s), 1, 2, 5, 6, 8, 9, 11, 12, 18, 19, 20, 21, 23, 24, 25, 27, 28, 86, 98, 101, 105, 112, 113, 115, 120, 121, 124, 168
services, 3, 4, 5, 6, 7, 8, 11, 12, 20, 21, 23, 57, 122, 124, 148, 164, 166, 183, 191, 192, 193, 194, 195, 196, 197, 198, 199, 200, 201, 202, 204, 205, 206, 207, 208, 210, 211, 213, 237, 259, 262, 269, 301
shape, 141, 142, 196
shortage, 75, 166, 260
signals, 113, 114, 176, 188
signs, 21, 26, 70, 141, 167, 193, 241
simulation(s), 41, 97, 98, 99, 105, 111
skin, 149, 236, 240, 248
smart healthcare, vii, viii, 2, 4, 5, 13, 163, 164, 165, 166, 167, 180, 183
smart nursing home, 192
Smart Technologies, 14, 17, 27
smoking, 113, 262, 265, 269, 283, 296
SMS, 258, 264, 265, 266, 267, 268, 269, 270, 272, 274, 275, 278, 301, 309, 316
software, 12, 15, 20, 28, 32, 38, 39, 41, 42, 44, 45, 50, 53, 56, 57, 58, 59, 60, 61, 62, 63, 64, 67, 68, 69, 72, 76, 80, 92, 112, 113, 116, 169, 232, 239, 272, 273, 274, 281
solution, 25, 54, 61, 70, 78, 85, 86, 87, 98, 114, 118, 142, 170, 203, 228, 243, 247
specialists, 7, 75, 164, 197, 199, 201, 203, 204, 205, 208, 235
species, 130, 232, 239, 241, 243, 245
speculation, 49, 51, 76
stakeholders, 32, 82, 108, 109, 117, 121, 262
state, 22, 50, 57, 107, 114, 116, 134, 164, 172, 173, 192, 211, 214, 221, 239, 261, 262, 270
statistics, 155, 224, 281
stock, 34, 45, 46, 71, 73, 75, 204
storage, 11, 110, 115, 118, 125, 193, 232
structure, 33, 35, 55, 68, 74, 82, 130, 169, 173, 201, 234, 272, 273, 282
subjectivity, 49, 52, 281
supervisor(s), 43, 45, 51
supplier(s), 8, 81, 121, 191, 194, 195, 200, 201, 202, 206, 207, 208, 211
supply chain, 34, 57, 89, 94, 101, 102, 118, 122, 259
survival, 162, 240, 247
sustainability, 295, 298, 300, 301
symptoms, 139, 142, 148, 167, 221, 240, 241, 260, 266

T

Tanzania, 229, 250, 252, 253
target, 11, 32, 76, 104, 107, 110, 192, 265, 271, 272, 273, 274, 295
techniques, viii, 7, 23, 57, 58, 60, 76, 77, 83, 84, 85, 86, 90, 127, 153, 164, 165, 166, 167, 172, 173, 175, 176, 177, 178, 179, 180, 182, 183, 188, 217, 219, 222, 223, 225, 226, 227, 231, 232, 233, 236, 239, 241, 250, 253, 301
technology/technologies, vii, viii, ix, 4, 9, 11, 12, 13, 17, 18, 19, 20, 21, 22, 23, 27, 26, 28, 36, 44, 52, 56, 57, 58, 78, 82, 83, 87, 98, 99, 101, 102, 105, 107, 108, 109, 110, 114, 117, 118, 119, 120, 121, 122,

124, 126, 127, 128, 153, 163, 166, 167, 182, 183, 185, 192, 200, 214, 225, 228, 232, 235, 237, 244, 252, 254, 258, 259, 260, 263, 264, 270, 294, 301, 319
telephone(s), 205, 259, 267, 276, 301
temperature, 10, 25, 103, 110, 294
testing, 53, 55, 59, 61, 67, 72, 81, 105, 107, 113, 147, 175, 177, 274, 318
therapy, 89, 112, 113, 122, 130, 140, 151, 199, 207
thoughts, 40, 59, 69, 75, 180, 197
tissue, 130, 143, 156
trade, 37, 50, 202, 211
training, 44, 53, 99, 109, 115, 165, 168, 172, 175, 177, 200, 205, 224, 233, 243, 244, 247, 252, 294, 318
transactions, 117, 118, 119, 124, 125
transformation(s), 38, 72, 97, 107, 108, 109, 119, 167, 259
transmission, 12, 121, 123, 194, 195, 202, 247, 267
transparency, 117, 118, 120, 121
transportation, 3, 75, 121, 193, 232
treatment, 8, 86, 99, 100, 116, 129, 139, 140, 144, 147, 149, 150, 152, 155, 156, 157, 166, 167, 171, 176, 183, 191, 195, 198, 201, 203, 206, 209, 243, 252, 259, 260, 262, 298
trial, 99, 160, 167, 215, 248, 252, 258, 278, 295
twins, viii, 97, 98, 99, 100, 101, 102, 103, 104, 105, 106, 107, 108, 109, 110, 111, 112, 116, 117, 118, 119, 121, 122, 123, 124, 125, 126, 127

U

urban, 34, 58, 245, 282, 283
USA, 265, 266, 267, 297

V

variables, 50, 74, 84, 111, 227, 285, 286, 287
variations, 89, 101, 145, 159, 264, 276
vector, 90, 239, 248, 250, 251, 254, 255
viruses, 173, 183, 221, 222, 223
vision, 108, 124, 126, 133, 134, 135, 137, 138, 139, 142, 143, 144, 145, 147, 148, 152, 153, 155, 156, 254
visualization, 57, 85, 139
vulnerability, 71, 72, 77, 142

W

water, 89, 226, 227
wear, 105, 135, 137, 138, 148, 151, 266
wearable devices, viii, 17, 18, 19, 20, 21, 26, 29, 167, 209
web, 19, 32, 36, 37, 43, 56, 57, 66, 69, 70, 77, 78, 80, 81, 89, 95, 127, 167, 198, 200, 205, 267
weight management, 260, 265, 269
well-being, 8, 98, 108, 114, 115, 125, 261, 262, 263, 284, 285, 286, 287, 291, 293, 298, 299
workers, 7, 174, 224, 232, 247
workflow, 99, 104, 106, 248
World Health Organization (WHO), 127, 128, 194, 201, 204, 244, 252, 259, 261, 270, 316
worldwide, 2, 75, 118, 205, 206, 238, 244, 262, 264, 265, 266, 301